# GLUCOCRINOLOGY
The Relationship between Glucose and Endocrine Function

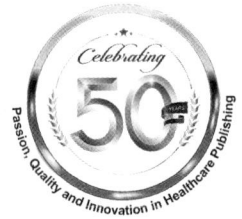

# GLUCOCRINOLOGY
The Relationship between Glucose and Endocrine Function

*Editors*

**Sanjay Kalra** MD DM
Consultant
Department of Endocrinology
Bharti Hospital
Karnal, Haryana, India

**Gagan Priya** MD DM
Consultant Endocrinologist
Department of Endocrinology
Fortis Hospital and Ivy Hospital
Mohali, Punjab, India

*Forewords*
**Emanuel Christ**
**Vivien Lim**

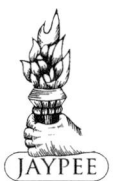

**JAYPEE BROTHERS MEDICAL PUBLISHERS**
The Health Sciences Publisher
New Delhi | London

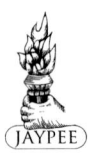 **Jaypee Brothers Medical Publishers (P) Ltd**

**Headquarters**
Jaypee Brothers Medical Publishers (P) Ltd
4838/24, Ansari Road, Daryaganj
New Delhi 110 002, India
Phone: +91-11-43574357
Fax: +91-11-43574314
Email: jaypee@jaypeebrothers.com

**Overseas Offices**
J.P. Medical Ltd
83 Victoria Street, London
SW1H 0HW (UK)
Phone: +44 20 3170 8910
Fax: +44 (0)20 3008 6180
Email: info@jpmedpub.com

Website: www.jaypeebrothers.com
Website: www.jaypeedigital.com

© 2020, Jaypee Brothers Medical Publishers

The views and opinions expressed in this book are solely those of the original contributor(s)/author(s) and do not necessarily represent those of editor(s) of the book.

All rights reserved. No part of this publication may be reproduced, stored or transmitted in any form or by any means, electronic, mechanical, photocopying, recording or otherwise, without the prior permission in writing of the publishers.

All brand names and product names used in this book are trade names, service marks, trademarks or registered trademarks of their respective owners. The publisher is not associated with any product or vendor mentioned in this book.

Medical knowledge and practice change constantly. This book is designed to provide accurate, authoritative information about the subject matter in question. However, readers are advised to check the most current information available on procedures included and check information from the manufacturer of each product to be administered, to verify the recommended dose, formula, method and duration of administration, adverse effects and contraindications. It is the responsibility of the practitioner to take all appropriate safety precautions. Neither the publisher nor the author(s)/editor(s) assume any liability for any injury and/or damage to persons or property arising from or related to use of material in this book.

This book is sold on the understanding that the publisher is not engaged in providing professional medical services. If such advice or services are required, the services of a competent medical professional should be sought.

Every effort has been made where necessary to contact holders of copyright to obtain permission to reproduce copyright material. If any have been inadvertently overlooked, the publisher will be pleased to make the necessary arrangements at the first opportunity. The **CD/DVD-ROM** (if any) provided in the sealed envelope with this book is complimentary and free of cost. **Not meant for sale.**

Inquiries for bulk sales may be solicited at: jaypee@jaypeebrothers.com

*Glucocrinology: The Relationship between Glucose and Endocrine Function / Sanjay Kalra, Gagan Priya*

*First Edition*: **2020**

ISBN: 978-93-88958-67-7

*Printed at: Samrat Offset Pvt. Ltd.*

**Dedicated to**
*Our Parents*
*Mrs Sudesh Kalra and Mr Hans Raj Kalra*
*Mrs Satish Kaur and Mr Balbir Singh Saini*

# Contributors

## Editors

**Sanjay Kalra** MD DM
Consultant
Department of Endocrinology
Bharti Hospital
Karnal, Haryana, India

**Gagan Priya** MD DM
Consultant Endocrinologist
Department of Endocrinology
Fortis Hospital and Ivy Hospital
Mohali, Punjab, India

## Contributing Authors

**A Prem Kumar** MD DM
Consultant Endocrinologist
SKS Hospital
Salem, Tamil Nadu, India

**Abilash Nair** MD DM
Assistant Professor
Department of Endocrinology
Government Medical College
Thiruvananthapuram, Kerala, India

**Abraham Alex Kodiatte** MD DNB
Senior Resident
Department of Medicine
Christian Medical College and Hospital
Ludhiana, Punjab, India

**Akshata Desai** American Board Certified in Endocrinology, Diabetes and Metabolism
Consultant Endocrinologist
Apex Hospital
Jalandhar, India

**Ali Latheef** MD
Department of Medicine
Indira Gandhi Memorial Hospital
Male, Maldives

**Alpesh Goyal** MD DM
Assistant Professor
Department of Endocrinology
All India Institute of Medical Sciences
New Delhi, India

**Altamash Shaikh** DNB MNAMS DNB
Consultant Endocrinologist
Department of Medicine, Saifee Hospital,
Mumbai, Maharashtra, India

**Ameya Joshi** MD DM
Consultant In Charge
Department of Endocrinology
Bhaktivedanta Hospital and Research Institute
Thane, Maharashtra, India

**Andrew E Uloko** BM BCh FMCP FACE
Professor of Medicine
Consultant Physician and Endocrinologist
Head of Endocrinology, Diabetes and
Metabolism, Department of Medicine
College of Health Sciences
Bayero University Kano,
Aminu Kano Teaching Hospital
Kano, Nigeria

**Ankia Coetzee** MBChB MMed FCP MPhil Certificate (Endo and Metab)
Consultant Endocrinologist
Department of Internal Medicine, Division of Endocrinology, Stellenbosch University
Faculty of Medicine and Health Sciences
Cape Town, South Africa

**Beatrice Anne** MD DM
Assistant Professor
Department of Endocrinology
Nizam's Institute of Medical Sciences
Hyderabad, Telangana, India

**Belinda George** MD DM
Associate Professor
Department of Endocrinology
St John's Medical College Hospital
Bengaluru, Karnataka, India

**C Jayakumari** MD DNB
Additional Professor
Government Medical College
Thiruvananthapuram, Kerala, India

**Darvin V Das** MD DNB
Assistant Professor
Government Medical College
Thiruvananthapuram, Kerala, India

**Dayakshi DK Abeyaratne** MD
Clinical Fellow in Endocrinology
Diabetes and Endocrinology Unit
National Hospital of Sri Lanka
Colombo, Sri Lanka

**Deep Dutta** MD DM DNB Specialty Certificate (Endo and Diab) FRCP (Edin)
Director
CEDAR Superspeciality Center
New Delhi, India

**Dina Shrestha** MD
Consultant Endocrinologist
Norvic International Hospital and
Medical College
Kathmandu, Nepal

**Emmy Grewal** MD DM
Consultant Endocrinologist
Ivy Multispeciality Hospital
Mohali, Punjab, India

**Ganesh HK** MD DM
Consultant Endocrinologist
AJ Hospital and Research Centre
Mangaluru, Karnataka, India

**Indira Maisnam** MD DM
Consultant Endocrinologist and Faculty
Department of Endocrinology
RG Kar Medical College
Kolkata, West Bengal, India

**Jaikrit Bhutani** MBBS
Resident, Department of Medicine
Post Graduate Institute of Medical Sciences
Rohtak, Haryana, India

**Jubbin Jagan Jacob** MD DNB MNAMS
Professor and Head
Endocrine and Diabetes Unit
Department of Medicine
Christian Medical College and Hospital
Ludhiana, Punjab, India

**Khalid Sheikh** MSc Diab PG Dip (Endocrinology)
Specialist, Department of Internal Medicine
Royal Oman Police Hospital
Muscat, Oman

# Contributors

**Kirtida Sandeep Acharya** MBChB MRCP (Ire)
National Chair Diabetes Kenya
Consultant Endocrinologist, MP Shah Hospital
Nairobi, Kenya

**Lakshmana Perumal Nandhini** MD DM
Assistant Professor
Department of Endocrinology
St John's Medical College
Bengaluru, Karnataka, India

**Mohammad Wali Naseri** MD PGD
Associate Professor
Department of Endocrinology Metabolism
and Diabetes
Kabul University of Medical Sciences
Kabul, Afghanistan

**Nandini Prasad** MD
Senior Resident, Department of Endocrinology
Government Medical College
Thiruvananthapuram, Kerala, India

**Ndeye M Ndour Mbaye** MD PhD
Professor
Department of Internal Medicine
Cheikh Anta Diop University
Dakar, Senegal

**Nikhil Gupta** MD MPH DABIM FACE
Endocrinologist
CanMed Multispeciality Clinics
Toronto, Canada

**Om J Lakhani** MD DNB
Consultant Endocrinologist
Department of Endocrinology
Zydus Hospital
Ahmedabad, Gujarat, India

**Partha Pratim Chakraborthy** MD DM DNB
Tutor, Department of Endocrinology and
Metabolism, Kolkata Medical College
Kolkata, West Bengal, India

**Perla A Carrillo-González** MD
Department of Endocrinology
ISSSTE Regional Hospital Lic. Adolfo López
Mateos
Mexico City, Mexico

**PK Jabbar** MD DNB (Medicine) DM DNB
(Endocrinology) FRCP (Glas)
Professor and Head
Department of Endocrinology
Government Medical College
Thiruvananthapuram, Kerala, India

**Roberta Lamptey** MSC Diab PGDD FWACP
FGCP MBChB
Consultant
Department of Family Medicine
Korle Bu Teaching Hospital
Accra, Ghana

**S Abbas Raza** American Board of Internal
Medicine, American Board of Diabetes,
Endocrinology and Metabolism
Endocrinologist
Shaukat Khanum Cancer Hospital and
Research Centre
Lahore, Pakistan

**Sakthivel Sivasubramanian** MD DM
Consultant Endocrinologist
The Hormone Clinic
Tiruchirappalli, Tamil Nadu, India

**Sambit Das** MD DM PGD (Endocrinology)
Consultant Endocrinologist
Apollo Hospitals
Bhubaneswar, Odisha, India

**Sameer Aggarwal** MD DM
Head
Department of Endocrinology and
Metabolism
Apex Plus Superspeciality Hospital
Rohtak, Haryana, India

**Sandeep Chaudhary** MD DM
Specialist
Department of Endocrinology
NMC Specialty Hospital
Al Nahda, Dubai, UAE

**Saptarshi Bhattacharya** MD DM FACE
Senior Consultant and Head
Department of Endocrinology
Max Superspeciality Hospital
Patparganj, Delhi, India

**Senthil Senniappan** MD MRCPCH FRCPCH MSC CCT PhD
Consultant Pediatric Endocrinologist and Honorary Senior Lecturer
Alder Hey Children's Hospital
Liverpool, United Kingdom

**Shahjada Selim** MD FACE FRSM
Assistant Professor
Department of Endocrinology and Metabolism, Bangabandhu Sheikh Mujib Medical University
Shahbag, Dhaka, Bangladesh

**Silver K Bahendeka** MD PhD
Consultant Endocrinologist
Mother Kevin Post Graduate Medical School
Martyrs University, St Francis Hospital
Kampala, Uganda

**Soumya S** MD
Senior Resident, Department of Endocrinology
Government Medical College
Thiruvananthapuram, Kerala, India

**Sunil K Kota** MD DNB
Consultant Endocrinologist
Diabetes and Endocare Clinic
Berhampur, Odisha, India

**Than Than Aye** MMedSc DTM&H (London) MRCP (UK) DMedSC FRCP (Edin, Lond)
Professor Emeritus
Department of Endocrinology
University of Medicine 2
Yangon, Myanmar

**Vishal Bhatia** MD FACE
Director
Department of Endocrinology, Diabetes and Metabolism
St Vincent Hospital
Associate Professor
Department of Internal Medicine and Division of Endocrinology
Indiana University School of Medicine
Evansville, USA

# Foreword

In addition to the reproductive system, hormones regulate the availability of energy for different situation (i.e. famine and feast, physical exercise, sleep, fasting, eating etc.) in order to adapt and finally survive. Energy is provided by the degradation of carbohydrates, fat and proteins through their respective metabolic pathways. Therefore, the endocrine system (including all hormones) is the key regulator of metabolism and some metabolites regulate hormones leading to regulatory circles. In a healthy subject with an intact endocrine system and regulatory circles, a stable energy balance (energy availability and energy consumption) can be observed with a stable body weight and metabolic parameters over time. On the other hand, autonomous hormone secretion, impairing the regulatory circles and metabolism, very often results in an impaired energy balance and, therefore, a change in body weight and metabolic parameters.

Glucose is a marker of insulin action at the tissue level. The main target tissues of insulin action are skeletal muscle, adipose tissue and liver. In a healthy person, glucose levels are tightly regulated within a small normal range, mainly by insulin and its counter regulatory hormones (glucagon, cortisol, catecholamines and growth hormone), thereby allowing for an adequate supply of glucose to the peripheral tissues. An increased level of glucose has to be considered as an impaired insulin action, an increased action of counter regulatory hormones or a combination of both conditions, whereas a decrease in glucose levels may be due to inadequate insulin secretion, an impaired action of counter regulatory hormones or a combination of both.

"Glucocrinology"—the topic of this book—is defined as the relationship between the endocrine system and glucose metabolism. Importantly, it not only examines the physiological and pathophysiological role of the entire endocrine system on glucose metabolism by summarizing the most important mechanisms of action of all the hormones, but also explores the effect of glucose metabolism on the endocrine system in a bidirectional way (regulatory circles).

In 4 sections and 22 chapters, authors at the cutting edge of science summarize the effect of all endocrine hormones on glucose homeostasis and the effect of glucose metabolism on the endocrine system. This manuscript extends the "glucose-insulin" focused image of diabetes to a global endocrine disease thereby reassembling Endocrinology and Diabetology, which falsely tend to be treated separately.

For me as the secretary-treasurer of the International Society of Endocrinology (ISE) it is a particular honor and pleasure to write the foreword for this book. Similar to "Glucocrinology", which includes the role of the global endocrine system in regulating glucose metabolism, ISE tries to reach out to the global endocrine community to improve the endocrine knowledge.

I congratulate all the authors and the editors for this wonderful piece of work and I am sure that the readers will appreciate it.

**Emanuel Christ** MD PhD
Secretary-Treasurer
International Society of Endocrinology
Head of Interdisciplinary Endocrinology
University Hospital of Basel
Switzerland

# Foreword

We live in exciting times where the knowledge of our chosen topic of interest—Endocrinology—increases by leaps and bounds. The study of it is wide, given that it spans many glands and systems and hitherto unsuspected and undetected linkages are being teased out every day.

At the same time, diabetes is one of the major conditions under our purview as endocrinologists. Its prevalence is increasing worldwide, not least of which is in Asia and Southeast Asia. At press time, about 1 in 11 people suffer from diabetes worldwide and in some countries the numbers are even greater. In addition, the prevalence seems to be increasing at a tremendous rate. The implications of a patient afflicted with diabetes is wide and far-reaching and contributes greatly to a nation's healthcare burden. It is no surprise therefore that endocrinologists and diabetologists worldwide would band together to try to fight this epidemic of our time.

Meanwhile, it is not uncommon to be suffering from endocrine disorders. As such the overlap between these two conditions is great and it is apt then that this book explores the interlinking influence of glucose metabolism on endocrine systems and vice-versa—coined as Glucocrinology. At the same time, the book lays bare the associations of various endocrine disorders with glucose metabolism and diabetes itself. This knowledge would no doubt enable us to give better care customized to the particular patient.

Kudos are to be given to the various authors who managed to bring forth their knowledge, translating it into clear prose that is a delight to read and sheds light on this new field of Glucocrinology.

**Vivien Lim** MRCP (UK) MMed FAMS
Specialist in Endocrinology
Immediate Past President Endocrine Metabolic Society of Singapore
Vivien Lim Endocrinology Specialist Centre
Gleneagles Medical Centre
Singapore

# Preface

The science of endocrinology and metabolism focuses on the integrated role of various endocrine axes and protein-energy metabolism in the maintenance of homeostasis. Dysfunction of the endocrine and metabolic systems impacts multiple organ systems, and influences long-term health of the individual. Physiological alterations and various pathological states in the endocrine-metabolic milieu impact the individual across the life-span, right from pre-conception till death.

An epidemic of endocrinopathy is sweeping across the world today, and has led to a heightened interest in the subject. Indeed, "Endocrinology and Metabolism" is one of the most rapidly advancing fields of modern medicine. The most prevalent endocrine dysfunction today is dysglycemia, including impaired glucose tolerance and diabetes mellitus. While there is extensive research and discussion regarding the multifaceted pathophysiology of diabetes, the endocrine aspects of this hormonal disease have not been highlighted adequately. This has led to an under-appreciation and under-recognition of the fact that dysglycemia is an endocrine disease.

The novel concept of "Glucocrinology" seeks to address this lacuna. It highlights the challenges and complexity of the endocrine relationships of glucose homeostasis, both in health and disease. Written by eminent authors from all continents, "Glucocrinology" is a book which will change the way we think about, approach and deal with diabetes. The structured layout of the book discusses each gland, covering its impact on glucose physiology, and its bidirectional relationship with diabetes, metabolic syndrome and hypoglycemia. It goes on to cover the concept of glucovigilance in endocrine disease, and endovigilance in diabetes. The need for endocrine pharmacovigilance, and important topics such as bone and reproductive health are given special attention. Wall structured sections explain the concept of glucocrinology in a basic and beautiful manner, making it easy to understand for the endocrinologist and non-endocrinologist alike. Students, clinicians and researchers will benefit from the lucid descriptions and explanations shared in this book.

**Sanjay Kalra**
**Gagan Priya**

# Contents

## Section 1 — The Scope of Glucocrinology

1. **Glucocrinology: Definition and Domains** — 3
   *Sanjay Kalra, Gagan Priya*

2. **Glucocrinology of Hypothalamus and Pituitary** — 11
   *Nandini Prasad, Abilash Nair, PK Jabbar, Ali Latheef*

3. **Glucocrinology of Thyroid** — 27
   *Emmy Grewal, Gagan Priya, Ndeye M Ndour Mbaye*

4. **Glucocrinology of Parathyroid and Bone Mineral Metabolism** — 41
   *Ameya Joshi, Perla A Carrillo-González*

5. **Glucocrinology of Adrenal Cortex** — 53
   *Gagan Priya, Than Than Aye*

6. **Glucocrinology of Adrenal Medulla** — 71
   *Ganesh HK, Kirtida Sandeep Acharya*

7. **Glucocrinology of Pancreas** — 79
   *Sakthivel Sivasubramanian, Partha Pratim Chakraborthy, Senthil Senniappan*

8. **Glucocrinology of Reproductive System: Male** — 97
   *Om J Lakhani, Khalid Sheikh*

9. **Glucocrinology of Reproductive System: Female** — 108
   *Lakshmana Perumal Nandhini, Dayakshi DK Abeyaratne, Gagan Priya*

## Section 2 — Glucovigilance in Endocrinology

10. **Metabolic Syndrome in Endocrinopathy** — 123
    *Jubbin Jagan Jacob, Abraham Alex Kodiatte, Vishal Bhatia*

11. **Endocrine Syndromes in Diabetes** — 135
    *Alpesh Goyal, Saptarshi Bhattacharya, Shahjada Selim*

12. **Hypoglycemia in Endocrinopathies** — 148
    *Belinda George, Ankia Coetzee*

| | | |
|---|---|---|
| 13. | Glucovigilance in Endocrine Therapy<br>*Altamash Sheikh, Sandeep Chaudhary* | 161 |
| 14. | Glucovigilance Across Stages of Life<br>*Beatrice Anne, Roberta Lamptey, Gagan Priya* | 174 |

## Section 3  Endovigilance in Diabetes

| | | |
|---|---|---|
| 15. | Endovigilance in Refractory Hyperglycemia<br>*A Prem Kumar, Sanjay Kalra* | 193 |
| 16. | Hypoglycemia in Diabetes: Endocrine Perspectives<br>*Akshata Desai, Andrew E Uloko* | 204 |
| 17. | Endovigilance in Diabetes Therapy<br>*Sameer Aggarwal, Jaikrit Bhutani, Dina Shrestha* | 217 |
| 18. | Endovigilance in Diabetic Vasculopathy<br>*Soumya S, Darvin Vamadevan Das, C Jayakumari, Sanjay Kalra* | 227 |

## Section 4  Specific Issues in Glucocrinology

| | | |
|---|---|---|
| 19. | Adipose Tissue Health in Diabetes<br>*Indira Maisnam, Nikhil Gupta, Gagan Priya* | 247 |
| 20. | Bone Health in Diabetes<br>*Deep Dutta, Mohammad Wali Naseri,*<br>*Indira Maisnam, Gagan Priya* | 265 |
| 21. | Sexual Dysfunction in Diabetes<br>*Sunil K Kota, Sambit Das, S Abbas Raza* | 278 |
| 22. | Reproductive Health in Diabetes<br>*Sambit Das, Sunil K Kota, Silver K Bahendeka* | 290 |

*Index*     299

# SECTION 1

## The Scope of Glucocrinology

# CHAPTER 1

# Glucocrinology: Definition and Domains

*Sanjay Kalra, Gagan Priya*

## INTRODUCTION

Glucose and energy metabolism are embedded in endocrinology, and hormonal function is an integral regulator of metabolism. Insulin and glucagon, the two key regulators of glucose physiology, maintain blood glucose concentration within a relatively narrow range. In addition, several other endocrine players, including glucagon-like polypeptide-1 (GLP-1), gastric inhibitory polypeptide (GIP), glucocorticoids, growth hormone (GH) and insulin-like growth factor-1 (IGF-1) influence glucose homeostasis through myriad mechanisms. They affect insulin secretion, body weight and body fat distribution, adipose tissue health, liver glucose output, and skeletal muscle and adipose tissue insulin sensitivity.

The interplay between these regulatory (insulin, GLP-1) and counter-regulatory (glucagon, cortisol, GH, IGF-1, epinephrine) hormones ensures a ready supply of fuel to all tissues during fasting period, and peripheral uptake and storage of excess nutrients during postprandial period. The endocrine system also regulates lipid and protein metabolism, appetite and satiety and resting metabolic rate. During periods of nutrient excess, energy is stored in adipose tissue; thereby maintaining blood glucose and lipid fractions within normal range to protect cellular machinery from glucotoxicity and lipotoxicity. During periods of nutrient deficit, this energy is mobilized as fuel for cells.

Recent research also suggests that several other hormones, that are not traditionally associated with metabolic regulation, such as prolactin, vitamin D, parathyroid hormone (PTH), bone-specific peptides (osteocalcin, osteoprotegerin, bone morphogenetic protein 7, lipocalin 2), estrogen, progesterone and testosterone, may also impact glucose and energy homeostasis by influencing insulin sensitivity and/or secretion.

Therefore, several endocrine disorders can be associated with abnormal glucose and lipid homeostasis, hypertension, metabolic syndrome and cardiovascular disease. Disorders such as acromegaly, Cushing's syndrome, hyperthyroidism, pheochromocytoma, primary hyperparathyroidism, and primary hyperaldosteronism may cause secondary diabetes. Other disorders such as hypothyroidism, adrenal insufficiency, and hypopituitarism may increase the risk of hypoglycemia.

In turn, metabolic health also influences the functioning of various endocrine axes. The classic example of this is the progressive decline in β-cell function, as well as increased insulin resistance, that occurs in diabetes due to glucotoxicity and lipotoxicity. Diabetes is also associated with alterations in hypothalamic–pituitary–adrenal (HPA) axis, hypothalamic–pituitary–thyroid (HPT) axis, hypothalamic–pituitary–gonadal (HPG) axis, bone mineral metabolism and skeletal health, renin–angiotensin–aldosterone system and catecholamine secretion.

It is, therefore, abundantly clear that endocrinology and metabolism are not separate disciplines, but a comprehensive subject that must always be considered together. This relationship is crystallized in the term glucocrinology, defined as "the study of medicine that relates to the relationship of glycemia with the endocrine system".[1]

## BIDIRECTIONAL RELATIONSHIP

Endocrine system and metabolism, therefore, have a bidirectional relationship. This statement rings even louder in today's era of comprehensive care, where the emphasis is on personalized, patient-centric care. It is now imperative to focus on comprehensive clinical evaluation, to identify pathophysiology specific to the individual's glycemic patterns, microvascular health, lipid and cardiovascular health, bone health and gonadal health. This implies identification of secondary causes of diabetes, including endocrinopathies or endocrine disorders that may coexist with diabetes and influence its course. Redressal of endocrine disorder in such circumstances is likely to have rewarding metabolic effects. In addition, addressing multisystem and endocrine issues is considered integral to, and not distinct from, personalized diabetes care. While adequate emphasis is already placed on obesity management, microvascular and macrovascular health, this concept also includes the management of sexual dysfunction, functional hypogonadism, bone quality and fracture risk, thyroid dysfunction, and growth and pubertal disorders in children.

The endocrine health of an individual determines metabolic health and vice-versa. This bidirectional relationship means that endocrinology and metabolism cannot be segregated as distinct disciplines. In addition, endocrine and metabolic health together influence every organ system in tandem, be it the cardiovascular, cerebrovascular, renal or hepatic health.

## HISTORICAL PERSPECTIVES

The close synchrony between endocrine function and metabolism has been reflected throughout the history of medicine. Glucocrinology has a noble history, marked by seminal discoveries and milestones. The Nobel Prize for Medicine was won in 1947 by CF Cori and GT Cori for their work on the catalytic conversion of glycogen. In the same year, BA Houssay was coawarded the prize for his work on the role of anterior pituitary hormones in sugar metabolism. EC Kendall, T Reichstein and PS Hench followed with a Nobel Prize in 1950, for discovering the adrenal cortex hormones. In 1953, H Krebs and F Lipmann won the prize for elucidating Kreb's cycle, while EW Sutherland Fr won it in 1971 for finding the mechanism of action of hormones through cycle adenosine monophosphate (cAMP). R Yalow was awarded the Nobel Prize in Physiology or Medicine in 1977 for the development of radioimmunoassays of peptide hormones and without a surprise, insulin was the first hormone to be assayed. Further discoveries related to peptide hormones of the brain (R Guillemin, AV Schally 1977) and dopamine (A Carlsson, P Greengard, E Kandel, 2000) have also been deemed worthy of the Nobel Prize. This list symbolizes the importance of endocrinology in glucose metabolism.[2,3]

This significance is such that the Nobel Prize in Chemistry has also been awarded to endocrinology-focused researchers. Vigneaud (1953), Sanger (1958) and Leloir (1970) have won the prize for their work on oxytocin, insulin and sugar nucleotides.[3,4]

## NEGLECTED BASICS

Over the past few years, diabetes management has improved in many ways. Once limited to reduction of hyperglycemia, diabetes care now includes cardiorenal safety and benefit in its ambit.[5] The welcome interest in cardiovascular and renal health in diabetes, however, distracts attention from a basic fact: *"Diabetes is an endocrine disorder".*

Diabetes is a complex syndrome.[6] Lack of attention to the etiopathophysiology of diabetes may lead to unacceptable errors and unsatisfactory outcomes. A lack of knowledge of the endocrine contribution to glucose metabolism may cause errors in diagnosis and treatment. The differential diagnosis between type 2 diabetes mellitus and diabetes secondary to endocrinopathy, for instance, can be made only if one is aware of the hormonal aspects of diabetes. Similarly, possible etiologies of refractory hyperglycemia, or unexplainable hypoglycemia, may be missed if endocrine causes are not ruled out.[7] Various endocrine systems such as reproductive function and bone health may be affected by diabetes and require specific evaluation and therapy. The pharmacologic treatment of hyperglycemia may need modification in the presence of endocrine or metabolic comorbidity—this, too, demands that the diabetes care professional understands the nuances of endocrinology.

## EXPANDING FRONTIERS

It is these aspects of health and disease which the concept of glucocrinology seeks to address. Far from being a glucocentric science, endocrinology seeks to provide accurate, comprehensive and patient-centered care to person with diabetes. The philosophy of glucocrinology is to achieve these aims, by integrating the study of hormonal physiology and pathology into modern diabetology discourse.

The canvas of endocrinology is an infinite one. Including in its ambit, the study of hormones in health and disease, it provides a framework for the understanding of human physiology and pathophysiology. Similarly, the study of glucose metabolism has expanded to explore novel, hitherto unexplored facets. These developments, occurring in parallel with the emergence of the diabetes pandemic, have facilitated better management of the syndrome.

## DEFINING GLUCOCRINOLOGY

Glucocrinology is almost infinite in its expanse as suggested in Table 1. However, it becomes easy to grasp if studied in a systematic manner. To do so, an inclusive definition is required, which can serve as an umbrella for an all-inclusive learning rubric.

Glucocrinology has earlier been described as "the study of medicine that relates to the relationship of glycemia with the endocrine system".[1] We expand this definition

**TABLE 1**  Glucocrinology: Scope and breadth.

| Pathophysiological considerations | |
|---|---|
| *Endocrine factors in diabetes* | |
| Endocrine disease may cause secondary diabetes | • Acromegaly<br>• Hypothalamic obesity<br>• Hyperthyroidism<br>• Primary hyperparathyroidism<br>• Cushing's syndrome<br>• Primary hyperaldosteronism<br>• Glucagonoma<br>• Somatostatinoma<br>• Pancreatic diabetes—pancreatitis, fibrocalculous pancreatopathy, pancreatic cancer |
| Endocrine disease may be associated with refractory hyperglycemia | • Acromegaly<br>• Cushing's syndrome<br>• Hyperthyroidism<br>• Pheochromocytoma<br>• Glucagonoma |
| Endocrine disease may be associated with metabolic syndrome | • Acromegaly<br>• Growth hormone deficiency<br>• Hyperprolactinemia<br>• Hypothyroidism<br>• Primary hyperaldosteronism<br>• Congenital adrenal hyperplasia<br>• Cushing's syndrome<br>• PCOS<br>• Hypogonadism<br>• Primary hyperparathyroidism<br>• Vitamin D deficiency |
| Metabolic disease may coexist with diabetes | • Obesity<br>• Dyslipidemia<br>• Nonalcoholic fatty liver disease |

*Continued*

*Continued*

| | |
|---|---|
| Diabetes syndromes associated with other endocrine disorders | • Polyglandular autoimmune endocrinopathy<br>• Maturity-onset diabetes of the young<br>• Lipodystrophy<br>• Multiple endocrine neoplasia<br>• Neonatal diabetes<br>• Mitochondrial diabetes<br>• Turner syndrome<br>• Klinefelter syndrome<br>• Wolfram syndrome<br>• Down syndrome<br>• Bardet–Biedl syndrome<br>• Huntington's chorea<br>• Friedreich's ataxia |
| *Endocrine factors in hypoglycemia* | |
| Endocrine diseases causing spontaneous hypoglycemia | • Endogenous hyperinsulinism—insulinoma, noninsulinoma pancreatogenous hyperinsulinism, insulin autoimmune syndrome<br>• Hypopituitarism<br>• Hypothyroidism<br>• Adrenal insufficiency<br>• Glycogen storage diseases<br>• Hereditary fructose intolerance<br>• Fatty acid oxidation defects |
| Endocrine diseases increasing the risk of hypoglycemia in diabetes | • Hypopituitarism<br>• Hypothyroidism<br>• Adrenal insufficiency<br>• Growth hormone deficiency<br>• Celiac disease |
| **Alterations in endocrine function in diabetes** | |
| Diabetes is associated with disturbances in hormones regulating metabolism, resulting in progression of diabetes and complications | • Impaired insulin secretion and insulin action<br>• Glucagon dysfunction—hyperglucagonemia or impaired glucagon secretion<br>• Impaired counter-regulatory hormone response<br>• Impaired incretin secretion<br>• Abnormal adipocytokine profile—increased proinflammatory cytokines<br>• Increased activity of renin–angiotensin–aldosterone axis<br>• Increased signaling through mineralocorticoid receptors |
| Diabetes may lead to endocrine complications | • Sexual dysfunction— male and female<br>• Functional hypogonadism<br>• Delayed puberty and early menarche<br>• PCOS and ovulatory dysfunction<br>• Impaired spermatogenesis<br>• Subfertility<br>• Osteoporosis, poor bone quality, fractures |

*Continued*

*Continued*

| Pharmacological considerations | |
|---|---|
| Glucose-lowering drugs may have endocrine effects | • Metformin: Reduces TSH, may increases bone density, reduces biochemical hyperandrogenism and improves ovulation in PCOS, lactic acidosis<br>• Pioglitazone: Reduces bone density, increases fracture risk, reduces biochemical hyperandrogenism and improves ovulation in PCOS, increases weight, body fat redistribution<br>• Insulin: Weight gain, hypoglycemia risk, bone anabolic effect, but increased fall risk<br>• Sulfonylureas: Weight gain, hypoglycemia risk, may have beneficial effect on bone, but increase fall risk, hyponatremia (chlorpropamide), increase in thyroid volume<br>• GLP-1R agonist: Weight loss, improve bone health, reduce hyperandrogenism and improve ovulation in PCOS, pancreatitis, thyroid C-cell hyperplasia<br>• DPP-4 inhibitors: Weight neutral, neutral effect on bone, pancreatitis<br>• SGLT-2 inhibitors: Weight loss, reduce BMD, increased fall and fracture risk |
| Endocrine therapies may have glucose-lowering effects | • Surgical excision of endocrine tumors—acromegaly, Cushing's syndrome, primary hyperparathyroidism, primary hyperaldosteronism, glucagonoma<br>• Medical management of hyperprolactinemia— bromocriptine, cabergoline<br>• Medical management of acromegaly—pegvisomant, bromocriptine, cabergoline<br>• Medical management of Cushing's syndrome—ketoconazole, mifepristone, metyrapone<br>• Treatment of hyperthyroidism —antithyroidal drugs, radioiodine ablation, surgery<br>• Testosterone replacement in male hypogonadism<br>• Weight loss drugs—orlistat, phentermine-topiramate, lorcaserin, naltrexone-bupropion<br>• Bariatric surgery<br>• Treatment of vitamin D deficiency |
| Endocrine therapies under evaluation in diabetes management | • Bromocriptine<br>• Bariatric surgery<br>• 11β-hydroxysteroid dehydrogenase 1 inhibitors<br>• Selective glucocorticoid receptor modulators<br>• Metreleptin<br>• FGF21 analogs<br>• β3-adrenergic agonists<br>• Brown adipose tissue transplant |
| Endocrine therapies that may increase the risk of hyperglycemia | • Glucocorticoids<br>• Somatostatin analogs—octreotide, lanreotide<br>• Pasireotide<br>• Growth hormone<br>• Epinephrine, norepinephrine<br>• Oral contraceptives<br>• Diazoxide |
| Endocrine therapies may increase the risk of hypoglycemia, requiring downtitration of antidiabetic agents | • Surgical removal of acromegaly, Cushing's syndrome, pheochromocytoma<br>• Tapering of glucocorticoid doses<br>• Bariatric surgery |

(BMD: bone mineral density; DPP-4: dipeptidyl peptidase-4; FGF21: fibroblast growth factor 21; GLP-1R: glucagon-like peptide-1 receptor; PCOS: polycystic ovary syndrome; SGLT-2: sodium-glucose cotransporter-2; TSH: thyroid-stimulating hormone) as *"the study of the relationship between the endocrine system and glucose metabolism, in health and disease".* This multifaceted, multidirectional relationship includes the changes in glucose metabolism seen in endocrine disease and with endocrinotropic drugs, as well as the alterations in endocrine function noted with dysglycemia and glucose-modifying interventions.

Glucocrinology is justified by the common origins of endocrine disorders and dysglycemia, as seen in genetic endocrine syndromes and auto immune polyendocrinopathy. Even in a healthy individual, physiological changes in the endocrine environment, as noted across various phases of life, are associated with alterations in glucose physiology. Novel investigative markers and therapeutic interventions, such as glucagon-like peptide-1 receptor (GLP-1R) agonists, dipeptidyl peptidase 4 (DPP-4) inhibitors, bromocriptine, osteocalcin, fibroblast growth factor 23 (FGF23) and 11 β-hydroxysteroid dehydrogenase type 1 inhibitors (11βHSD1) reinforce the rationale for studying glucocrinology.[1]

To critics, the term glucocrinology may suggest promotion of a glucocentric approach. In fact, it conveys the very opposite. The philosophy of glucocrinology is to ensure that glucose dynamics is studied in the right perspective, beyond mere glycemia, keeping all related biochemical and physiological functions in mind. By analyzing mutual harmony with endocrine and other metabolic physiology, glucocrinology promotes a holistic viewpoint of diabetes management.

## THE FRAMEWORK

Here in, we present an overview of the thought process followed while crafting this book. The book is structured in four sections with 22 chapters, each written by leaders in the field. The first section, "Scope of Glucocrinology" follows the traditional format of endocrinology, covering each gland at a time. These chapters—"Glucocrinology of (a particular) Endocrine Axis" (e.g. hypothalamus–pituitary, thyroid, adrenal and others) provide the foundation for subsequent sections of the book.

A uniform chapter layout has been followed to ensure easy readability. Each author team introduces the effect of the gland on glucose and metabolism, and focuses on the bidirectional relationship between glucose metabolism and endocrine axis. The team then discusses glucose physiology in relation to the particular gland, highlights the necessary glucovigilance in disorders of that endocrine axis, and then describes the vigilance specific to this gland that is required in individuals with diabetes.

Both basic science and clinical perspectives are provided, to meet the requirements of students, researchers and clinical practitioners. These chapters discuss what happens to insulin sensitivity, insulin secretion and glucose dynamics in disorders of that endocrine axis. They also cover risks and challenges of metabolic syndrome and diabetes in disorders of that axis, and explore the need for regular screening for dysglycemia as well. The last section of the same chapter covers the alterations in that endocrine system which occurs in individuals with diabetes.

Two distinct, clinically relevant aspects of glucocrinology are glucovigilance in endocrinology, and endovigilance in diabetes.[8] Endocrine disorders are often associated with alterations in insulin sensitivity, some are associated with insulin resistance and/or impairment of insulin secretion. Many endocrinopathies are characterized by dysglycemia. Some can lead to secondary diabetes or worsen glycemic control in pre-existing diabetes. Others may cause hypoglycemia or increase the risk of hypoglycemia in a diabetic individual.

The section on "Glucovigilance in Endocrinology" expands upon the importance of assessing and managing metabolic syndrome and hypoglycemia in endocrine diseases, identification of various endocrine syndromes associated with diabetes and glucose metabolism with various endocrinotropic drugs, as well as unique glucometabolic challenges that may present across various stages of life. The section "Endovigilance in Diabetes" delves into endocrine causes of refractory hyperglycemia as well as hypoglycemia, and endocrine aspects of diabetes pharmacotherapy and diabetes vasculopathy.

The last part "Specific Issues in Glucocrinology" is equally relevant for the diabetes care professional, as it covers specific endocrine issues including adipose tissue, bone, sexual and reproductive health. Indeed, adipose tissue dysfunction is an important player in the pathogenesis of diabetes and there is an urgent need to focus on therapies that address adiposopathy.

## A NEW BEGINNING

Glucocrinology provides a 360° viewpoint of the complex relationship between the various endocrine glands and glucose metabolism. The bidirectional relationship between endocrine system and metabolism is elaborated on. With an increasing focus on targets and therapeutic strategies including pharmacological approach in diabetes care, the fact that diabetes is an endocrine disorder is often overlooked. We reiterate the need to understand diabetes in the context of the discipline of endocrinology and metabolism and approach the disorder from a truly holistic view. By doing so, the book hopes to facilitate provision of comprehensive and seamless diabetes and endocrine care to the society that we serve.

## REFERENCES

1. Kalra S, Priya G, Gupta Y. Glucocrinology. J Pak Med Assoc. 2018;68(6):963-5.
2. All Nobel Prizes in Physiology or Medicine. Available from https://www.nobelprize.org/prizes/lists/all-nobel-laureates-in-physiology-or-medicine [Last accessed April 2019].
3. Kalra S, Unnikrishnan AG, Jacob J. Endocrinology @ the nobels. Indian J Endocrinol Metab. 2012;16 (Suppl 2): S138-S139.
4. All Nobel Prizes in Chemistry. Available from https://www.nobelprize.org/prizes/lists/all-nobel-prizes-in-chemistry [Last accessed April 2019].
5. Cefalu WT, Kaul S, Gerstein HC, et al. Cardiovascular outcomes trials in type 2 diabetes: where do we go from here? Reflections from a diabetes care editors' expert forum. Diabetes care. 2018;41(1):14-31.
6. Zaccardi F, Webb DR, Yates T, et al. Pathophysiology of type 1 and type 2 diabetes mellitus: a 90-year perspective. Postgrad Med J. 2016;92(1084):63-9.
7. Lamos EM, Younk LM, Davis SN. Hypoglycemia. Endocrine and Metabolic Medical Emergencies: A Clinician's Guide. London: Wiley Blackwell; 2018. pp. 506-30.
8. Kalra S, Khandelwal D. Thyrovigilance in diabetes; glucovigilance in thyroidology. J Pak Med Assoc. 2018;68(6):966-7.

# CHAPTER 2

# Glucocrinology of Hypothalamus and Pituitary

*Nandini Prasad, Abilash Nair, PK Jabbar, Ali Latheef*

## INTRODUCTION

The central nervous system plays a very important role in the regulation of peripheral insulin sensitivity and glucose homeostasis and this was recognized very early. In the 1850s, physiologist Claude Bernard observed that manipulation of the floor of the fourth ventricle in the hindbrain of experimental animals caused hyperglycemia and glucosuria. In the early 1950s, Jean Mayer proposed the "glucostatic theory", which implied the brain could detect glucose fluctuations, and by the mid-1960s electrophysiological recordings uncovered glucose-sensing neurons in the hypothalamus.

Disorders of the hypothalamus and pituitary axis are associated with alterations in glucose homeostasis. Acromegaly, Cushing's disease, and hyperprolactinemia are often associated with hyperglycemia while hypopituitarism, growth hormone (GH) deficiency, central hypothyroidism and secondary adrenal insufficiency increase the risk of hypoglycemia. At the same time, alterations in hypothalamic–pituitary function have been documented in individuals with diabetes. In this chapter, we will discuss the bidirectional relationship between hypothalamic–pituitary axis and glucose homeostasis. We further elaborate on the need for glucovigilance in hypothalamic and pituitary disorders and the need for hypothalamic and pituitary vigilance in diabetes.

## GLUCOSE PHYSIOLOGY IN RELATION TO HYPOTHALAMUS AND PITUITARY

### Role of the Hypothalamus in Glucose and Energy Regulation

The brain uses 60–70% of the total glucose. It predominantly expresses the high-affinity glucose transporters, GLUT-1 and GLUT-3, allowing effective glucose transport. Thus, the brain does not depend on insulin for glucose uptake, even though insulin

# SECTION 1: The Scope of Glucocrinology

is a key signaling molecule. Because the brain is the most avid glucose consumer, it is reasonable that it executes surveillance functions. Although glucose sensing is a complex distributed process, extensive research has recognized the hypothalamus as a key center of these networks.[1] The hypothalamic nuclei involved in glucose regulation include the arcuate nucleus (ARH), ventromedial nucleus (VMH) and lateral hypothalamic nucleus (LHN).

- *Arcuate nucleus*: The ARH is located at the floor of the third ventricle at the level of the base of pituitary stalk. Pro-opiomelanocortin (POMC), agouti-related peptide (AgRP) and neuropeptide Y (NPY) are expressed in the ARH and play a vital role in the control of energy homeostasis as they regulate appetite and feeding behavior.[1] Post-transcriptional processing of POMC leads to generation of a melanocyte-stimulating hormone (MSH), that acts via melanocortin-3 and -4 receptors (MC3R and MC4R) to reduce energy intake and increase energy expenditure. Acute activation of AgRP neurons resulted in impaired systemic insulin sensitivity and glucose tolerance. The insulin-stimulated glucose uptake was reduced selectively in the brown adipose tissue (BAT), likely through re-programming the gene expression profile toward a myogenic signature. Acute induction of myostatin partially explained the insulin resistance downstream of AgRP-neuron stimulation. AgRP activation also stimulated increased appetite and energy intake.[1]
- *Ventromedial nucleus*: The VMN senses leptin and glucose and has a crucial role in detecting hypoglycemia and initiating the physiological counter-regulatory responses including the release of glucagon and epinephrine.[1]
- *Lateral hypothalamic nucleus*: The LHN consists of a heterogeneous structure of neuronal population, including the well described orexin and melanin-concentrating hormone (MCH) neurons. The primary orexinergic nucleus widely projects to the remainder of the hypothalamus, in particular to the posterior hypothalamus, ARH and paraventricular hypothalamic nucleus.[1] This area is implicated in arousal, appetite and reward.

Energy intake and expenditure are closely regulated and hypothalamus plays a vital role in this central energy regulation, through an extensive bidirectional cross-talk with metabolically active tissues. It directly senses nutrient status and also receives peripheral inputs via leptin, ghrelin and insulin and in turn, regulates appetite and energy expenditure. Insulin acts via hypothalamus to regulate hepatic glucose output and peripheral glucose metabolism. While leptin has predominant anorectic effects, it also regulates glucose homeostasis through the hypothalamus and leptin deficiency is associated with insulin resistance and hyperglycemia.

## Molecular Mechanisms of Central Glucose Sensing

The molecular mechanisms underlying neuronal glucose sensing are diverse and not completely understood. Glucose-sensing neurons respond to increase in extracellular glucose by either increasing their activity (glucose-excited or GE) or decreasing their activity (glucose-inhibited or GI).[2] GI neurons are activated by a decrease in glucose concentration. GE neurons are located in VMH, ARC and paraventricular nuclei, while GI neurons are present in LH, ARC and paraventricular nuclei.

Depolarization in GE neurons operates similarly to pancreatic β-cells.[2] GE neurons take up glucose via GLUT2; glucose is then phosphorylated by glucokinase and subsequent oxidation leads to adenosine triphosphate (ATP) production. Increased intracellular ATP/ADP ratio mediates closure of potassium-sensitive ATP (KATP) channels and membrane depolarization that in turn stimulates neurotransmitter release. GI neurons also rely on glucokinase, though it is not essential for glucose sensing. The cellular energy sensor 5′-adenosine monophosphate-activated protein kinase (AMPK) has been proposed to play a relevant role in glucose sensing. In the VMN, low glucose levels depolarize GI neurons via closure of chloride channel through a mechanism mediated by AMPK and nitric oxide.[2] In addition to GI neurons that respond to fluctuations in glucose via its metabolism, the activity of some GI neurons including those expressing orexin in the lateral hypothalamus is modulated directly by the glucose molecule itself.[3]

The diversity of brain regions, neuronal types and molecular mechanisms involved in glucose sensing underscores the complexity and heterogeneity of this fundamental biological process and suggests the existence of intricate neurocircuits. According to these inputs, the hypothalamus conveys multiple effector mechanisms to precisely adjust the metabolic output of peripheral tissues, thus preserving glucose homeostasis. These effects involve the main metabolic tissues, including the liver, skeletal muscle, adipose tissue, sympathetic nervous system and pancreas.

### Hypothalamic control of pancreatic function

Several hypothalamic nuclei (ARC, VMN and LH) communicate with the brainstem (nucleus of tractus solitarius and dorsal motor nucleus of the vagus) via the paraventricular nucleus, the raphe group in the pons and the ventral zone of the periaqueductal gray (PAG) in the midbrain.[4] Brainstem structures, in turn, innervate pancreatic islets via the vagus and/or spinal cord. Sympathetic and parasympathetic pathways thereby regulate the secretion of insulin and glucagon. Parasympathetic neurons stimulate insulin release, while sympathetic neurons have an inhibitory effect. Glucagon release is increased by both sympathetic and parasympathetic nerve endings.

## Role of Anterior Pituitary in Glucose Regulation

The importance of the anterior pituitary gland in carbohydrate metabolism was established early by the work of Houssay and his group.[4] Two major hormones which regulate glucose levels are GH and cortisol. In addition, prolactin and sex steroids also influence insulin sensitivity.

### Growth Hormone

Growth hormone is an antagonist to the metabolic actions of insulin. GH mediates physiological effects on glucose metabolism both directly, by inducing gluco-neogenesis, glycogenolysis and lipolysis and promoting insulin resistance in the liver and the periphery; and indirectly, via insulin-like growth factor-1 (IGF-1) stimulation that facilitates insulin action. GH inhibits insulin-induced suppression of hepatic gluconeogenesis, thus increasing glucose production. On the other hand, the known lipolytic effects of GH provide free fatty acids (FFA) from the adipose tissue; leading to glucose-fatty acid substrate competition and decreased glucose utilization in the muscle.[5] The increase in FFA production is one of the factors leading to increased gluconeogenesis and to the development of insulin resistance. Nocturnal GH secretion in diabetic patients was suggested to play a role in the hyperglycemia during early morning hours, known as dawn phenomenon.

Therefore, chronic GH excess can induce hyperglycemia by increasing endogenous glucose production and decreasing peripheral glucose disposal in muscle. Conversely, under physiologic conditions, IGF-1 improves glucose homeostasis and enhances insulin sensitivity, primarily in skeletal muscles. Indeed, exogenous IGF-1 administration has been shown to promote glucose uptake in peripheral tissues and to reduce serum glucose levels not only in healthy individuals but also in those with severe insulin resistance[6] and type 2 diabetes mellitus (T2DM).

## Adrenocorticotrophic Hormone and Glucocorticoids

Glucocorticoids (GCs) are secreted from the adrenal cortex under control of the hypothalamus–pituitary–adrenal axis. GCs play an important role in glucose metabolism as well as in lipid and protein metabolism and significantly contribute to the energy homeostasis. The most important physiological role of GCs on metabolism is displayed during the postprandial period, when they behave as contrainsular hormones. GCs stimulate lipolysis and proteolysis to provide substrates for oxidative metabolism and gluconeogenesis and inhibit glycogen synthesis.

The metabolic effects of GCs, including the actions directed to the regulation of glucose metabolism are exerted in the liver and the skeletal muscle, which is responsible for the great majority of postprandial glucose uptake from the circulation and lodge the largest store of glycogen. However, GCs have significant effects on adipose tissue as well. The effects of GCs on metabolism are discussed in the chapter "Glucocrinology of Adrenal Cortex".

## Prolactin

While prolactin is best known for the initiation and maintenance of lactation in premenopausal women, it is a major stimulus for the β-cell adaptation during gestation. Maternal prolactin increases concurrently to insulin during the second half pregnancy and stimulates β-cell proliferation, insulin production and insulin secretion.[7] Elevated prolactin levels during lactation period have been associated with improved insulin sensitivity in the postpartum period.

# GLUCOVIGILANCE IN HYPOTHALAMIC–PITUITARY DISORDERS

## Glucovigilance in Hypothalamic Disorders

The hypothalamus in the brain exerts essential role in glucose regulation by sensing circulating metabolic signals (e.g. nutrients, insulin and leptin) and instructing various neuroendocrine and neural pathways to control peripheral glucose metabolism as previously described.

## Hypothalamic Obesity

In a healthy individual, energy intake and energy expenditure are balanced so that body weight is optimally maintained. Any disturbance in the hypothalamic energy-regulating pathways, whether congenital or acquired, can lead to hypothalamic obesity, which is associated with morbid obesity, insulin resistance and diabetes.[8] The causes of hypothalamic obesity are enlisted in Table 1.

Hypothalamic obesity is usually characterized by increased appetite and less satiety and reduced energy expenditure. This results in a positive energy balance and rapid weight gain. Leptin resistance has been found to occur in individuals with exogenous obesity as well. In addition, defective signaling of hypothalamic neurons also results in disturbed glucose homeostasis and hyperglycemia. However, diet may influence the effect of insulin on hypothalamus and a high fat diet was found to blunt the central effects of insulin.

## Glucovigilance in Pituitary Disorders

### Acromegaly

Chronic GH excess in acromegaly is associated with reduced glucose uptake in muscle and fat and increased gluconeogenesis. Insulin resistance is accompanied

**TABLE 1** Causes of hypothalamic obesity.

|  | Causes |
|---|---|
| Single-gene mutations | • Leptin, leptin receptor, cocaine-amphetamine regulated transcript, POMC, prohormone convertase-1, MC4R, brain-derived neurotrophic factor (TrkB), single-minded 1 (Sim-1) |
| Genetic syndromes | • Prader–Willi syndrome<br>• Bardet–Biedl syndrome<br>• Rapid-onset obesity with hypothalamic dysfunction, hypoventilation and autonomic dysregulation (ROHHAD) syndrome |
| Trauma | • Head trauma<br>• Neurosurgery<br>• Cranial radiotherapy<br>• Cerebral aneurysm |
| Tumors | • Craniopharyngioma, meningioma, glioma, ganglioneuroma, chordoma, ependymoma<br>• Angiosarcoma, endothelioma<br>• Cholesteatoma<br>• Epidermoid, germinoma, hamartoma<br>• Pituitary macroadenoma, pinealoma, teratoma<br>• Metastases, leukemias, lymphomas |
| Inflammatory | • Sarcoidosis, tuberculosis, arachnoiditis, histiocytosis X, encephalitis, langerhans cell histiocytosis |
| Psychotropic drugs | • Antidepressants, mood stabilizers, antipsychotics |

(MC4R: melanocortin 4 receptor; POMC: pro-opiomelanocortin)

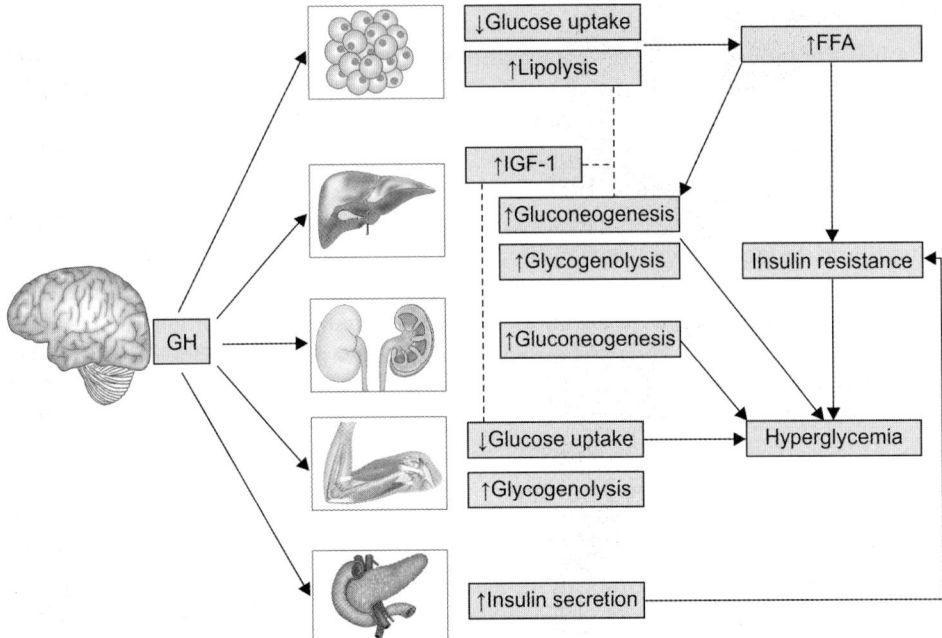

(FFA: free fatty acids; IGF-1: insulin-like growth factor-1)

**FIG. 1:** Mechanisms of hyperglycemia related to chronic growth hormone excess in acromegaly.[15]

by a compensatory rise in insulin secretion but abnormal glucose tolerance develops when this compensation is inadequate. The net effect is an increased risk of hyperglycemia and secondary diabetes. Figure 1 depicts the pathophysiological mechanisms resulting in hyperglycemia due to acromegaly. In contrast to T2DM, individuals with acromegaly have a lower amount of visceral fat and insulin resistance is mainly related to GH/IGF-1 excess. The dysfunction of visceral fat, rather than the total amount, plays a relevant role in determining insulin resistance and impairment of glucose metabolism in patients with acromegaly.

The prevalence of impaired glucose tolerance (IGT) or impaired fasting glucose (IFG) ranges from 6% to 45% and from 7% to 22%, respectively, while overt diabetes has been reported in 16–56% of acromegaly patients.[9] Acromegaly patients often develop diabetes at a younger age as compared to general population. The risk for diabetes increases with the severity and the duration of GH excess.

In addition, acromegaly is associated with hypertension in 30–40% patients. This results from GH-induced increase in renal tubular reabsorption of sodium and water with an increase in plasma volume; and due to increased cardiac output and peripheral vascular resistance. GH excess also results in increased lipolysis, increased circulating FFAs and dyslipidemia. Acromegaly is associated with impaired myocardial function, biventricular hypertrophy, impaired cardiac contractility and vascular dysfunction, often presenting as acromegalic cardiomyopathy. All of these factors result in a significantly increased risk of cardiovascular disease and mortality. In acromegaly, diabetes is actually a major determinant of mortality, and only 30% of patients with diabetes at the time acromegaly is diagnosed appear to survive over 20 years.

## CHAPTER 2: Glucocrinology of Hypothalamus and Pituitary

### *Diagnosis of acromegaly in individuals with diabetes*

Diagnosis of acromegaly is based on the measurement of both GH and IGF-1. GH levels correlate with the presence and activity of GH-secreting adenoma, while IGF-1 levels indicate the peripheral activity of GH. From a clinical point of view, both GH and IGF-1 levels have been shown to predict mortality risk in acromegaly. While a significantly high basal GH level may indicate acromegaly, the biochemical diagnosis rests on the demonstration of unsuppressed GH during an oral glucose tolerance test (OGTT). In normal individuals, GH levels decline rapidly due to inhibition of GH-releasing hormone (GHRH) and/or stimulation of somatostatin secretion. However, there is a paradoxical rise in GH levels or GH remains nonsuppressed in individuals with GH-producing pituitary adenomas. According to the current consensus guidelines, acromegaly is diagnosed if IGF-1 levels (determined by a reliable standardized assay) are above the age-adjusted normal range and GH levels during OGTT are higher than 0.4 mg/L, as measured by ultrasensitive assays.

The diagnostic approach to acromegaly in patients with coexistent diabetes could be challenging.[9] It has been demonstrated that the pulsatile secretion of GH is maintained in T2DM and enhanced in individuals on insulin therapy. The suppression of GH secretion during OGTT is independent of plasma glucose concentrations, but it was shown to be closely correlated with whole-body insulin sensitivity. The suppressive action of circulating glucose on central GH release was shown to be 50% lower in insulin resistant subjects compared with those with normal insulin sensitivity.

Even if the individual has diabetes, GH suppression test with OGTT may be needed for the evaluation of acromegaly as the effects of rapid glucose increase during an OGTT may not be reproduced by chronic hyperglycemia.[9] However, in patients with overt diabetes, particularly those on antidiabetic therapies or with significant hyperglycemia, an OGTT may not be indicated for safety reasons. In these patients, besides random GH >1 ng/mL, diagnosis relies on serum IGF-1. However, interpretation of IGF-1 levels may also be difficult in this clinical setting.

To overcome these potential diagnostic pitfalls, dynamic tests with galanin and thyrotropin-releasing hormone (TRH) have been proposed. Galanin was found to paradoxically decrease circulating GH levels in patients with active acromegaly and the results were not influenced by coexistent disorders of glucose metabolism. Therefore, when the biochemical diagnosis of a patient with suspected acromegaly and diabetes is not clear cut, a confirmatory galanin test may be recommended.[9] But it is not routinely available in several countries including India.

### *Effect of treatment of acromegaly on glycemic control*

- *Surgery and radiotherapy:* Transsphenoidal surgery is considered the first line approach to treatment in acromegaly. In a recent study, surgical treatment of acromegaly resulted in improved glycemic control in both cured and not cured patients.[10] However, once β-cell function is impaired, abnormal glucose metabolism can persist even after cure. In radiotherapy, glycemic status correlated with post-treatment GH level.[11]
- *Effect of medical therapy:* Medical management of acromegaly can have varied effects on glycemic control and depends on the pharmacological agent, as discussed here:

- *Somatostatin analogs*: Somatostatin analogs (SSAs) including octreotide and lanreotide can affect glucose homeostasis by reducing pancreatic insulin and glucagon secretion. It has been suggested that, over the long-term, the decreased insulin secretion could be counterbalanced by the improvement of insulin sensitivity due to reduced GH secretion.[12] As they have an impact on glucose metabolism, periodic glucose monitoring is recommended in these patients.
- *Pasireotide*: It is a multi-receptor ligand SSA which, compared to octreotide, displays a 30-, 5- and 40-times higher binding affinity to somatostatin receptor-1 (SSTR-1), SSTR-3 and SSTR-5, respectively and a 2.5-times lower affinity to SSTR-2. Pasireotide can result in significant hyperglycemia, which is due to its differential effect on SSTRs. Glucagon-producing α-cells predominantly express SSTR-2, whereas insulin-producing β-cells mainly express SSTR-2 and SSTR-5. Pasireotide, by binding with high affinity to SSTR-5, suppresses insulin secretion, whereas the inhibitory effect on glucagon secretion is only modest.[12] This insulin-glucagon imbalance results in rise in blood glucose levels. Pasireotide can result in significant hyperglycemia, requiring frequent monitoring of blood glucose values and titration of insulin and other antidiabetic therapies.[12] In diabetic patients, hyperglycemic treatment should be optimized before starting pasireotide. Incretin drugs including glucagon-like polypeptide-1 (GLP-1) receptor agonists and dipeptidyl peptidase 4 (DPP4) inhibitors reduce glucagon secretion while increasing insulin secretion and are particularly useful for hyperglycemia resulting from pasireotide.[12]
- *Pegvisomant*: Pegvisomant (PEG) is a genetically-engineered GH-analog which antagonizes the effect of GH at the GH receptor, leading to reduced IGF-1 production. When compared to first-generation SSAs, PEG shows a better impact on glucose homeostasis and insulin-sensitivity, as evidenced by studies in patients switched from octreotide to PEG therapy.[13] While several studies have demonstrated the positive impact of PEG on fasting plasma glucose (FPG), IGT, HbA1c levels and insulin-sensitivity, the effect on FFA is still controversial. Some studies have reported a decrease in FFA levels during PEG treatment.[14] Considering the overall positive impact on glucose homeostasis, PEG treatment represents a good option in patients with uncontrolled diabetes and resistance or poor response to first-generation SSAs.
- *Dopamine agonists*: Bromocriptine and cabergoline are dopamine agonists, which, by binding to the D2 receptor in the pituitary tumor, can suppress GH secretion. They can be used for the treatment of acromegaly as monotherapy or, more frequently, in combination with SSAs. Bromocriptine can exert a positive impact on glucose metabolism via a direct effect on central nervous system and also by reducing gluconeogenesis.

### Management of diabetes in acromegaly

Even though the control of GH hypersecretion significantly improves the metabolic complications of acromegaly, diabetes maintains a higher prevalence in acromegaly patients in remission compared to general population, therefore individuals with acromegaly need long-term follow-up even after remission has been attained.[15]

There are no specific recommendations for the treatment of acromegaly-associated diabetes. All antidiabetic drugs can be used in individuals with acromegaly following the stepwise approach generally recommended for individuals with T2DM. Many patients with significant hyperglycemia require insulin for management. Following surgery for pituitary adenoma, most patients who undergo disease remission will have improvement in insulin sensitivity, requiring down-titration of pharmacological treatment for hyperglycemia.

## Cushing's Disease

Adrenocorticotrophic hormone (ACTH)-producing pituitary adenomas are the most common cause of endogenous Cushing's syndrome. Cushing's disease is characterized by impaired glucose homeostasis and secondary diabetes. In fact, the prevalence of diabetes and IGT in Cushing's syndrome can be as high as 50% and 70%, respectively.[16]

Chronic GC excess results in increased gluconeogenesis in the liver and skeletal muscle, by both inducing the expression of enzymes of gluconeogenesis and increasing the availability of substrates for the same from enhanced proteolysis and lipolysis. In addition, there is decreased peripheral glucose uptake and reduced glycogen synthesis, further contributing to hyperglycemia. The effects of GC excess on glucose metabolism are depicted in Figure 2. It is noteworthy that the onset of insulin resistance is related to either a direct effect of GCs on insulin receptor signaling pathway or an indirect effect of GCs altering the insulin function through the changes in lipid and protein metabolism.[16]

GC-induced diabetes is discussed in greater details in the chapter "Glucocrinology of Adrenal Cortex" and here briefly described are the relevant aspects related to management of Cushing's disease and secondary diabetes.

### Clinical presentation

Patients with glucocorticoid-induced diabetes manifest poorly controlled diabetes and can have typical features of hypercortisolism, such as hypokalemia, facial plethora, easy bruising, reddish purple striae, proximal myopathy, prominent dorsocervical fat pad, sexual dysfunction in men and menstrual disorders, acne and hirsutism in women. They may suffer from coexistent complications of hypercortisolism such as hypertension, recurrent infections, ischemic cardiac disease, fragility fractures and neuropsychiatric disorders which may have a synergistic impact on quality of life and survival of patients with Cushing's disease. The risk of mortality is double in Cushing's disease than in the general population; diabetes, hypertension and uncontrolled hypercortisolism have been reported to predict the risk of death.[17]

### Diagnosis of diabetes in Cushing's disease

Diagnosis of glucocorticoid-induced diabetes is based on measurement of FPG, HbA1c and plasma glucose values on OGTT. A significant proportion of patients may have normal FPG and have predominantly postprandial hyperglycemia. Therefore, OGTT has greater sensitivity in detection of GC-induced hyperglycemia.

# SECTION 1: The Scope of Glucocrinology

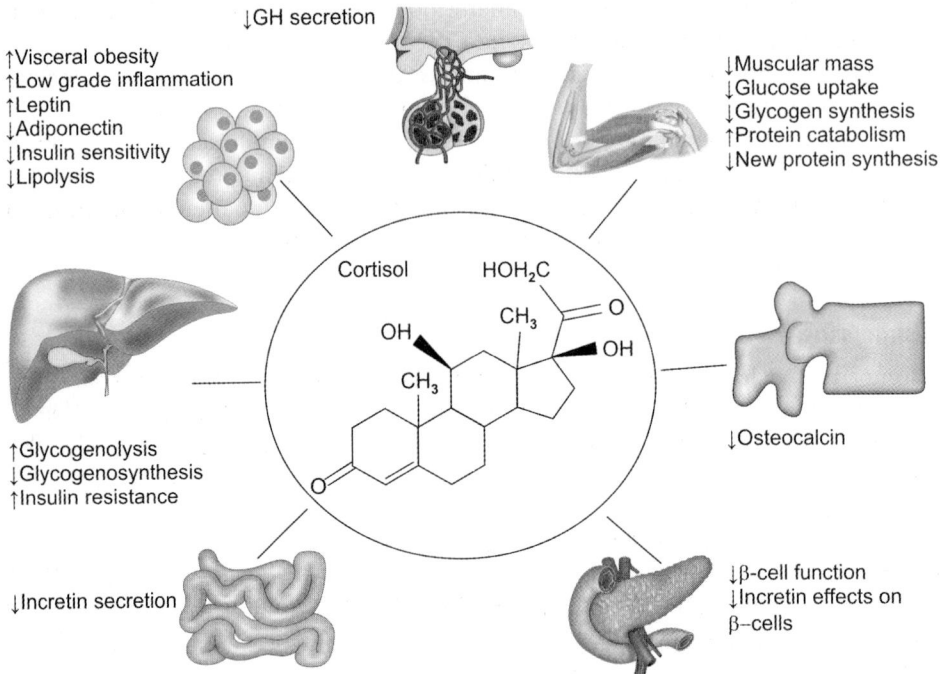

**FIG. 2:** Mechanisms of hyperglycemia due to chronic glucocorticoid excess.[19]

## Effect of treatment of Cushing's disease on glycemic status

Reduction in serum cortisol levels is associated with improved insulin sensitivity and overall positive effect on glycemic control.

- *Surgery:* The first-line approach remains transsphenoidal surgery with a mean remission rate of 77.8% when performed by an experienced neurosurgeon. Normalization of cortisol levels after surgery is generally followed by an improved glycemic control, but insulin resistance and cardiovascular risk may persist, particularly in patients with a genetic predisposition and/or persistent visceral adiposity.[18] There is a risk for postoperative hypoglycemia following pituitary surgery due to sudden fall in cortisol levels, requiring careful titration of insulin and other medications.
- *Effect of medical management of Cushing's disease on glycemic status:* Various pharmacological agents can have varied effect on glycemic control[18] as discussed here:
  - *Pasireotide:* It can cause significant hyperglycemia and requires close blood glucose monitoring, as discussed earlier.
  - *Dopamine agonist:* Bromocriptine and cabergoline can have a favorable effect on glucose metabolism.
  - *Retinoic acid:* It inhibits the expression of POMC in ACTH-producing and has been considered another potential option for Cushing's disease treatment. Retinol active metabolites are able to stimulate insulin secretion, enhance

mRNA expression of GLUT2, and promote lipolysis in adipocytes by activating PPARγ, thereby having a favorable effect on glycemic status.[19]
- *Ketoconazole:* It inhibits GC synthesis and has a positive effect on glycemic control.[18]
- *Mifepristone:* It is a glucocorticoid receptor (GR) antagonist that is associated with improved insulin resistance, especially in the first 6 weeks of treatment initiation. The early rapid improvement in glycemic control is probably due to direct blockade of GC effects.[19]

## Management of diabetes in Cushing's disease

Improvement in glycemic control parallels reduction in cortisol levels. Therefore, correction of hypercortisolism is an important therapeutic goal. Treatment of diabetes in individuals with Cushing's disease is similar as T2DM, with an increased focus on optimization of protein intake and increased physical activity. However, glucocorticoid-induced myopathy may greatly limit their physical activity. Metformin remains the first line drug, but insulin may be required in a large number of patients. Pioglitazone is limited by side effects related to fluid retention, weight gain, heart failure and osteoporosis. Insulin secretagogues can be considered; however, careful dose titration is needed following surgery or medical management as amelioration of hypercortisolism may increase the risk of hypoglycemia. Incretin-based drugs have been reported to be useful in GC-induced diabetes, and have been found to be particularly useful in pasireotide-induced diabetes. These aspects of management are elaborated on in the chapter "Glucocrinology of Adrenal Cortex".

## Hyperprolactinemia

Chronic hyperprolactinemia, due to prolactin-secreting pituitary adenomas, is associated with increased food intake and weight gain, therefore promoting obesity. Prolactin-induced increase in appetite has been mainly linked to the functional blockade of dopaminergic tone. In fact, dopaminergic tone plays a key role in increasing energy expenditure and reducing food intake and its suppression has been considered a potential mechanism contributing to hyperphagia and weight gain in patients with hyperprolactinemia, together with the increased hypothalamic levels of the appetite-stimulating hormones NPY and corticotropin-releasing hormone (CRH).[20]

In addition to the effects of hyperprolactinemia on modulation of food intake, it also affects adipocyte function and insulin secretion.[20] Men and women with chronic hyperprolactinemia have been demonstrated to display postprandial hyperinsulinemia and exaggerated insulin secretory response to glucose. Metabolic syndrome has been reported in approximately one-third of patients with hyperprolactinemia, ranging from 23% to 50% in different series.[21]

## Effect of dopamine agonists on glycemic control

Dopamine agonists are the first-line drugs in the management of symptomatic hyperprolactinemia. They can have a favorable effect on glycemic control by an effect on insulin action. Bromocriptine quick release (QR) decreased plasma glucose levels and improved glucose tolerance in both diabetic and nondiabetic subjects, and is approved for use in diabetes management. In a double blinded placebo-controlled study in individuals with diabetes, there was significant reduction in HbA1c levels when cabergoline 0.5 mg per week was added to ongoing antidiabetic medications.[22] Fasting insulin levels and HOMA-β correlated with the dose of cabergoline.

In addition, cabergoline was also shown to reduce the prevalence of metabolic syndrome by up to 5% in patients treated for 6–60 months.[20] This benefit occurs due to significant decrease in body weight and improvement in lipid and glycemic profile resulting from reduction in prolactin levels. Bromocriptine QR also has a favorable cardiovascular risk profile but long-term studies of its efficacy and safety are lacking. In patients with hyperprolactinemia, dopamine agonists may result in weight reduction, improved glycemic and lipid control and reduced cardiovascular risk; but at present evidence is insufficient to consider them as front-line drugs for the management of T2DM.[23]

### Metformin in drug induced hyperprolactinemia

Metformin effectively crosses the blood-brain barrier and attains relatively high concentrations in the pituitary. Pituitary gland seems to be an important target for metformin action and modulates the function of lactotrophs to reduce prolactin levels. Metformin reduces the synthesis and release of prolactin by affecting dopaminergic regulation of lactotroph function. However, the effect of metformin on prolactin secretion is only seen if there is enhanced secretion and the reduction in prolactin levels occurs only at higher doses of metformin.[24] Metformin may be a useful option in drug-induced hyperprolactinemia, especially associated with the use of anti-psychotic medications where dopamine agonists can aggravate psychosis.

### Growth Hormone Deficiency

Growth hormone deficiency in adulthood manifests as visceral adiposity, insulin resistance, dyslipidemia and hyperglycemia, which contribute to increased cardiovascular morbidity and mortality. Because IGF-1 has anti-inflammatory properties and is important for glucose uptake in peripheral tissues, metabolic disturbances in GH-deficient adults can be explained by the IGF-1 deficit.[25] A deprivation of GH-induced lipolysis and subsequent increased visceral adiposity are also involved in increased circulating FFAs and insulin resistance in these patients. Most of the metabolic disturbances, including visceral adiposity, sarcopenia, hypertension and dyslipidemia were reported to be relieved after GH treatment.

### Effect of growth hormone replacement on glucose homeostasis

Most of the studies on evaluation of the metabolic effects of GH therapy have demonstrated increased insulin resistance, indicated by increased fasting insulin and homeostasis model assessment of insulin resistance (HOMA-IR) levels.[25] Therefore, there have been concerns about the risk of glucose intolerance and diabetes with long-term use of GH.

However, most studies have not reported any significant effect of GH replacement on fasting and postprandial glucose and HbA1c levels.[25] Studies in children and adolescents also suggested that GH administration may induce insulin resistance in short-term treatment, but its long-term consequences have not been fully determined yet. International cohort studies indicate that GH therapy may increase the incidence of T2DM in children and adolescents with predisposing risk factors; therefore, it is prudent to monitor glycemic status during and after GH administration.[26] More recently, no increase in the long-term risk of diabetes was reported in subjects treated with GH for idiopathic isolated GH deficiency, idiopathic short stature or short stature in children born short for gestational age, regardless of sex.[27] There was no added risk of gestational diabetes in women treated with GH during childhood when compared to the general population. These results are reassuring as they suggest that GH treatment does not increase the risk of diabetes, but further studies are required to confirm their validity.

### Hypopituitarism

Hypopituitarism may have variable effect on glucose homeostasis. Untreated GH deficiency, central hypothyroidism and central hypogonadism, as well as over-treatment of adrenal insufficiency, are associated with insulin resistance and may predispose to the development of diabetes.

However, anterior pituitary also plays a key role in the physiological response to hypoglycemia. Cortisol and GH are important counter-regulating hormones that act in concert with glucagon and epinephrine to regulate blood glucose levels. A deficiency of either the counter-regulatory hormones or the factors that control their production and secretion may predispose to hypoglycemia. Individuals with hypopituitarism, therefore, may present with recurrent hypoglycemia, that improves with appropriate hormone replacement.

## HYPOTHALAMIC–PITUITARY VIGILANCE IN DIABETES

Hyperglycemia and long-standing diabetes may also affect the functioning of various hypothalamic–pituitary–end organ axis. In this section, we discuss the alterations in hypothalamic and pituitary function that occur in individuals with type 1 diabetes mellitus (T1DM) or T2DM.

### Growth Hormone Axis

Adequate glycemic control is required for optimal growth and development of children with T1DM. Growth failure has been reported in children with long-standing poor glycemic control. This was especially true prior to the widespread use of intensive insulin regimens in the management of T1DM.

Many pathophysiologic processes, including malnutrition, chronic intermittent acidosis, increased glucocorticoid production, hypothyroidism, impaired calcium balance and end-organ unresponsiveness to either GH or IGF, may contribute to this growth failure.[28] IGF-1 and insulin-like growth factor binding protein 3 (IGFBP3) levels are diminished with enhanced GH production in poorly controlled diabetes, reflecting acquired GH insensitivity. However, most children with T1DM, even those with marginal control, grow quite normally, especially in prepubertal years, but growth velocity can decrease during puberty.

## Hypothalamic–Pituitary–Thyroid Axis

Metabolic decompensation in diabetic patients leads to the impaired secretion of TSH and thyroid hormones and a blunted response of TSH and thyroid hormones to TRH. This may result in subtle abnormalities in thyroid function tests.[29] In addition, metformin can lower TSH levels through its effect on hypothalamus, but does not affect circulating T3 and T4 concentrations. The effect of diabetes on thyroid physiology is discussed in greater detail in the chapter "Glucocrinology of Thyroid".

## Hypothalamic–Pituitary–Adrenal Axis

The hypothalamic–pituitary–adrenal (HPA) function is upregulated in uncontrolled or poorly controlled diabetes. Alterations in HPA axis in diabetes may be the result of insulin deficiency and/or hyperglycemia and insulin administration was associated with normalized pituitary and adrenal activity.[30] Interestingly, central components of the HPA axis remained upregulated. Chronic hyperglycemia has been shown to be a major factor in some of the long-term complications associated with diabetes, including neurodegeneration[31] and impairment of glucose counter-regulatory mechanisms.

Insulin-induced hypoglycemia is a potent activator of the HPA axis, and results in increased secretion of CRH and ACTH. ACTH in turn increases the secretion of cortisol from the adrenal cortex. The stress response is terminated via glucocorticoid negative feedback through occupation of GR by glucocorticoids.

Dysregulation of basal HPA function in diabetes may stem from the complex metabolic changes that occur in diabetes and there may be a blunting of the counter-regulatory response to hypoglycemia. On the other hand, even a partial improvement in plasma glucose can restore the HPA response to hypoglycemia in diabetic rats. This indicates that optimal glucose control is crucial for the maintenance of HPA responses to insulin-induced hypoglycemia.

## Hypothalamic–Pituitary–Gonadal Axis

The incidence of diabetes among men attending infertility clinics was estimated to be 0.3%, and about 1% of subfertile male patients may have diabetes.[32] Diabetic men had significantly low serum testosterone with low LH and FSH, hypoalbuminemia, hypercholesterolemia and hypertriglyceridemia. Low serum testosterone could be due to decreased synthesis or increased metabolic clearance.[32] In addition, women with diabetes also have significant reproductive dysfunction. While poorly controlled T1DM is associated with hypothalamic amenorrhea, T2DM in women has a significant overlap with polycystic ovary syndrome (PCOS).[32] The effects of diabetes on hypothalamic–pituitary–gonadal axis are discussed in the chapter "Reproductive Dysfunction in Diabetes".

## CONCLUSION

The hypothalamus and pituitary gland work in close collaboration with metabolically active tissues to regulate energy balance and glucose homeostasis. Disorders of hypothalamus due to a wide variety of congenital or acquired factors may result in obesity and diabetes. In addition, acromegaly, hyperprolactinemia and Cushing's disease resulting from hormone-secreting pituitary adenoma are associated with hyperglycemia and secondary diabetes. Management of these disorders with surgery, radiation or pharmacological agents is associated with improved glycemic control resulting from amelioration of hormone excess. However, certain pharmacological agents such as pasireotide, octreotide and lanreotide may worsen hyperglycemia requiring close monitoring. On the other hand, dopamine agonists, pegvisomant and ketoconazole have a favorable impact on glycemic control.

Hypopituitarism is associated with increased risk of hypoglycemia and deficits of anterior pituitary function should be excluded in individuals presenting with unexplained hypoglycemia. On the other hand, diabetes itself is associated with alterations in hypothalamic–pituitary function. Therefore, it is abundantly clear that there is a need for glucovigilance in the endocrine clinic when treating individuals with hypophyseal-pituitary disorders and there is a need for endovigilance of hypothalamic–pituitary function in the diabetes clinic.

# REFERENCES

1. Tena-Sempere M. Neuroendocrinology in 2016: Neuroendocrine control of metabolism and reproduction. Nat Rev Endocrinol. 2017;13(2):67-8.
2. Routh VH, Hao L, Santiago AM, et al. Hypothalamic glucose sensing: making ends meet. Front Syst Neurosci. 2014;8:236.
3. Fioramonti X, Chrétien C, Leloup C, et al. Recent advances in the cellular and molecular mechanisms of hypothalamic neuronal glucose detection. Front Physiol. 2017;8:875.
4. Rosario W, Singh I, Wautlet A, et al. The brain-to-pancreatic islet neuronal map reveals differential glucose regulation from distinct hypothalamic regions. Diabetes. 2016;65(9):2711-23.
5. Rizza RA, Mandarino LJ, Gerich JE. Effects of growth hormone on insulin action in man. Mechanisms of insulin resistance, impaired suppression of glucose production, and impaired stimulation of glucose utilization. Diabetes. 1982;31(8 Pt 1):663-9.
6. Zenobi PD, Glatz Y, Keller A, et al. Beneficial metabolic effects of insulin-like growth factor I in patients with severe insulin-resistant diabetes type A. Eur J Endocrinol. 1994;131(3):251-7.
7. Huang C, Snider F, Cross JC. Prolactin receptor is required for normal glucose homeostasis and modulation of beta-cell mass during pregnancy. Endocrinology. 2009;150(4):1618-26.
8. Abuzzahab MJ, Roth CL, Shoemaker AH. Hypothalamic Obesity: Prologue and Promise. Horm Res Paediatr. 2019;18:1-9.
9. Frara S, Maffezzoni F, Mazziotti G, et al. Current and Emerging Aspects of Diabetes Mellitus in Acromegaly. Trends Endocrinol Metab. 2016;27(7):470-83.
10. Helseth R, Carlsen SM, Bollerslev J, et al. Preoperative octreotide therapy and surgery in acromegaly: associations between glucose homeostasis and treatment response. Endocrine. 2016;51(2):298-307.
11. Barrande G, Pittino-Lungo M, Coste J, et al. Hormonal and metabolic effects of radiotherapy in acromegaly: long-term results in 128 patients followed in a single center. J Clin Endocrinol Metab. 2000;85:3779-85.
12. Paragliola RM, Salvatori R. Novel Somatostatin Receptor Ligands Therapies for Acromegaly. Front Endocrinol (Lausanne). 2018;9:78.
13. Barkan AL, Burman P, Clemmons DR, et al. Glucose homeostasis and safety in patients with acromegaly converted from long-acting octreotide to pegvisomant. J Clin Endocrinol Metab. 2005;90(10):5684-91.
14. Rose DR, Clemmons DR. Growth hormone receptor antagonist improves insulin resistance in acromegaly. Growth Horm IGF Res. 2002;12:418-24.
15. Ferraù F, Albani A, Ciresi A, et al. Diabetes Secondary to Acromegaly: Physiopathology, Clinical Features and Effects of Treatment. Front Endocrinol (Lausanne). 2018;9:358.

16. Andrews RC, Walker BR. Glucocorticoids and insulin resistance: old hormones, new targets. Clin Sci (Lond). 1999;96(5):513-23.
17. Mazziotti G, Gazzaruso C, Giustina A. Diabetes in Cushing syndrome: basic and clinical aspects. Trends Endocrinol Metab. 2011;22:499-506.
18. Mazziotti G, Formenti AM, Frara S, et al. Diabetes in Cushing Disease. Curr Diab Rep. 2017;17(5):32.
19. Barbot M, Ceccato F, Scaroni C. Diabetes Mellitus Secondary to Cushing's Disease. Front Endocrinol (Lausanne). 2018;9:284.
20. Auriemma RS, De Alcubierre D, Pirchio R, et al. The effects of hyperprolactinemia and its control on metabolic diseases. Expert Rev Endocrinol Metab. 2018;13(2):99-106.
21. Andersen M, Glintborg D. Metabolic Syndrome in Hyperprolactinemia. Front Horm Res. 2018;49: 29-47.
22. Bahar A, Kashi Z, Daneshpour E, et al. Effects of cabergoline on blood glucose levels in type 2 diabetic patients: a double-blind controlled clinical trial. Medicine (Baltimore). 2016;95(40):e4818.
23. Garber AJ, Blonde L, Bloomgarden ZT, et al. The role of bromocriptine-QR in the management of type 2 diabetes expert panel recommendations. Endocr Pract. 2013;19(1):100-6.
24. Krysiak R, Kowalcze K, Szkrobka W, et al. The effect of metformin on prolactin levels in patients with drug-induced hyperprolactinemia. Eur J Intern Med. 2016;30:94-8.
25. Groop L, Segerlantz M, Bramnert M. Insulin sensitivity in adults with growth hormone deficiency and effect of growth hormone treatment. Horm Res. 2005;64:45-50.
26. Kim SH, Park MJ. Effects of growth hormone on glucose metabolism and insulin resistance in human. Ann Pediatr Endocrinol Metab. 2017;22(3):145-52.
27. Poidvin A, Weill A, Ecosse E, et al. Risk of Diabetes Treated in Early Adulthood After Growth Hormone Treatment of Short Stature in Childhood. J Clin Endocrinol Metab. 2017;102(4):1291-8.
28. Jackson RL, Holland E, Chatman ID, et al. Growth and maturation of children with insulin dependent diabetes mellitus. Diabetes Care. 1978;1(2):96-107.
29. Biondi B, Kahaly GJ, Robertson RP. Thyroid Dysfunction and Diabetes Mellitus: Two Closely Associated Disorders. Endocr Rev. 2019;40(3):789-824.
30. Chan O, Inouye K, Akirav EM, et al. Hyperglycemia does not increase basal hypothalamo-pituitary-adrenal activity in diabetes but it does impair the HPA response to insulin-induced hypoglycemia. Am J Physiol Regul Integr Comp Physiol. 2005;289(1):R235-46.
31. Chan O, Chan S, Inouye K, et al. Molecular regulation of the hypothalamo-pituitary-adrenal axis in streptozotocin-induced diabetes: effects of insulin treatment. Endocrinology. 2001;142(11): 4872-9.
32. Gandhi J, Dagur G, Warren K, et al. The Role of Diabetes Mellitus in Sexual and Reproductive Health: An Overview of Pathogenesis, Evaluation, and Management. Curr Diabetes Rev. 2017; 13(6):573-81.

# CHAPTER 3

# Glucocrinology of Thyroid

*Emmy Grewal, Gagan Priya, Ndeye M Ndour Mbaye*

## INTRODUCTION

Thyroid hormones (THs) are important regulators of glucose and energy metabolism, and by action on liver, adipose tissue, skeletal muscle and pancreas, they influence insulin sensitivity and carbohydrate metabolism. Therefore, any alteration in thyroid physiology can have clinically meaningful impact on pancreatic function as well as glucose homeostasis. Several studies have documented an increased prevalence of thyroid disorders in people with diabetes and vice versa.

Both disorders mutually influence each other and evidence suggests a pivotal role of insulin resistance in underlining the relation between type 2 diabetes mellitus (T2DM) and thyroid dysfunction. In addition, type 1 diabetes mellitus (T1DM) and autoimmune thyroid disease (AITD) share common genetic susceptibility loci. Untreated thyroid disorders affect glycemic control in individuals with diabetes; on the other hand, diabetes affects thyroid function tests to variable extent. Both hyperthyroidism and hypothyroidism have been associated with insulin resistance, a major pathophysiological defect in T2DM. Concomitant occurrence of diabetes and thyroid disorders can impact the clinical presentation and influence diagnosis and management of both.

This chapter sums up the interdependent relationship between thyroid physiology and glucose homeostasis in health and disease. This will guide clinicians on the optimal screening and management of these conditions.

## GLUCOSE PHYSIOLOGY IN RELATION TO THYROID

Thyroid hormones exert profound effects on the regulation of glucose homeostasis and lipid metabolism.[1] These effects are mediated both through the central nervous system and via direct interaction of THs with peripheral target organs such as liver, white adipose tissue (WAT) and brown adipose tissue (BAT), pancreatic β-cells and skeletal muscle. TH action is exerted primarily by binding with high affinity nuclear thyroid hormone receptors (TRs), α and β. TRα is abundant in brain, kidneys, gonads,

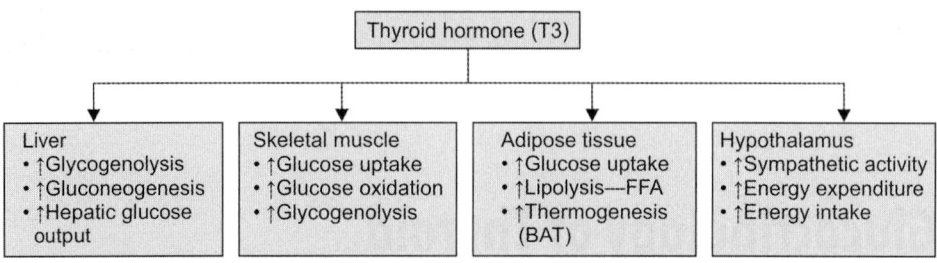

(BAT: brown adipose tissue; FFA: free fatty acid)

**FLOWCHART 1:** Effect of thyroid hormones on glucose and energy metabolism.

muscle and heart; whereas, TRβ expression is relatively high in pituitary and liver. The differential expression of these isoforms within tissues is responsible for TH specificity.

Thyroid hormones regulate glucose homeostasis in several ways, as depicted in Flowchart 1 and discussed further in text.

## Increase Hepatic Glucose Production

Thyroid hormones exert an important role in hepatic glucose metabolism with a stimulating effect on hepatic glucose production in vivo and in vitro.[2] THs stimulate glycogenolysis as well as gluconeogenesis by increasing the availability of alanine, a metabolic intermediate of the gluconeogenic pathway, and upregulating the expression of phosphoenolpyruvate carboxykinase (PEPCK), which is a critical enzyme for gluconeogenesis. Both lipogenesis and lipolysis are stimulated by triiodothyronine (T3); increased lipolysis results in an increase in free fatty acids (FFA) that also stimulates hepatic gluconeogenesis. T3 acts centrally on T3-sensitive neurons in paraventricular hypothalamus to increase hepatic glucose production via sympathetic stimulation.

## Maintain Pancreatic Beta-cell Function

Pancreatic islets contain TRα1 and TRβ1 which are important for normal islet development. In culture studies, T3 is required for the transition of islets to glucose-responsive insulin-secreting cells and their proliferation; physiological T3 maintains islet structure and prevents streptozotocin-induced islet cell deterioration.[3] However, hyperthyroidism leads to impaired insulin secretion secondary to reduced β-cell mass and dysregulation of ATP-sensitive potassium (KATP) channels and L-type $Ca^{2+}$ channels in the insulin secretory pathway.[4] In pancreatic α-cells, TH enhances glucagon secretion.

## Regulation of Glucose Metabolism in Skeletal Muscle and Adipose Tissue

Thyroid hormone has insulin antagonistic effects in liver; whereas, it acts synergistically with insulin in peripheral tissues. In skeletal muscle, T3 increases basal and insulin-stimulated glucose uptake by increased expression of glucose transporter-4 (GLUT-4), adenosine monophosphate–activated protein kinase (AMPK), and acetyl coenzyme A (acetyl CoA) carboxylase. In adipose tissue, TH stimulates lipolysis and increases serum FFA level, which causes insulin resistance. TH may also influence carbohydrate metabolism via its interaction with adipocytokines and gut hormones. A correlation between leptin and TH levels has been demonstrated in several studies. However, results have also been discordant. Adipose tissue and skeletal muscle secrete adipokines and myokines, respectively, which can modulate insulin sensitivity in these tissues. Both hypothyroidism and hyperthyroidism can interfere with the normal adipocyte-myocyte crosstalk, thus contributing to insulin resistance.[5]

## Increased Energy Expenditure—Peripheral and Central Effects

Thyroid hormones influence thermogenesis by regulating transcription factors involved in adipogenesis of WAT (white adipose tissue) and BAT (brown adipose tissue), appetite regulation, and glucose and lipid metabolism and oxidation. T3 in BAT upregulates mitochondrial uncoupling protein 3 (UCP3), which leads to increased energy expenditure and basal metabolic rate. Centrally, T3 decreases AMPK activity in the hypothalamus which in turn, increases sympathetic nervous system (SNS) activation of BAT. Whereas thyrotropin-releasing hormone (TRH) has a direct anorectic effect, on the other hand T3 stimulates food intake at the level of the hypothalamus.[6] TRH neurons in the hypothalamus also express TH nuclear receptors and melanocortin 4 receptor (MC4R), which is a key receptor involved in central energy regulation. Activation of MC4R leads to increased energy expenditure and decreased food intake. T3 decreases the expression of MC4R as well as decreases the hypothalamic sensitivity of pro-opiomelanocortin (POMC) and agouti-related peptide (AgRP) signaling, and both processes help in conserving energy in hyperthyroid states.[6] Hyperthyroidism leads to dysregulation of the hypothalamic neuropeptide system, including increased neuropeptide Y (NPY) and AgRP expression, and decreased POMC expression in the arcuate nucleus. Despite increased appetite, hyperthyroidism is usually associated with a variable decrease in body weight, due to the increase in total energy expenditure.[6]

## GLUCOVIGILANCE IN THYROID DISORDERS

Thyroid disorders are associated with significant changes in insulin sensitivity, weight and body fat, blood pressure, and glucose and lipid metabolism. Both hypothyroidism and hyperthyroidism may be associated with impaired glucose metabolism and dysglycemia.

### Hypothyroidism

Serum thyroid-stimulating hormone (TSH) has been positively associated with hyperglycemia and insulin resistance in euthyroid subjects in several studies.[7,8] Longitudinal studies suggest that even subtle changes in the levels of serum TSH, thyroxine (T4) and T3 within the physiological range can induce insulin resistance or diabetes. In a longitudinal study, the risk of incident T2DM was significantly increased with each 1 mU/L increment of serum TSH; individuals in the highest tertile of TSH change had a greater risk of incident T2DM [hazard ratio (HR): 1.44, 95% confidence interval (CI): 1.04–1.98, p = 0.027] in comparison with individuals in the lowest tertile.[9] In a population-based prospective cohort study of 8,452 participants over 7.9 years, higher TSH levels even within the reference range were associated with a higher diabetes risk (HR 1.13; 95 % CI 1.08–1.18, per logTSH); and in prediabetics, the risk of progression to diabetes was 1.13 times higher for every doubling of TSH levels (95 % CI 1.03–1.24).[10] The pathogenic mechanism responsible for insulin resistance may be related to leptin resistance at hypothalamus, decreased GLUT-4 receptors, increased circulating FFA and chronic inflammation.

In addition, hypothyroidism shares common comorbidities with diabetes including higher prevalence of obesity, hypertension, endothelial dysfunction and dyslipidemia [raised total and low-density lipoprotein (LDL) cholesterol and reduced high-density lipoprotein (HDL) cholesterol], and cardiovascular risk. In fact, low normal TH levels and high normal TSH even in euthyroid range is associated with hyperlipidemia and insulin resistance. Levothyroxine (LT4) replacement therapy may improve insulin sensitivity. Additionally, LT4 replacement, at least partially, ameliorates other cardiovascular risk factors including hypertension, dyslipidemia and endothelial dysfunction. Therefore, glucovigilance is needed when treating patients with hypothyroidism.

## Hyperthyroidism

Hyperthyroidism may be associated with glucose intolerance in a significant proportion of patients. In a study of 38 patients with hyperthyroidism without previous history of diabetes, oral glucose tolerance test (OGTT) revealed a prevalence of glucose intolerance in 39.4%, of which 31.5% had impaired glucose tolerance (IGT) and 7.9% had diabetes. Insulin sensitivity significantly improved after attaining euthyroid status with treatment of hyperthyroidism, despite an increase in body weight.[11] In another observation case-control study from Dhaka, glucose intolerance was detected in 72.3% of 65 patients with thyrotoxicosis (45 Graves' disease and 20 toxic multinodular goiter), suggesting that Asian Indians may be particularly susceptible. A significant positive correlation was detected between plasma glucose and free T4 (FT4) levels.[12]

Hyperthyroidism leads to enhanced glucose absorption from gastrointestinal tract due to increased gastrointestinal mobility resulting from TH excess. However, THs may also directly activate $Na^+/K^+$-ATPase; increased sodium flux causing increased sodium-glucose cotransporter-1 (SGLT-1) activity that in turn contributes to increased intestinal glucose absorption.[13]

Glucose intolerance results from increased hepatic insulin resistance as well as increased endogenous glucose production. THs increase gluconeogenesis in liver through direct effect as well as indirectly by increasing glucagon and catecholamine levels. Gluconeogenesis is increased in both subclinical and overt hyperthyroidism. In adipose tissues, TH stimulates lipolysis and increases serum FFA level which causes insulin resistance. On the other hand, GLUT-4 expression and glucose uptake in skeletal muscle are increased in hyperthyroidism.

In pancreatic β-cells, TH stimulates insulin secretion, although TH excess leads to β-cell apoptosis as well as increased degradation of insulin. The half-life of insulin is reduced in hyperthyroidism secondary to an increased rate of degradation and an enhanced release of biologically inactive insulin precursors.[14] In pancreatic α-cells, TH enhances glucagon secretion. Via sum of these effects on glucose metabolism by TH, excess TH can cause dysglycemia and secondary diabetes or glucose intolerance.

Individuals with thyrotoxicosis require an OGTT for detection of glucose intolerance as glycated hemoglobin (HbA1c) may underdiagnose a significant proportion of thyrotoxicosis-associated glucose intolerance. In a study of 310 patients with newly diagnosed Graves' disease, 33.2% had prediabetes by HbA1c criteria compared to 41.3% by OGTT. Overt diabetes was diagnosed using HbA1c in only 4.5% compared to 11.3% by OGTT.[15] Amelioration of thyrotoxicosis can result in improvement in glucose intolerance. In 119 patients with Graves' disease, glycemic abnormalities partially improved with antithyroidal drugs with lowering of serum T4 and T3 concentrations.[16] In another study of 64 hyperthyroid patients, glucose intolerance improved in most after correction of hyperthyroidism, though those with overt diabetes remained hyperglycemic.[17]

## THYROVIGILANCE IN DIABETES

Hyperglycemia may lead to significant alterations in TH levels. While on the one hand, hyperglycemia is associated with reduced peripheral conversion of T4 to T3 resulting in a low T3 state, the nocturnal peak of TSH is also blunted in diabetics. Interpretation of thyroid functions may be challenging in acute hyperglycemic emergencies which are associated with reduced total T4 levels due to decreased protein binding and reduced T3 levels due to decreased peripheral conversion of T4 to T3. Additionally, sick patients can also have impaired TSH secretion. Subtle abnormalities in thyroid functions may improve with improvement of glycemic control.

In addition, several studies have demonstrated a high prevalence of thyroid dysfunction in individuals with T1DM and T2DM, and the thyroid disorder may affect both glycemic control and cardiovascular risk. Clinical features of thyroid dysfunction often overlap with diabetes and diagnosis of thyroid dysfunction can be missed in the absence of active case finding. This calls for a need for thyrovigilance in diabetes care and diabetes care providers should be aware of the inter-relationship between diabetes and thyroid dysfunction. These facets of thyrovigilance in individuals with diabetes are discussed in this section.

### Thyroid Dysfunction in Patients with Type 1 Diabetes Mellitus

Autoimmune thyroid disease remains the most frequent autoimmune disorder associated with T1DM and occurs in 17–30% of adults with T1DM.[18] Cross-sectional studies have reported a prevalence of hypothyroidism in 12–24% females and approximately 6% males with T1DM with an increased prevalence in patients with positive antithyroid peroxidase (anti-TPO) antibodies; the prevalence of anti-thyroid antibodies have been reported to be 16–18.7%.[19]

Hyperthyroidism has lower prevalence, with rate of approximately 1.7% in patients with T1DM and 0.3% in patients with T2DM.[19] However, hyperthyroidism prevalence is higher than in nondiabetic individuals. Hyperthyroidism in T1DM is associated with younger age, shorter diabetes duration, female sex and reduced body mass index.

Individuals with T1DM develop thyroid disorders at an earlier age as compared to the general population and AITD onset is associated with more aggressive presentation of diabetes and poorly controlled diabetes.

## Common Genetic Susceptibility of Type 1 Diabetes Mellitus and Thyroid Disease

Autoimmune thyroid disease and T1DM are autoimmune diseases which share common genetic susceptibility loci within the human leukocyte antigen (HLA) and other genes involved in immune regulation. Concomitant occurrence of T1DM and AITD without autoimmune Addison's disease is denominated as autoimmune polyglandular syndrome type 3 variant or APS3. T1DM and AITD may also co-exist within the very rare juvenile APS1 (encompassing autoimmune hypoparathyroidism and primary hypogonadism) as well as within the APS adult type 2 with Addison's disease as primary endocrine component. However, both in APS1 and 2, AITD and T1DM neither define the diagnosis nor are they the major endocrine components. For APS3, disease susceptibility genes are the HLA on chromosome 6, the protein tyrosine phosphatase nonreceptor type 22 or PTPN22 (chromosome 1), the cytotoxic T lymphocyte antigen 4 or CTLA4 (chromosome 2), the forkhead box P3 or FOXP3 (X chromosome), and the interleukin-2 receptor alpha or *IL-2Rα* gene region (chromosome 10).[20] These genes are involved in immune regulation and T-cell activation within the immunological synapse. Among the HLA, haplotype HLA-DR3-DQB1*0201 is the primary haplotype conferring susceptibility to both T1DM and AITD within families.

## Thyroid Dysfunction in Patients with Type 2 Diabetes Mellitus

The interaction of thyroid status and T2DM is complex. In the National Health and Nutrition Examination Survey (NHANES) III study, a survey of 17,353 subjects representing the US population, hypothyroidism and hyperthyroidism were found in 4.6% and 1.3% of subjects, respectively with a higher prevalence of thyroid disorders in the diabetic compared to nondiabetic individuals, especially in patients with positive thyroid peroxidase antibodies (TPO-Abs).[21]

Subclinical hypothyroidism (SCH) and overt hypothyroidism are the most common forms of thyroid disorder. The prevalence of hypothyroidism in T2DM ranges between 6% and 20% in epidemiologic studies across different ethnic groups depending upon age, gender and iodine intake.[22,23] A significant increased risk of hypothyroidism was observed in patients with T2DM over 65 years of age with an odds ratio (OR) of 4.2, with higher risk in women versus men (OR 4.82 vs. 2.60), and with presence or absence of thyroid autoantibodies (OR 4.26 vs. 2.93).[24]

Higher levels of circulating insulin associated with insulin resistance have shown a proliferative effect on thyroid tissue resulting in larger thyroid size with increased formation of nodules.[25] The prevalence of hyperthyroidism in T2DM does not seem to be different than general population.

## Pathophysiological Link between Type 2 Diabetes Mellitus and Hypothyroidism

The co-occurrence of T2DM and hypothyroidism is unlikely to be a chance finding. It has also been reported that the prevalence of thyroid autoimmunity is higher in people with T2DM, especially in females. However, unlike T1DM, a genetic link between T2DM and AITD has not been well characterized. A polymorphism of type 2 deiodinase (DIO2) gene (*Thr92Ala*) has been found to be associated with increased risk of T2DM. In a meta-analysis of 11,000 individuals, it was reported that deiodinase polymorphisms may play a role as intracellular T3 regulates insulin sensitivity.[22]

Hyperglycemia may itself impact the hypothalamic–pituitary–thyroid (HPT) axis in many ways. In individuals with diabetes, the nocturnal TSH peak is blunted or abolished, and TSH response to TRH is impaired. Reduced T3 levels have been observed in uncontrolled diabetics. This "low T3 state" could be explained by impairment of peripheral conversion of T4 to T3, which normalizes with improvement in glycemic control. An abnormal TH pattern is attributed to the presence of thyroid hormone binding inhibitor (THBI), an inhibitor of the extrathyroidal conversion enzyme (5′-deiodinase) of T4 to T3, and to dysfunction of the HPT axis.

Additionally, long-term complications of diabetes such as chronic kidney disease (CKD) may also impact thyroid functions variably. A high prevalence of hypothyroidism has been reported in individuals with CKD. They may have greater iodine retention, which predisposes them to thyroid dysfunction due to Wolff–Chaikoff effect. Metabolic acidosis also results in TH alterations with elevated TSH and low T4 and T3. However, current evidence seems insufficient to explain the mechanisms underlying the correlation between thyroid dysfunction and T2DM.

## Should all Individuals with Diabetes be Screened for Thyroid Dysfunction?

- *Screening in T1DM*: In case of T1DM, guidelines recommend that thyroid antibody test and thyroid function tests should be considered at the time of diagnosis and TSH should be repeated annually if TPO-Abs are initially negative and more frequently (up to every 6 months) if TPO-Abs are positive or if there are symptoms of thyroid dysfunction such as goiter, poor height velocity in children, menstrual dysfunction or unexplained glycemic variation[26]
- *Screening in T2DM*: The necessity of a screening program for thyroid dysfunction in T2DM is a controversial issue because current evidence is insufficient to assess the benefits of such screening. The specific tests for screening (TSH alone, TSH and TPO-Ab, or TSH and FT4), the exact interval of periodic screening, and the cost-benefit ratio are also undetermined. The American Thyroid Association recommends that all adults should be screened by the measurement of serum TSH concentration, beginning at age of 35 years and every 5 years thereafter.[27] Since hypothyroidism is frequently observed in patients with T2DM and many patients may be asymptomatic even in the presence of overt hypothyroidism and symptoms of thyroid disorders may be masked by a poor metabolic control, there should be a low threshold for thyroid function evaluation in diabetic individuals.

SECTION 1: The Scope of Glucrinology

## Hypothyroidism and Diabetes

The glucrinological considerations in relation to hypothyroidism in diabetes are enumerated in Table 1 and discussed further in text.

### Changes in Glycemic Control

Hypothyroidism is characterized by insulin resistance due to delayed peripheral glucose uptake and assimilation. Hypothyroidism is also associated with chronic inflammation that may further contribute to insulin resistance. Proinflammatory adipocytokines such as tumor necrosis factor-α (TNF-α) and ghrelin have been found

**TABLE 1** Glucrinological considerations in hypothyroidism and diabetes.

| | |
|---|---|
| Prevalence of hypothyroidism in diabetes | • Increased prevalence of AITD in type 1 diabetes mellitus<br>• Increased prevalence of hypothyroidism (overt and subclinical in type 2 diabetes mellitus) |
| Effect of hypothyroidism on glucose homeostasis and metabolic health in diabetes | • Worsening of insulin resistance<br>• Reduced insulin clearance<br>• Decreased intestinal glucose absorption<br>• Decreased gluconeogenesis and glycogenolysis<br>• Reduced growth hormone and cortisol response to hypoglycemia<br>• Increased endothelial dysfunction<br>• Increased arterial stiffness<br>• Hyperlipidemia—raised total and LDL cholesterol |
| Clinical considerations | • Increased risk of hypoglycemia<br>• Recurrent unexplained hypoglycemia<br>• Common comorbidities—obesity, hypertension, dyslipidemia<br>• Increased cardiovascular risk<br>• Increased risk of microvascular complications (diabetic kidney disease) |
| Therapeutic considerations | • Reduced dose requirement of antidiabetic medications to avoid hypoglycemia<br>• Dose requirements of antidiabetic medications may increase after adequate levothyroxine replacement<br>• Levothyroxine replacement reduces occurrence of hypoglycemia and improves insulin sensitivity<br>• Levothyroxine replacement may partially improve dyslipidemia, hypertension, and cardiovascular risk. Evidence of benefit is uncertain for subclinical hypothyroidism<br>• Levothyroxine dose requirements may be higher in diabetic individuals<br>• Metformin suppresses TSH levels; no effect on free T3 or free T4 levels<br>• GLP-1R agonists are contraindicated in individuals at risk of medullary thyroid cancer |

(AITD: autoimmune thyroid disease; GLP-1R: glucagon-like polypeptide-1 receptor; LDL: low-density lipoprotein; T3: triiodothyronine; T4: thyroxine; TSH: thyroid-stimulating hormone)

to be elevated in hypothyroidism. Therefore, hypothyroid individuals may have a high prevalence of metabolic syndrome.

However, there is impaired glucose absorption from the gastrointestinal tract due to delayed gastric emptying. Liver and muscle gluconeogenesis and glycogenolysis are reduced and hepatic glucose output is decreased or normal. In addition, though insulin secretion has been reported to be normal, increased, or reduced; insulin half-life is prolonged due to decreased renal clearance of insulin.[28] Hypothyroidism is associated with low growth hormone (GH) and cortisol response to insulin-induced hypoglycemia. Basal as well as stimulated GH levels have been found to be reduced in individuals with overt hypothyroidism, and they may have relative adrenal insufficiency. Therefore, the hypothalamic–pituitary–adrenal response to hypoglycemia may be blunted. Therefore, the net effect of hypothyroidism in diabetic individuals on treatment is an increased risk of hypoglycemia.

### Clinical Presentation

Patients with uncontrolled hypothyroidism may present with recurrent hypoglycemia. Unexplained and recurrent hypoglycemic episodes in a diabetic individual should prompt evaluation of thyroid functions. Since the counter-regulatory hormone release may be blunted leading to less symptoms of hypoglycemia, a higher index of suspicion is required to detect hypoglycemic events. Hypothyroidism may necessitate a downtitration of antidiabetic drugs including insulin doses due to transient decreased insulin requirements. Thyroid dysfunction may also impact glycemic assessment. There may occur spurious elevations in HbA1c due to altered red-cell lifespan.

Signs and symptoms of hypothyroidism such as fatigue, tiredness or change in appetite, obesity, hypertension, and dyslipidemia remain nonspecific and may be present in a significant proportion of diabetic individuals. In addition, edema, pallor, dry skin and other physical signs of hypothyroidism may closely overlap those seen in CKD or congestive heart failure. Therefore, the diagnosis of hypothyroidism may get delayed in individuals with diabetes and the diabetes care provider needs to be thyrovigilant.

### Effect on Diabetic Complications

Both diabetes and hypothyroidism are associated with increased cardiovascular risk with increased prevalence of obesity, hypertension, dyslipidemia, and endothelial dysfunction. Untreated hypothyroidism may magnify the cardiovascular risk in diabetes. Hypothyroidism also impacts kidney functions due to intra-renal vasoconstriction, decreased cardiac output and increased tubulo-glomerular feedback, with reduction in single-nephron glomerular filtration rate (GFR). Severe hypothyroidism is associated with reduced GFR, which is reversed with LT4 replacement.

### Levothyroxine Treatment

Once the hypothyroid patient with diabetes is initiated on thyroid replacement therapy, amelioration of recurrent hypoglycemia is noted and an increase in insulin dose and antidiabetic medications may be necessary. At the same time, LT4 treatment may normalize fasting hyperinsulinemia and significantly improve insulin sensitivity in patients with overt and SCH and insulin resistance. LT4 may also lead to significant improvement in dyslipidemia, hypertension and other cardiovascular risk factors. However, uncontrolled diabetes may impair the effectiveness of LT4 treatment in patients with hypothyroidism, and they may require higher doses of LT4.

## Effect of Metformin on Thyroid Function

Some antidiabetic drugs can also affect thyroid function and impact the HPT axis. Recent studies have shown that serum TSH levels were decreased with metformin and effects were reversible after its withdrawal.[29] A meta-analysis in 206 patients showed that metformin reduced TSH levels in both overt and SCH, while there was no change in euthyroid patients.[30] The TSH lowering effect of metformin can also be observed in diabetic patients with thyroid disorder when treating with thyroxine. This decline in serum TSH levels was not associated with change in serum FT4 and free T3 (FT3) levels, negating potential effect of metformin on LT4 absorption. The mechanism postulated is that as metformin crosses blood–brain barrier and reaches high concentration in pituitary, and inhibition of hypothalamic AMPK might be responsible for central TSH suppression.[31] Although the effect of metformin is yet to be clearly established, literature suggests that TSH levels should be monitored in diabetic patients with overt and SCH during treatment with metformin.

## Glucagon-like Polypeptide-1 Receptor Agonists and Risk of Medullary Thyroid Carcinoma

Glucagon-like polypeptide-1 receptor (GLP-1R) agonists have been associated with increased plasma calcitonin levels and progressive development of C-cell hyperplasia; high dosages of liraglutide (45 times the human dosages) caused C-cell carcinoma in rodent models.[32] But monkey and human thyroid gland, have lower levels of GLP-1R expression and do not respond to GLP-1R agonists with an acute release of calcitonin. The LEADER (Liraglutide Effect and Action in Diabetes: Evaluation of Cardiovascular Outcome Results) Trial, a population-based randomized control trial, did not show any effect of GLP-1R activation on serum calcitonin, C-cell hyperplasia, or C-cell malignancy in humans over 3.5–5 years suggesting that the findings previously reported in rodents may not apply to humans.[32]

## Subclinical Hypothyroidism and Diabetes

Individuals with T2DM are more likely to have SCH when compared with healthy population. A meta-analysis of 17 studies showed a prevalence of SCH in individuals with T2DM of 4.69–18.86%, with a 1.93-fold increased risk as compared to non-diabetics.[33] However, SCH needs to be reconfirmed on repeat testing since many borderline thyroid function abnormalities may be transient. In addition, the rate of progression from SCH to overt hypothyroidism does not seem to be different in diabetic individuals when compared to nondiabetics. Whether SCH has a significant impact on glycemic control is also debated. Few studies in individuals with T1DM reported increased risk of recurrent hypoglycemia in the presence of SCH.

Subclinical hypothyroidism has been variably associated with increased diabetic complications. SCH is associated with hypertension, dyslipidemia, metabolic syndrome, and increased cardiovascular risk in both diabetic and nondiabetic populations. It may therefore, contribute to the cardiovascular risk in diabetes, but this is debatable as there is lack of evidence that LT4 replacement reduces cardiovascular risk. SCH was associated with an increased risk of diabetic microvascular complications. The OR for diabetic nephropathy was 1.74 (95% CI 1.34–2.28), that for diabetic retinopathy was 1.42 (95% CI 1.21–1.67), for diabetic peripheral neuropathy was 1.87 (95% CI 1.06–3.28), and for peripheral arterial disease was 1.85 (95% CI 1.35–2.54). And, overall OR for diabetic complications was 1.74 (95% CI 1.34–2.28).[33] Furthermore, SCH may be associated with increased vascular stiffness, endothelial dysfunction and hypercoagulability which lead to increased risk of peripheral arterial disease.

However, a cause-and-effect relationship between subclinical thyroid dysfunction and diabetic complications is not established as most of the evidence comes from observational studies. It is unclear whether LT4 replacement would offer any benefits beyond reduction of hypoglycemic events.

## Hyperthyroidism and Diabetes

The glucocrinological considerations in relation to hyperthyroidism in diabetes are enumerated in Table 2 and discussed further in text.

Hyperthyroidism alters glucose metabolism, potentially resulting in the deterioration of metabolic control.[19] TH excess results in increased gluconeogenesis,

**TABLE 2** Glucocrinological considerations in diabetes and hyperthyroidism.

| | |
|---|---|
| Prevalence of hyperthyroidism in diabetes | • Slightly higher prevalence than general population, especially in type 1 diabetes mellitus |
| Effect of hyper-thyroidism on glucose homeostasis and metabolic health in diabetes | • Increased gluconeogenesis and glycogenolysis<br>• Increased intestinal glucose absorption<br>• Increased insulin clearance<br>• Increased lipolysis<br>• Systolic hypertension, tachycardia and raised cardiac output |
| Clinical considerations | • Worsening of glycemic control<br>• More catabolic features<br>• Acute hyperglycemic emergencies including diabetic ketoacidosis<br>• Increased risk of high output failure and atrial fibrillation<br>• Osmotic symptoms due to hyperglycemia may mask the symptoms of thyrotoxicosis and vice versa—need for vigilance |
| Therapeutic considerations | • Increased dose requirement of antidiabetic medications that may be reduced after attaining euthyroid state<br>• Antithyroidal drugs and definitive treatment improve glycemic control<br>• Pioglitazone may worsen thyroid-associated ophthalmopathy<br>• Antithyroid drugs (carbimazole, methimazole) may cause autoimmune hypoglycemia in rare cases |

glycogenolysis, hepatic glucose output and lipolysis. While insulin sensitivity is reduced, insulin clearance is increased. Therefore, concomitant thyrotoxicosis can lead to worsening of glycemic control in diabetic individuals and even precipitation of acute hyperglycemic emergencies such as diabetic ketoacidosis (DKA) due to increased lipolysis. In fact, DKA and hypoglycemia are more common in type 1 diabetic patients with concomitant hyperthyroidism. Insulin dose requirement may increase in patients with diabetes after the occurrence of hyperthyroidism. Amelioration of thyrotoxicosis results in improved glycemic control and antidiabetic medications may require retitration in hyperthyroid subjects after the control of thyroid dysfunction.

Hyperthyroidism is also associated with tachycardia, arrhythmias, high-output heart failure and systolic hypertension, which may further add to the cardiovascular risk in diabetes. Both overt hyperthyroidism and subclinical hyperthyroidism are associated with atrial fibrillation and increased cardiovascular mortality as well as osteoporosis. Studies have not reported any difference in the rates of micro- or macrovascular complications, however.

Acute hyperglycemia and hypermetabolic state in thyrotoxicosis have significant symptom overlap (weight loss, fatigue, myalgias) and if the clinician is not vigilant, the diagnosis of hyperthyroidism may be missed. Acute hyperglycemia is also associated with lower levels of T4 and T3, which may further mislead the clinician about the severity of underlying thyrotoxicosis.

For reasons not well understood, diabetic subjects with Graves' orbitopathy have been reported to have higher incidence of dysthyroid optic neuropathy. Few studies have shown exacerbation of Graves' ophthalmopathy after initiation of pioglitazone.[34] Thiazolidinediones stimulate proliferator-activated receptor-gamma which is expressed in orbital adipose and connective tissues and increased expression in active stages of thyroid-associated orbitopathy was reported in diabetic patients. Thus, pioglitazone should be used with caution in clinically active Graves' ophthalmopathy.

## CONCLUSION

Diabetes mellitus and thyroid disorders are very common diseases; they may occur concurrently in several individuals. A higher prevalence of thyroid dysfunction in both T1DM and T2DM compared with nondiabetics has been documented throughout literature suggesting a close inter-relationship between these two common endocrinopathies. Both hypothyroidism and hyperthyroidism may impact glycemic control and cardiovascular risk in diabetic individuals, and this is partially ameliorated with appropriate management of the underlying thyroid disorder. Systematic approach to thyroid testing in diabetic subjects is favorable and universally recommended in T1DM; however, no definitive guidelines exist regarding screening for thyroid dysfunction in T2DM. Finally, while overt thyroid dysfunction should always be treated, it remains uncertain which individuals with SCH would benefit from LT4 replacement. Glucovigilance in the management of thyroid disorders and thyrovigilance in diabetes care is required in the wake of a rising burden of metabolic and endocrine disorders.

## REFERENCES

1. Brent GA. Mechanisms of thyroid hormone action. J Clin Invest. 2012;122(9):3035-43.
2. Mullur R, Liu YY, Brent GA. Thyroid hormone regulation of metabolism. Physiol Rev. 2014;94(2): 355-82.
3. Verga FC, Mangialardo C, Madaro L, et al. Thyroid hormone T3 counteracts STZ induced diabetes in mouse. PLoS One. 2011;6(5):e19839 .
4. Karbalaei N, Noorafshan A, Hoshmandi E. Impaired glucose-stimulated insulin secretion and reduced β-cell mass in pancreatic islets of hyperthyroid rats. Exp Physiol. 2016;101(8):1114-27.
5. Santini F, Marzullo P, Rotondi M, et al. Mechanisms in endocrinology: The crosstalk between thyroid gland and adipose tissue: signal integration in health and disease. Eur J Endocrinol. 2014;171(4):R137-52.
6. Iwen KA, Oelkrug R, Brabant G. Effects of thyroid hormones on thermogenesis and energy partitioning. J Mol Endocrinol. 2018;60(3):R157-70.
7. Roos A, Bakker SJ, Links TP, et al. Thyroid function is associated with components of the metabolic syndrome in euthyroid subjects. J Clin Endocrinol Metab. 2007;92:491-6.
8. Mehran L, Amouzegar A, Tohidi M, et al. Serum free thyroxine concentration is associated with metabolic syndrome in euthyroid subjects. Thyroid. 2014;24:1566-74.
9. Jun JE, Jee JH, Bae JC, et al. Association between changes in thyroid hormones and incident type 2 diabetes: A seven-year longitudinal study. Thyroid. 2017;27(1):29-38.
10. Chaker L, Ligthart S, Korevaar TI, et al. Thyroid function and risk of type 2 diabetes: a population-based prospective cohort study. BMC Med. 2016;14(1):150.
11. Roubsanthisuk W, Watanakejorn P, Tunlakit M, et al. Hyperthyroidism induces glucose intolerance by lowering both insulin secretion and peripheral insulin sensitivity. J Med Assoc Thai. 2006;89 (Suppl 5):S133-40.
12. Paul DT, Mollah FH, Alam MK, et al. Glycemic status in hyperthyroid subjects. Mymensingh Med J. 2004;13(1):71-5.
13. Matosin-Matekalo M, Mesonero JE, Delezay O, et al. Thyroid hormone regulation of the Na+/glucose cotransporter SGLT1 in Caco-2 cells. Biochem J. 1998;334:633-40.
14. O'Meara NM, Blackman JD, Sturis J, et al. Alterations in the kinetics of C-peptide and insulin secretion in hyperthyroidism. J Clin Endocrinol Metab. 1993;76(1):79-84.
15. Yang L, Shen X, Yan S, et al. HbA1c in the diagnosis of diabetes and abnormal glucose tolerance in patients with Graves' hyperthyroidism. Diabetes Res Clin Pract. 2013;101(1)28-34.
16. Komiya I, Yamada T, Sato A, et al. Effects of antithyroid drug therapy on blood glucose, serum insulin, and insulin binding to red blood cells in hyperthyroid patients of different ages. Diabetes Care. 1985;8(2):161-8.
17. Hamada N, Ito K, Mimura T, et al. Factors predicting the course of diabetes mellitus in hyperthyroid patients. Horm Metab Res. 1986;18(4):260-3.
18. Shun CB, Donaghue KC, Phelan H, et al. Thyroid autoimmunity in type 1 diabetes: systematic review and meta-analysis. Diabet Med. 2014;31:126-35.
19. Umpierrez GE, Latif KA, Murphy MB, et al. Thyroid dysfunction in patients with type 1 diabetes: a longitudinal study. Diabetes Care. 2003;26(4):1181-5.
20. Dittmar M, Kahaly GJ. Genetics of the autoimmune polyglandular syndrome type 3 variant. Thyroid. 2010;20(7):737-43.
21. Hollowell JG, Staehling NW, Flanders WD, et al. Serum TSH, T4, and thyroid antibodies in the United States population (1988 to 1994): National Health and Nutrition Examination Survey (NHANES III). J Clin Endocrinol Metab. 2002;7(2):489-99.
22. Al-Geffari M, Ahmad NA, Al-Sharqawi AH, et al. Risk factors for thyroid dysfunction among type 2 diabetic patients in a highly diabetes mellitus prevalent society. Int J Endocrinol. 2013;41:7920.
23. Nair A, Jayakumari C, Jabbar PK, et al. Prevalence and associations of hypothyroidism in Indian patients with type 2 diabetes mellitus. J Thyroid Res. 2018;2018:5386129.
24. Song F, Bao C, Deng M, et al. The prevalence and determinants of hypothyroidism in hospitalized patients with type 2 diabetes mellitus. Endocrine. 2017;55(1):179-85.

25. Tang Y, Yan T, Wang G, et al. Correlation between insulin resistance and thyroid nodule in type 2 diabetes mellitus. Int J Endocrinol. 2017;2017:1617458.
26. Kordonouri O, Maguire AM, Knip M, et al. ISPAD Clinical Practice Consensus Guidelines 2006-2007. Other complications and associated conditions. Pediatr Diabetes. 2007;8(3):171-6.
27. Ladenson PW, Singer PA, Ain KB, et al. American Thyroid Association guidelines for detection of thyroid dysfunction. Arch Intern Med. 2000;160(11):1573-5.
28. Okajima F, Ui M. Metabolism of glucose in hyper and hypothyroid rats in vivo. Glucose turnover values and futile cycle activities obtained with 14 C and 3H labeled glucose. Biochem J. 1979;182:565-75.
29. Cappelli C, Rotondi M, Pirola I, et al. TSH-lowering effect of metformin in type 2 diabetic patients: differences between euthyroid, untreated hypothyroid, and euthyroid on LT4 therapy patients. Diabetes Care. 2009;32(9):1589-90.
30. Lupoli R, Di Minno A, Tortora A, et al. Effects of treatment with metformin on TSH levels: a meta-analysis of literature studies. J Clin Endocrinol Metab. 2014;99(1):E143-8.
31. Chau-Van C, Gamba M, Salvi R, et al. Metformin inhibits adenosine-5'-monophospate-activated kinase activation and prevents increase in neuropeptide Y expression in cultured hypothalamic neurons. Endocrinology. 2007;148:507-11.
32. Hegedüs L, Sherman SI, Tuttle RM, et al. No evidence of increase in calcitonin concentrations or development of C-cell malignancy in response to liraglutide for up to 5 years in the LEADER trial. Diabetes Care. 2018;41(3):620-2.
33. Han C, He X, Xia X, et al. Subclinical hypothyroidism and type 2 diabetes: A systematic review and meta-analysis. PLoS One. 2015;10(8):e0135233.
34. Valyasevi RW, Harteneck DA, Dutton CM, et al. Stimulation of adipogenesis, peroxisome proliferator-activated receptor gamma (PPARgamma), and thyrotropin receptor by PPAR gamma agonist in human orbital preadipocyte fibroblasts. J Clin Endocrinol Metab. 2002;87(5):2352-8.

# CHAPTER 4

# Glucocrinology of Parathyroid and Bone Mineral Metabolism

Ameya Joshi, Perla A Carrillo-González

## INTRODUCTION

The endocrine system is composed of glands that secrete hormones directly into circulation to regulate the function of distant target organs. Diabetes mellitus (DM) affects all organs in the body and one of the major focus of management of DM is the prevention, detection and treatment of this involvement of multiple organ systems. While a lot has been discussed about the involvement of cardiac, neurologic, renal, gastrointestinal and ophthalmic systems (the well-known micro- and macrovascular disease), relatively little is described about the relationship of endocrine system per se with DM. Glucocrinology is the study of medicine that relates to the relationship between glucose physiology and the endocrine system. In this chapter, we explore the bidirectional relationship between bone mineral metabolism and glucose homeostasis, in health and disease.

### Bone Mineral Metabolism and Vitamin D/Parathyroid System

Bones provide strength and support for the body, and serve as an attachment for skeletal muscles. Bone is an extremely active organ at the metabolic level and is relevant in the regulation of several endocrine functions. Bones are the major source of calcium, act as a buffer against acidosis and adsorb toxins. Calcium, phosphate and magnesium are minerals vital to the functioning of all cells. Parathormone (PTH) and vitamin D (Vit D) are the major regulators of mineral metabolism. PTH and Vit D form a tightly controlled feedback cycle, PTH being a major stimulator of Vit D synthesis in the kidney while Vit D exerts negative feedback on PTH secretion. The major function of PTH and major physiologic regulator is circulating ionized calcium. The effects of PTH on gut, kidney and bone serve to maintain serum calcium within a tight range. PTH has a reciprocal effect on phosphate metabolism. In contrast, Vit D has a stimulatory effect on both calcium and phosphate homeostasis, playing a key role in providing adequate mineral for normal bone formation. Both hormones act in concert with the more recently discovered fibroblast growth factor 23 (FGF23) and klotho, hormones involved predominantly in phosphate metabolism, which also participate in this closely-knit feedback circuit.

## GLUCOSE PHYSIOLOGY IN RELATION TO BONE MINERAL METABOLISM

Calcium is an important second messenger in many intracellular processes, including both first-phase and second-phase insulin secretion. A rise in intracellular calcium is required for insulin release from β-cells by exocytosis. Functional impairment of voltage-gated calcium channels has been documented in individuals with type 2 diabetes mellitus (T2DM), which may mediate the insulin secretory defects.[1]

Calcium also affects the affinity and sensitivity of insulin receptor to insulin in target tissues, especially skeletal muscle. Intracellular calcium is involved in the insulin-stimulated glucose uptake into myocytes. In addition, the multiple hormones that regulate liver glycogenolysis, gluconeogenesis and glucose oxidation do so by calcium-signaling mechanisms.[2] Animal models of T2DM and obesity have demonstrated abnormal cellular calcium homeostasis.[2] Furthermore, abnormal intracellular calcium homeostasis may also be the link between insulin resistance (IR) and hypertension.

### Role of Vitamin D in Glucose Homeostasis

Vitamin D is present in the body in several forms like cholecalciferol, ergocalciferol and calcitriol [1,25(OH)$_2$D], which is the active form which acts on the cells affecting transcription. Its primary role is ensuring adequate absorption of dietary calcium. Vit D exerts autocrine and paracrine effects such as direct intracellular effects via its receptors and the local production of 1,25-dihydroxyvitamin D3 [1,25(OH)$_2$D3], especially in muscle and pancreatic β-cells. 1,25(OH)$_2$D also acts as a hormone causing immunomodulatory effect on gene transcription at the cellular level. Indeed, it can downregulate mechanisms connected with adaptive immunity, induce immunological tolerance and decrease autoaggression-related inflammation.[3] These properties provide the basis for a preventive and therapeutic role of Vit D.

Recent research suggests that Vit D also regulates metabolism, and influences both insulin secretion and insulin action. This has been depicted in Table 1. Vit D promotes pancreatic β-cell function via direct genomic action, regulating the transcription of target genes via Vit D responsive elements. Thus, it enhances insulin secretion and synthesis and promotes β-cell survival by inhibiting cytokine-induced β-cell apoptosis.[3] Further, Vit D regulates calbindin (a cytosolic Ca-binding protein in β-cells) and intracellular calcium. Hence, it acts as a modulator of depolarization-stimulated insulin release.[4] Calcium is needed for insulin secretion by β-cells. Vitamin D deficiency (VDD) or defects in activation/action and resultant hypocalcemia have been shown to be associated with reduced glucose-stimulated insulin secretion.

Chronic inflammation is one of the important factors responsible for IR and T2DM. Macrophages and dendritic cells express the enzymes vitamin D-25-hydroxylase and 1α-hydroxylase and can produce 1,25(OH)$_2$D.[3] Several studies have supported the role of Vit D and 1,25(OH)$_2$D as anti-inflammatory agents. The

**TABLE 1** Effects of vitamin D [1,25(OH)₂D] on glucose homeostasis.

|  | β-cell function | Insulin sensitivity |
|---|---|---|
| Rapid nongenomic effects | • Regulates intracellular calcium to modulate insulin release | • Increases insulin gene transcription and insulin synthesis<br>• Anti-inflammatory effects<br>• Reduces β-cell apoptosis by downregulation of Fas pathway<br>• Increases calbindin that acts as a buffer for intracellular calcium—regulates intracellular calcium |
| Genomic effects | • Regulates intracellular calcium—improved insulin sensitivity<br>• Reduces the activity of renin–angiotensin system by inhibiting secretion of renin | • Increases insulin receptor gene expression<br>• Increases activity of PPARδ, improved fatty acid metabolism<br>• Reduces expression of inflammatory cytokines |

(1,25(OH)₂D: calcitriol; PPARδ: peroxisome proliferator-activated receptor delta)

regulation of serum calcium via PTH and 1,25(OH)₂D following changes in dietary calcium and obesity has been proposed to mediate the effects of Vit D on IR.

Its effect on insulin sensitivity could also be due to the regulation of intracellular calcium levels within a narrow physiological range. In addition, Vit D modulates the expression of insulin receptors in adipose tissue and skeletal muscle.[4] By activating peroxisome proliferator-activated receptor delta (PPARδ), it also plays a role in fatty acid metabolism. Vit D is also a negative regulator of the renin–angiotensin–aldosterone system (RAAS) and it suppresses renin formation from the kidneys. VDD has been associated with IR.

## Role of Parathormone in Glucose Homeostasis

The role of PTH in glucose regulation is not completely clear. It increases the generation of 1,25(OH)₂D that influences both insulin secretion and sensitivity. However, high PTH as seen in primary or secondary hyperparathyroidism is associated with increased IR and greater prevalence of diabetes.

Parathormone in mice models have been shown to increase cytosolic calcium and impair insulin release through adenosine triphosphate (ATP)-dependent potassium channels. In addition, the rise in intracellular calcium also induces IR in target cells.[5] PTH stimulates cyclic adenosine monophosphate (cAMP) production in a calcium-dependent manner, and through activation of protein kinase C, it increases phosphorylation of insulin receptor substrate-1 (IRS-1). Resultant reduced expression of IRS-1 and glucose transporter 4 (GLUT4) are associated with decreased peripheral glucose uptake and IR.[5]

## Role of Osteokines in Glucose Homeostasis

Bone is an important endocrine organ that secretes several bone-specific proteins with widespread effects.[6] The osteokines that have important metabolic effects include osteocalcin (OC) and osteoprotegerin.

- *Osteocalcin*: OC is secreted by osteoblasts and stored in the bone extracellular matrix in its carboxylated form, which binds with high affinity to hydroxyapatite. Undercarboxylated OC is readily secreted into circulation. In the active undercarboxylated form, OC has been found to promote insulin expression and secretion via OC receptor on β-cells.[6] OC also stimulates insulin secretion indirectly by promoting the release of glucagon-like peptide-1 (GLP-1) in intestinal epithelial cells. Undercarboxylated OC also increases insulin sensitivity in muscle, adipose tissue, and liver and was found to increase glucose and fatty acid uptake in rodents.[6] The improvement in insulin sensitivity is mediated by means of upregulation of adiponectin, an adipokine that facilitates insulin sensitivity.
  Several cross-sectional studies of patients with T2DM have reported negative associations between higher serum levels of OC and fasting plasma glucose and hemoglobin A1c (HbA1c) and a higher risk for prediabetes and T2DM among individuals with lower baseline serum levels of OC. Weight reduction and aerobic exercise are associated with increase in OC levels[6]
- *Lipocalin-2*: The osteoblast-derived lipocalin-2 (LCN2) has been found to regulate appetite through hypothalamic action. This increase in LCN2 seems to contribute to postprandial satiety, as restoration of LCN2 levels in *Lcn2* null mice corrected the rebound hyperphagia induced by fasting.[7] The LCN2 levels are higher in normal weight individuals and lower in obese individuals. When rodents were administered by exogenous LCN2, they experienced reduced food intake, body weight and fat mass, along with improved glucose tolerance, insulin secretion and energy expenditure
- *Bone morphogenetic protein 7*: Osteocyte-secreted molecules such as bone morphogenetic protein 7 (BMP7) and sclerostin may also have a potential role in diabetes management. BMP7 has long been reported to reduce food intake and stimulate brown adipogenesis, thus improving energy metabolism.[7] BMP7 was positively linked with the insulin secretion index and fasting insulin, indicating that the protein may prompt insulin secretion and fasting insulin
- *Sclerostin*: Sclerostin has been shown to have positive associations with body mass index, fat mass and IR. Some studies have recorded elevated sclerostin levels in patients with impaired glucose regulation, type 1 diabetes mellitus (T1DM) and T2DM; although findings from other research on the topic have varied[7]
- *Osteoprotegerin (OPG)*: It is a glycoprotein of the tumor necrosis factor superfamily that prevents the binding of receptor activator for nuclear factor κB ligand (RANKL) to RANK, and inhibits osteoclastogenesis. OPG increases IR, inflammation, and proliferation of endothelial and vascular smooth muscle cells and may have a role in atherogenesis.[6] High serum OPG levels are associated with IR, metabolic syndrome (MS), and micro- and macrovascular complications in diabetes.

## Effects of Insulin on Bone

Insulin is an osteogenic hormone. It was earlier regarded that the anabolic effects of insulin may be mediated due to its homology with insulin-like growth factor-1 (IGF-1). However, insulin acts via insulin receptors on osteoblasts, with increase in osteoblast differentiation and proliferation, glucose uptake and collagen formation.

Thus, insulin results in an increase in bone mass.[8] It also reduces the expression of OPG and increases OC. With reduced OPG, differentiation of osteoclasts is increased. Resultant low pH in the resorption lacunae increases decarboxylation of OC, which has a positive effect on both insulin secretion and sensitivity.[8]

In addition, gastric inhibitory polypeptide (GIP) receptors are present in osteoblasts, osteoclasts, and osteocytes and it is believed to mediate postprandial reduction in bone resorption. Adiponectin also seems to influence bone by increasing proliferation of osteoblasts and reducing osteoclast formation. The net effect is an increase in bone mass.

While IGF-1 is a well-known anabolic agent in bone, evidence is beginning to accumulate that its homolog, insulin, also has some anabolic properties for bone. There is specific evidence that insulin may work to stimulate osteoblast differentiation, which in turn would enhance production of OC, the osteoblast-produced peptide that can stimulate pancreatic β-cell proliferation and skeletal muscle insulin sensitivity. It is uncertain whether insulin stimulates bone directly or indirectly by increasing muscle work and therefore, skeletal loading. We raise the question of the sequence of events that occurs with IR, such as T2DM. Evidence to date suggests that these patients have lower serum concentrations of OC, perhaps reduced skeletal loading and reduced bone strength as evidenced by microindentation studies.

## GLUCOVIGILANCE IN VITAMIN D DEFICIENCY, PARATHYROID DISORDERS AND BONE DISEASE

After noting the glucocrinological considerations of bone mineral metabolism, it is clear that aberrations in bone mineral metabolism will warrant for vigilance for glycemic abnormalities.

### Vitamin D Deficiency

Vitamin D deficiency has been linked to an increased risk of T1DM, T2DM and gestational diabetes mellitus (GDM).
- *Type 1 diabetes mellitus*: T1DM involves immune-mediated destruction of β-cells. Vitamin D receptor (VDR) is expressed in antigen-presenting cells (macrophages and dendritic cells) and activated T-cells. VDR is involved in the activation of several intracellular pathways involved in the proliferation, differentiation and function of cells of immune system (both innate and adaptive). $1,25(OH)_2D$ decreases the maturation of dendritic cells and also inhibits the release of proinflammatory cytokines, interleukin-12 (IL-12), IL-2, interferon-γ (INF-γ) and tumor necrosis factor-α (TNF-α). These immunomodulatory and anti-inflammatory effects of $1,25(OH)_2D$ can lead to the protection of target tissues, such as β-cells.[9]

    Vitamin D deficiency has been associated with an increased risk of T1DM in epidemiological studies. A higher incidence of T1DM has been reported in association with low sunlight exposure. At the same time, high doses of $1,25(OH)_2D$ were found to suppress insulitis and occurrence of hyperglycemia in T1DM nonobese mice.[9]

Studies suggest that Vit D supplementation may reduce the risk of T1DM. Supplementation in early life was associated with a 33% reduced risk of T1DM in the European Diabetes (EURODIAB) study. In a meta-analysis of eight studies, Vit D supplementation of infants was associated with a 29% risk reduction, but maternal supplementation did not reduce the risk in offspring.[10] However, this is not substantiated by large prospective studies. Structural analogs of Vit D, that are not associated with risk of hypercalcemia or tissue calcification, are under exploration for their potential role in the prevention of T1DM and other autoimmune diseases and in immunomodulatory therapy following islet cell transplantation[10]

- *Type 2 diabetes mellitus*: There exists a positive relationship between 25-hydroxyvitamin D [25(OH)D] levels and insulin sensitivity, and an inverse relationship with the risk of T2DM in cross-sectional studies. VDD is associated with obesity, IR, MS and T2DM. The Nurses' Health Study reported a 33% lower risk of T2DM in women with calcium intake of at least 1,200 mg and Vit D intake of 800 IU daily, compared to those with intake less than 600 mg and 400 IU, respectively. Higher calcium intake in Women's Health Study was also associated with lower prevalence of MS.[11]

  However, it is unclear whether VDD increases the risk of T2DM or occurs due to clustering of risk factors that increase the risk for both VDD and T2DM. Obesity is associated with increased sequestration of Vit D in adipose tissue. Poor dietary habits and sedentary lifestyle may also be contributory. Likewise, it is uncertain whether Vit D supplementation reduces the risk of diabetes.[12] Vit D has been shown to improve IR, reduce conversion from prediabetes to diabetes, and improve glycemic control in small studies. However, most of the studies done in this area are underpowered and there is lack of properly done randomized control trials.

  There is increasing evidence of an association of complications of T2DM with VDD, most notably with presence of diabetic peripheral neuropathy, diabetic kidney disease and macrovascular disease.[11] However, evidence that Vit D supplementation improves the risk of complications is lacking

- *Gestational diabetes mellitus*: VDD is common in pregnancy. Several studies have evaluated the potential role of Vit D supplementation in prevention of GDM. Observational studies provide conflicting evidence as to whether low serum 25(OH)D levels are associated with GDM. Two recent systematic reviews concluded that Vit D deficiency is associated with a higher risk of GDM.[13] Randomized controlled trial data remain limited. It will be important to understand whether supplementation with Vit D beyond what is contained in routine prenatal vitamins will prevent GDM or improve glucose tolerance for women with GDM.

To conclude, although hypovitaminosis D is a described risk factor for DM, a cause and effect relationship has not been determined. Moreover, there is insufficient evidence that Vit D supplementation reduces the occurrence or progression of diabetes and its complications. Therefore, at present, there are no specific recommendations for screening for DM in hypovitaminosis D.

## Primary Hyperparathyroidism

Primary hyperparathyroidism (PHPT) has been associated with IR, MS, impaired glucose tolerance (IGT) and diabetes. The main reason for IR seems to be hypercalcemia though hypophosphatemia has been attributed by some. IR not only increases DM risk but also may contribute to hypertension seen in PHPT. A high prevalence of diabetes has been reported in patients with PHPT across several cohorts. About 8% cases of PHPT had DM, which was higher than normal population. In a cohort of 105 consecutive patients with primarily asymptomatic PHPT, 40% had IGT and 15% overt diabetes on oral glucose tolerance test, compared to 25% and 5% of controls, respectively.[14] However, a higher prevalence of diabetes was not reported in a series of 609 patients with PHPT except for elderly subgroup.[15] Another group reported reduction in fasting and postmeal plasma glucose levels following parathyroidectomy.[16]

Therefore, all patients with PHPT should be screened for diabetes, with fasting and postmeal plasma glucose or oral glucose tolerance test. Glycemic control may improve in some patients following reduction of PTH levels after parathyroidectomy.[17] This may necessitate reduction in antidiabetic medications, including insulin. Hence, it is important to monitor glucose levels in diabetic patients who are undergoing surgery for PHPT as doses of insulin or oral antidiabetic medications may need to be reduced following parathyroidectomy.

Multiple endocrine neoplasia type 1 (MEN1) syndrome is characterized by PHPT in more than 90% patients and pancreatic islet cell tumors in 60–70% of patients. Of these, 40% are β-cell tumors or insulinomas. Any unprovoked hypoglycemia in a PHPT patient should raise the clinical suspicion of insulinoma and MEN1. Monitoring fasting glucose and insulin level is a routine part of protocol of monitoring of MEN1 patients, most of whom have PHPT.

## Hypoparathyroidism

Autoimmune hypoparathyroidism is more commonly associated with T1DM as a part of autoimmune polyglandular syndromes. Therefore, an attempt should be made to screen for other endocrinopathies in patients with hypoparathyroidism.

# OSTEOVIGILANCE IN DIABETES

With current medical advances, people with diabetes have improved survival and recent studies have shown that both T1DM and T2DM are associated with a significantly increased risk of vertebral, hip and all nonvertebral fractures due to osteoporosis. Altered bone quality appears to correlate with long standing and poorly controlled DM, suggesting the skeleton be viewed as a target for diabetic complications.

The risk of hip fractures was reported to be increased in individuals with T2DM, both men [relative risk (RR) 2.8, 95% confidence interval (CI) 1.2, 6.6] and women (RR 2.1, 95% CI 1.6, 2.7). The association between hip fractures and diabetes was even stronger for T1DM (RR 6.3, 95% CI 2.6, 15.1).[18] There was a weak association of diabetes with fractures at other sites. Not only is the fracture risk higher in diabetic patients, fractures are associated with worse outcomes compared to nondiabetic individuals, such as delayed healing, wound infections, longer hospital stay, postoperative cardiac events and mortality.[19]

## Factors Associated with Increased Fracture Risk in Diabetes

Several factors might influence the fracture risk in diabetes and these are discussed here and enlisted in Table 2.

As discussed earlier, diabetes has been associated with low Vit D levels that may impact long-term musculoskeletal health. In addition, hyperglycemia promotes adipogenesis rather than osteogenesis, impairs osteoblast growth, increases osteoblast apoptosis and inhibits osteoclastogenesis.[20] The sensitivity of osteoblasts and osteoclasts to insulin or hyperglycemia in individuals with T2DM, however, is undetermined. Osteoporosis is conventionally defined as low bone mass along with microarchitectural deterioration of bone. The bone disease correlates with levels of advanced glycosylation end products in diabetes. Indeed, longer disease duration and poor glycemic control are associated with greater risk.[20]

Both types of DM are associated with changes in bone turnover, but there are different patterns. Patients with T1DM have impaired osteoblastic bone formation, proven by low levels of bone-formation markers, like OC or alkaline phosphatase.[20] Most clinical studies investigating bone turnover markers (BTM) have reported lower bone turnover in T2DM. Bone resorption markers like C-terminal cross-linked

| TABLE 2 | Pathogenesis of increased fracture risk in diabetes. | |
|---|---|---|
| | **Type 1 diabetes mellitus** | **Type 2 diabetes mellitus** |
| Microarchitectural changes and bone strength | • ↓ cross-sectional bone area<br>• ↓ volumetric BMD (trabecular bone)<br>• Thin cortices and trabeculae<br>• ↑ trabecular separation | • ↑ cortical porosity<br>• ↓ bone material strength |
| Pathogenesis | • ↓ IGF-1<br>• Chronic hyperglycemia—accumulation of advanced glycation end products (AGEs)<br>• Microvascular bone damage | • ↓ IGF-1<br>• Obesity (↑ adipokines, inflammatory factors)<br>• Altered composition of marrow fat<br>• Low-grade chronic inflammation<br>• Chronic hyperglycemia—accumulation of AGEs<br>• Microvascular bone damage |
| Bone turnover | • Impaired osteoblastic bone formation<br>• Possibly increased bone resorption | • Decreased osteoblastic bone formation<br>• Decreased bone resorption |
| Neuropathy | Increased risk of falls | Increased risk of falls |
| Pharmacological | – | Antidiabetic drugs—thiazolidinediones, SGLT-2 inhibitors |

(BMD: bone mineral density; IGF-1: insulin-like growth factor-1; SGLT-2: sodium-glucose cotransporter-2)

telopeptide (CTX) of type I collagen and tartrate-resistant acid phosphatase 5b (TRAP5b) and PTH, and bone formation markers like P-procollagen type 1 amino-terminal propeptide (P1NP) and OC, are all decreased in T2DM.[20] Some markers are lower in patients with T2DM than in those with T1DM as is shown in Table 3.

In addition, concomitant presence of celiac disease worsens bone health in T1DM.[21] Insulin therapy, especially in T1DM, is associated with increased bone mass, indicating bone anabolic effects of insulin or the normalization of bone remodeling due to glycemic control, correction of acidosis, or increased body weight.[22]

Other factors associated with poor bone quality and fracture risk include comorbidities and complications, such as chronic kidney disease, peripheral and autonomic neuropathy, visual impairment, and an increased risk of falls. Antidiabetic medications may also have an effect on bone health. PPAR-γ agonists like pioglitazone drive differentiation of mesenchymal stem cells toward adipocytes rather than osteoblasts and are associated with an increased risk of osteoporosis and fractures. Bariatric surgery for the management of obese T2DM also contributes to bone loss by augmenting nutritional deficiencies, sarcopenia, altered adipokines, sex hormones, and central signaling pathways. Therefore, bone density should be regularly monitored in postbariatric surgery patients.[23]

## Prevention and Management of Fracture Risk in Diabetes

From the earlier discussion, it is clear that osteovigilance must be maintained in the diabetes clinic. A simple strategy would be to ensure adequate calcium and Vit D supplementation, nutrition and physical activity for optimal musculoskeletal health. Assessment of fracture risk using tools such as Fracture Risk Assessment Tool (FRAX) may be useful, but has been found to underestimate the risk of fractures in diabetic patients.[24]

**TABLE 3** Bone turnover markers in type 1 and type 2 diabetes mellitus.

| Bone markers in diabetes | | T1DM compared with controls | T2DM compared with controls |
|---|---|---|---|
| Bone formation | Osteocalcin | ↓ | ↓ |
| | Alkaline phosphatase | ↓ | =↑ |
| | P1NP | ↓ | ↓ |
| Bone resorption | CTX | ↓ | ↓ |
| | TRAP5b | ↓ | ↓ |
| | Pyridinoline | ↑ | ↓ |
| | Deoxypyridinoline | ↑ | ↓= |
| | PTH | ↓ | ↓ |
| | Sclerostin | = | ↑ |
| | s-RANKL | ↓= | NA |
| | OPG | ↓ | ↑ |

(CTX: C-terminal cross-linked telopeptide; NA: not assessed; OPG: osteoprotegerin; P1NP: procollagen type 1 amino-terminal propeptide; PTH: parathormone; s-RANKL: soluble receptor activator for nuclear factor κB ligand; T1DM: type 1 diabetes mellitus; TRAP5b: tartrate-resistant acid phosphatase 5b; =: no significant difference)

## SECTION 1: The Scope of Glucocrinology

Finally, since DM is associated with altered bone health and an increased risk of fractures, we have to be cautious about the effect that antidiabetic drugs may have on bone metabolism.[25] Table 4 summarizes the effects of various antidiabetic medications on bone health.

Fall prevention, optimization of glycemic control and management of comorbid conditions should be a priority. Impact of current therapies of osteoporosis on DM as well as their utility in DM-specific population has not been well-studied, though data of their efficacy has been largely reassuring. Bisphosphonates reduce the secretion of undercarboxylated OC, but did not have clinically meaningful effects on glycemic control in diabetic patients. Similarly, no negative effect on glucose levels or risk of diabetes has been reported with teriparatide or denosumab.[26]

**TABLE 4** Effects of antidiabetic medications on bone health.

| Antidiabetic medications | Effects on bone |
|---|---|
| Metformin | • Stimulates osteoblast differentiation through inducing AMPK/USF-1/SHP expression by increasing AMPK-dependent runt-related transcription factor 2 (RUNX2) expression<br>• Protects MG63 osteoblast-like cells against hyperglycemia by promoting type 1 collagen, osteocalcin and alkaline phosphatase |
| Sulfonylureas | • Stimulate proliferation and differentiation of osteoblast through activation of PI3K/Akt pathways<br>• Enhance the osteoblastic markers such as alkaline phosphatase and osteocalcin |
| Thiazolidine-diones | • PPARγ activation upregulates adipogenesis in the bone marrow and decreases osteogenesis by decreased stem cell differentiation into osteoblasts<br>• Enhance osteocyte apoptosis and sclerostin level<br>• Cause histomorphometric changes by affecting osteoblasts and osteoclasts |
| DPP-4 inhibitors | • Inhibit bone resorption markers such as serum CTX and improve bone loss |
| Glucagon-like peptide-1 receptor agonists | • Promote bone formation via Wnt signaling pathway<br>• Dual regulatory action on bone turnover by attenuating bone resorption through elevation of receptor activator for nuclear factor κB ligand/osteoprotegerin (RANKL/OPG) ratio and favors bone formation by increasing the expression of α-1 collagen, osteocalcin, alkaline phosphatase and RUNX2<br>• All in vitro effects with no reduction in fracture risk in large clinical studies |
| Sodium-glucose cotransporter-2 (SGLT-2) inhibitors | • Hyponatremia due to SGLT-2 inhibition may be associated with osteoporosis<br>• Increase the bone resorption markers CTX, PTH, and decreases 25-hydroxyvitamin D |
| Insulin | • Improves fracture healing by enhanced expression of vascular endothelial growth factor (VEGF)<br>• Anabolic effect on bone through increased IGF-1 and GLUT4 levels |

(AMPK: AMP-activated protein kinase; CTX: C-terminal cross-linked telopeptide; DPP-4: dipeptidyl peptidase-4; GLUT4: glucose transporter type 4; IGF-1: insulin-like growth factor-1; PPARγ: peroxisome proliferator-activated receptor gamma; PTH: parathormone; SHP: small heterodimer partner; USF-1: upstream stimulatory factor-1)

## CONCLUSION

Vitamin D, PTH and calcium are intricately involved in glucose metabolism regulation. Vit D has direct effect on insulin secretion and sensitivity and also regulates glucose homeostasis through immune modulation. Role of osteokines in glucose metabolism is increasingly being identified. Due to its impact on β-cell function and insulin sensitivity, VDD has been linked with the development of T1DM and T2DM. Association of VDD with complications of DM has also been documented, but there is insufficient evidence to suggest that Vit D supplementation reduces the risk or improves glycemic control. PHPT has been associated with IR, MS, and T2DM and glycemic control may improve after parathyroidectomy. In addition, individuals with autoimmune hypoparathyroidism may have T1DM.

The fracture risk is increased in individuals with diabetes and is associated with poor bone microarchitecture. A heightened vigilance for bone health, osteoporosis and fracture risk is needed in diabetes care. Good clinical practice demands conscious vigilance of bone metabolism parameters in patients with DM and its complications. More research is clearly needed to understand the complex interaction between bone mineral health and glucose homeostasis. Such research may provide with opportunities to develop drugs that target both glucose metabolism and skeletal health.

## REFERENCES

1. Jing X, Li DQ, Olofsson CS, et al. CaV2.3 calcium channels control second-phase insulin release. J Clin Invest. 2005;115(1):146-54.
2. Levy J, Zemel MB, Sowers JR. Role of cellular calcium metabolism in abnormal glucose metabolism and diabetic hypertension. Am J Med. 1989;87(6A):7S-16.
3. Kalra S. Recent advances in pathophysiology of diabetes: beyond the dirty dozen. J Pak Med Assoc. 2013;63(2):277-80.
4. El-Fakhri N, McDevitt H, Shaikh MG, et al. Vitamin D and its effects on glucose homeostasis, cardiovascular function and immune function. Horm Res Paediatr. 2014;81(6):363-78.
5. Rahimi Z. Parathyroid hormone, glucose metabolism and diabetes mellitus. J Parathyroid Dis. 2014;2(1):55-6.
6. Faienza MF, Luce V, Ventura A, et al. Skeleton and glucose metabolism: a bone-pancreas loop. Int J Endocrinol. 2015;2015:758148.
7. Han Y, You X, Xing W, et al. Paracrine and endocrine actions of bone-the functions of secretory proteins from osteoblasts, osteocytes, and osteoclasts. Bone Res. 2018;6:16.
8. Klein GL. Insulin and bone: Recent developments. World J Diabetes. 2014;5(1):14-6.
9. El-Fakhri N, McDevitt H, Shaikh MG, et al. Vitamin D and its effects on glucose homeostasis, cardiovascular function and immune function. Horm Res Paediatr. 2014;81(6):363-78.
10. Rak K, Bronkowska M. Immunomodulatory Effect of Vitamin D and Its Potential Role in the Prevention and Treatment of Type 1 Diabetes Mellitus-A Narrative Review. Molecules. 2018;24(1):E53.
11. Pittas AG, Lau J, Hu FB, et al. The role of vitamin D and calcium in type 2 diabetes. A systematic review and meta-analysis. J Clin Endocrinol Metab. 2007;92(6):2017-29.
12. Grammatiki M, Karras S, Kotsa K. The role of vitamin D in the pathogenesis and treatment of diabetes mellitus: a narrative review. Hormones (Athens). 2019;18(1):37-48.
13. Alzaim M, Wood RJ. Vitamin D and gestational diabetes mellitus. Nutr Rev. 2013;71(3):158-67.
14. Procopio M, Magro G, Cesario F, et al. The oral glucose tolerance test reveals a high frequency of both impaired glucose tolerance and undiagnosed Type 2 diabetes mellitus in primary hyperparathyroidism. Diabet Med. 2002;19(11):958-61.

15. Cardenas MG, Vigil KJ, Talpos GB, et al. Prevalence of type 2 diabetes mellitus in patients with primary hyperparathyroidism. Endocr Pract. 2008;14(1):69-75.
16. Khaleeli AA, Johnson JN, Taylor WH. Prevalence of glucose intolerance in primary hyperparathyroidism and the benefit of parathyroidectomy. Diabetes Metab Res Rev. 2007;23(1):43-8.
17. Procopio M, Borretta G. Derangement of glucose metabolism in hyperparathyroidism. J Endocrinol Invest. 2003;26(11):1136-42.
18. Janghorbani M, Van Dam RM, Willett WC, et al. Systematic review of type 1 and type 2 diabetes mellitus and risk of fracture. Am J Epidemiol. 2007;166(5):495-505.
19. Sellmeyer DE, Civitelli R, Hofbauer LC, et al. Skeletal Metabolism, Fracture Risk, and Fracture Outcomes in Type 1 and Type 2 Diabetes. Diabetes. 2016;65(7):1757-66.
20. Starup-Linde J, Lykkeboe S, Gregersen S, et al. Bone Structure and Predictors of Fracture in Type 1 and Type 2 Diabetes. J Clin Endocrinol Metab. 2016;101(3):928-36.
21. Joshi AS, Varthakavi PK, Bhagwat NM, et al. Coeliac autoimmunity in type I diabetes mellitus. Arab J Gastroenterol. 2014;15(2):53-7.
22. Joshi A, Varthakavi P, Chadha M, et al. A study of bone mineral density and its determinants in type 1 diabetes mellitus. J Osteoporos. 2013;2013:397814.
23. Kalra S, Gupta Y. Osteovigilance in diabetes. J Pak Med Assoc. 2018;68(9):1410-4.
24. Schacter GI, Leslie WD. DXA-Based Measurements in Diabetes: Can They Predict Fracture Risk? Calcif Tissue Int. 2017;100(2):150-164.
25. Starup-Linde J, Gregersen S, Frost M, et al. Use of glucose-lowering drugs and risk of fracture in patients with type 2 diabetes. Bone. 2017;95:136-142.
26. Schwartz AV, Schafer AL, Grey A, et al. Effects of antiresorptive therapies on glucose metabolism: results from the FIT, HORIZON-PFT, and FREEDOM trials. J Bone Miner Res. 2013;28(6):1348-54.

# CHAPTER 5

# Glucocrinology of Adrenal Cortex

*Gagan Priya, Than Than Aye*

## INTRODUCTION

The adrenal cortex secretes several steroidal hormones synthesized from a common precursor, cholesterol. These include glucocorticoids (GCs), mineralocorticoids (MCs) and adrenal androgens. Thus, adrenal cortex regulates diverse and multiple physiological functions, including regulation of glucose, lipid and protein metabolism, salt and water homeostasis, blood pressure regulation and pubarche. Altered adrenal cortical endocrine health can have a significant impact on glucose and energy homeostasis. Disorders of GC, MC and adrenal androgen pathways are associated with increased risk of diabetes and metabolic syndrome (MS) and similarly, abnormalities in adrenal physiology are demonstrated in metabolic disorders. In this chapter, we discuss this bidirectional relationship between adrenal cortical and metabolic health.

## GLUCOSE PHYSIOLOGY IN RELATION TO ADRENAL CORTEX

### Glucocorticoids—Effects on Glucose Homeostasis

Glucocorticoids are secreted from the zona fasciculata, under control of adrenocorticotropic hormone (ACTH) secreted by the anterior pituitary. Secretion of ACTH is further regulated by corticotropin-releasing hormone (CRH) and vasopressin, both of which are released from the hypothalamus. GCs, in turn, exert a negative feedback control of CRH and ACTH secretion.

Glucocorticoids are important counterregulatory stress hormones that have a significant impact on carbohydrate, lipid and protein metabolism. While they have myriad biological functions, the name "glucocorticoids" was coined due to their important role in glucose homeostasis. Their effect is mediated predominantly via nuclear glucocorticoid receptor (GR), but they also activate the mineralocorticoid receptor (MR).[1]

The effects of GCs on glucose physiology are mediated via multiple mechanisms, as enlisted in Table 1.

# SECTION 1: The Scope of Glucocrinology

**TABLE 1** Effects of glucocorticoids on glucose homeostasis and mechanisms of hyperglycemia in chronic glucocorticoid excess/Cushing's syndrome.

|  | Physiological effects of cortisol | Pathophysiological effects of cortisol excess |
|---|---|---|
| Liver | • Increased expression of enzymes of gluconeogenesis<br>• Increased glycogen synthesis and storage<br>• Increased triglyceride accumulation and lipogenesis | • Increased hepatic gluconeogenesis<br>• Hepatic insulin resistance<br>• Increased hepatic glucose output<br>• Increased hepatic steatosis |
| Skeletal muscle | • Reduced glucose uptake<br>• Reduced glucose oxidation<br>• Reduced glycogen synthesis<br>• Increased lipid accumulation<br>• Increased proteolysis | • Reduced peripheral glucose uptake and utilization<br>• Peripheral insulin resistance<br>• Increased ectopic fat deposition<br>• Decreased muscle mass/sarcopenia |
| Adipose tissue | • Increased lipolysis in peripheral adipose tissue depots<br>• Increased lipogenesis in visceral and ectopic tissue<br>• Increased circulating free fatty acids<br>• Abnormal adipokine secretion | • Increased central and ectopic fat with loss of extremity fat<br>• Peripheral insulin resistance |
| Pancreas | • Reduced glucose signaling<br>• Reduced insulin gene transcription<br>• Reduced insulin exocytosis<br>• Increased glucagon secretion<br>• Attenuated effect of incretins<br>• Increased expression of proapoptotic proteins and reduced expression of antiapoptotic proteins | • Impaired insulin secretion (direct)<br>• Initial rise in insulin secretion to compensate for insulin resistance followed by decreased secretion (long term)<br>• B-cell apoptosis |

- *Reduce peripheral glucose uptake and utilization*: GCs impair insulin-mediated cellular glucose uptake by directly interfering with postreceptor insulin signaling and membrane translocation of glucose transporter type 4 (GLUT4). In addition, they also reduce glucose oxidation. Therefore, they reduce peripheral glucose uptake and utilization by white adipose tissue (WAT) and skeletal muscle
- *Increase hepatic gluconeogenesis*: GCs increase hepatic gluconeogenesis, by both upregulating the expression of enzymes involved in gluconeogenesis and increasing the availability of gluconeogenic precursors (amino acids, glycerol and fatty acids) by increasing proteolysis and lipolysis.[2] GCs upregulate the expression of several gluconeogenic enzymes, including pyruvate carboxylase (PC), phosphoenolpyruvate carboxykinase (PEPCK), fructose-1,6-bisphosphatase (FBP1), phosphofructokinase 2/fructose bisphosphatase 2 (PFKFB2), glucose-6-phosphatase (G6PC) and glucose-6-phosphate transporter (*SLC37A4*). In addition, GCs have a permissive role on the effect of glucagon and epinephrine in inducing gluconeogenesis.[2] Adrenalectomized mice have been shown to have reduced glucagon, epinephrine and cyclic adenosine monophosphate (cAMP)-induced gluconeogenesis, which is restored with the administration of GCs

- *Tissue-specific effects on glycogen metabolism*: The effects of GCs on glycogen metabolism are tissue-specific. They increase catecholamine-induced glycogenolysis and reduce insulin-mediated glycogen synthesis in skeletal muscles, while in the liver, they promote glycogen synthesis and storage
- *Modulate insulin and glucagon secretion*: The effects on β-cell function are complex. Acute administration of GCs inhibits β-cell function by a direct dose-dependent effect that may involve reduced glucose sensing, reduced transcription of insulin gene, and reduced insulin exocytosis. This effect seems to be reversible.[3] GCs impair insulin secretion from pancreatic β-cells while the secretion of glucagon, another counterregulatory hormone, is increased. They may also attenuate the effect of incretin hormones on increasing insulin secretion and suppressing glucagon secretion. With chronic GC administration and endogenous GC excess, GC-induced insulin resistance is associated with initial compensatory β-cell hyperplasia and a rise in insulin secretion, and later failure to compensate for the insulin demands with resultant hyperglycemia. GCs also modulate the α2-adrenergic receptor-mediated inhibition of insulin secretion and may promote β-cell apoptosis, though the latter effect is debated[3]
- *Effect on lipid metabolism*: GCs regulate adipose tissue differentiation, distribution and function. GRα stimulation leads to increased activity of lipoprotein lipase (LPL) in adipose tissue, thereby increasing lipid mobilization and circulating free fatty acid (FFA) concentration.[2] While GCs promote lipolysis in the extremities, there is increased triglyceride accumulation and lipogenesis in upper body and visceral fat depots. The resultant increase in visceral fat and lipotoxicity further contributes to impaired insulin sensitivity
- *Effect on protein metabolism*: GCs inhibit postinsulin receptor signaling involving PKB/Akt and mammalian target of rapamycin (mTOR) pathways and thereby, suppress protein synthesis and increase protein degradation in skeletal muscle. This increases the availability of substrate for gluconeogenesis
- *Reduced secretion of osteocalcin*: GCs reduce the secretion of bone-derived osteocalcin, which is known to stimulate insulin sensitivity.

Thus, the net effect of GCs on carbohydrate and energy metabolism is antagonistic to insulin. By reducing peripheral glucose uptake and increasing hepatic gluconeogenesis, GCs create a metabolic milieu suitable for survival during stress, including fasting or starvation, by increasing the availability of glucose for the brain. While this is favorable in the short term, chronic GC excess can result in significant insulin resistance, visceral adiposity, hyperglycemia, dyslipidemia, hypertension and increased cardiovascular risk.[4]

## Mineralocorticoids—Effects on Glucose Homeostasis

Aldosterone is secreted from the zona glomerulosa and its secretion is regulated by the renin–angiotensin–aldosterone system (RAAS), sodium, potassium, extracellular fluid (ECF) status and ACTH. Aldosterone primarily regulates ECF volume and blood pressure by promoting sodium retention and potassium loss in the renal tubules.

The classic effects of aldosterone in regulation of ECF volume and potassium are primarily mediated via the MR. However, the MR has equal affinity for both aldosterone

| TABLE 2 | Effects of aldosterone on glucose homeostasis. |
|---|---|
| Mechanism of effect | Physiological role |
| Genomic effects mediated via MR | • MR regulates transcription of target genes including ENaC and serum- and glucocorticoid-induced protein kinase 1 (SGK1)<br>• Decreased glucose-6-phosphate dehydrogenase activity and activation of NAD(P)H oxidase—reduced oxidative stress |
| Rapid, nongenomic effects | • Activation of extracellular-regulated kinase/mitogen-activated protein kinase (ERK/MAPK) pathways<br>• Phosphorylation of c-Src, JNK and NF-κB<br>• Reduces insulin sensitivity<br>• Reduces glucose-stimulated insulin secretion |

(ENaC: epithelial sodium channels; MR: mineralocorticoid receptor)

and cortisol. In the kidney, colon, endothelium, and smooth muscle, MR is shielded from the effects of cortisol due to expression of 11β-hydroxysteroid dehydrogenase 2 (11βHSD2) that converts cortisol to inactive cortisone.[5] In brain and adipose tissue, most of the MR effects are mediated by cortisol.

In addition, aldosterone also has nongenomic effects in nonepithelial cells, including the regulation of intracellular cations and metabolic signaling, endothelial relaxation and redox state.[5] These effects are independent of their hemodynamic effects. Aldosterone also reduces insulin sensitivity in adipose tissue and skeletal muscle. In addition, it suppresses insulin signaling in vascular smooth muscle cells, cardiomyocytes and fibroblasts. Both GCs and MCs act through MRs in adipose tissue to increase the expression of inflammatory cytokines that contribute to insulin resistance and further stimulate increased aldosterone secretion. MCs also reduce glucose-stimulated insulin secretion, both directly and by causing hypokalemia. Aldosterone impairs first-phase insulin secretion. In addition, MC excess may contribute to islet cell inflammation and oxidative stress.[6] The effects of aldosterone on glucose homeostasis are enlisted in Table 2.

### Adrenal Androgens—Effect on Glucose Homeostasis

Adrenal androgens [dehydroepiandrosterone or DHEA, DHEA sulfate (DHEAS) and androstenedione] are secreted by zona fasciculata and reticularis. Their exact role is not well understood. Their action is primarily mediated via conversion to more potent sex steroids. In addition, DHEA may inhibit glucose-6-phosphate dehydrogenase and NADPH production and have antioxidant and anti-inflammatory properties.[7]

## GLUCOVIGILANCE IN DISORDERS OF ADRENAL CORTEX

### Endogenous Glucocorticoid Excess—Cushing's Syndrome

Milder forms of endogenous GC excess, called "subclinical" Cushing's syndrome, may be caused by small adrenal adenomas.

## Pathophysiology of Secondary Diabetes in Cushing's Syndrome

Chronic GC excess or Cushing's syndrome, whether endogenous or exogenous, can lead to insulin resistance and impaired insulin secretion. Endogenous Cushing's syndrome may result from ACTH-secreting tumors (pituitary adenoma or ectopic secretion) or ACTH-independent causes (adrenal adenoma, adrenal hyperplasia or adrenocortical carcinoma). Milder forms of endogenous GC excess, called "subclinical" Cushing's syndrome, may be caused by small adrenal adenomas.

Chronic GC excess is associated with impaired glucose homeostasis and hyperglycemia through several pathophysiological mechanisms, enlisted in Table 1 and depicted in Flowchart 1. GC excess results in increased hepatic glucose output and increased peripheral insulin resistance along with impaired β-cell function with reduced insulin secretion. GC excess is associated with increased visceral and ectopic fat, increased circulating FFAs and loss of muscle mass, further contributing to insulin resistance. There may be a compensatory rise in insulin secretion, but this fails to match the increased insulin demand with eventual occurrence of hyperglycemia. The defect in insulin secretion is at least partly reversible. In addition, elevated GCs can saturate 11βHSD2 enzyme, resulting in effects of cortisol through the MR also. MR activation further contributes to impaired insulin sensitivity in several tissues including the cardiovascular system, kidneys, adipose tissue, muscles and liver.[8]

## Clinical Phenotype of Diabetes in Cushing's Syndrome

Cushing's syndrome is associated with central obesity, insulin resistance and hyperglycemia, hypertension, dyslipidemia, proximal muscle weakness, hepatic steatosis and increased cardiovascular risk. Impaired fasting glucose (IFG), impaired glucose tolerance (IGT), or overt diabetes is present in 60–70% of individuals with Cushing's syndrome.[9] GC excess causes predominant postprandial hyperglycemia due to reduced peripheral glucose uptake, and may result in difficult-to-control diabetes.

The severity of diabetes often correlates with urinary free cortisol levels, but this association is not always seen. Several factors may contribute to the differences in interindividual susceptibility to hyperglycemia including age, lifestyle, genetic predisposition and the duration and degree of cortisol excess.[9]

## Subclinical Cushing's Syndrome

Almost 15–30% of patients with adrenal incidentalomas have underlying subclinical Cushing's syndrome on biochemical evaluation. While these individuals have chronic mild GC excess, they do not manifest typical clinical features of hypercortisolism. On the other hand, they may present with a phenotype similar to MS with insulin resistance, IGT, hypertension and dyslipidemia.[10] Many, but not all, studies have reported an increased prevalence of IGT and diabetes in these individuals, of almost up to 25%. Higher age, greater midnight cortisol levels, greater cortisol levels after overnight dexamethasone suppression test (ONDST), and larger adenomas are associated with greater incidence of diabetes. Surgical resection of adrenal tumor has been reported to result in improvement in weight, glycemic control and hypertension.[10] However, a clear cause-and-effect relationship between subclinical hypercortisolism and

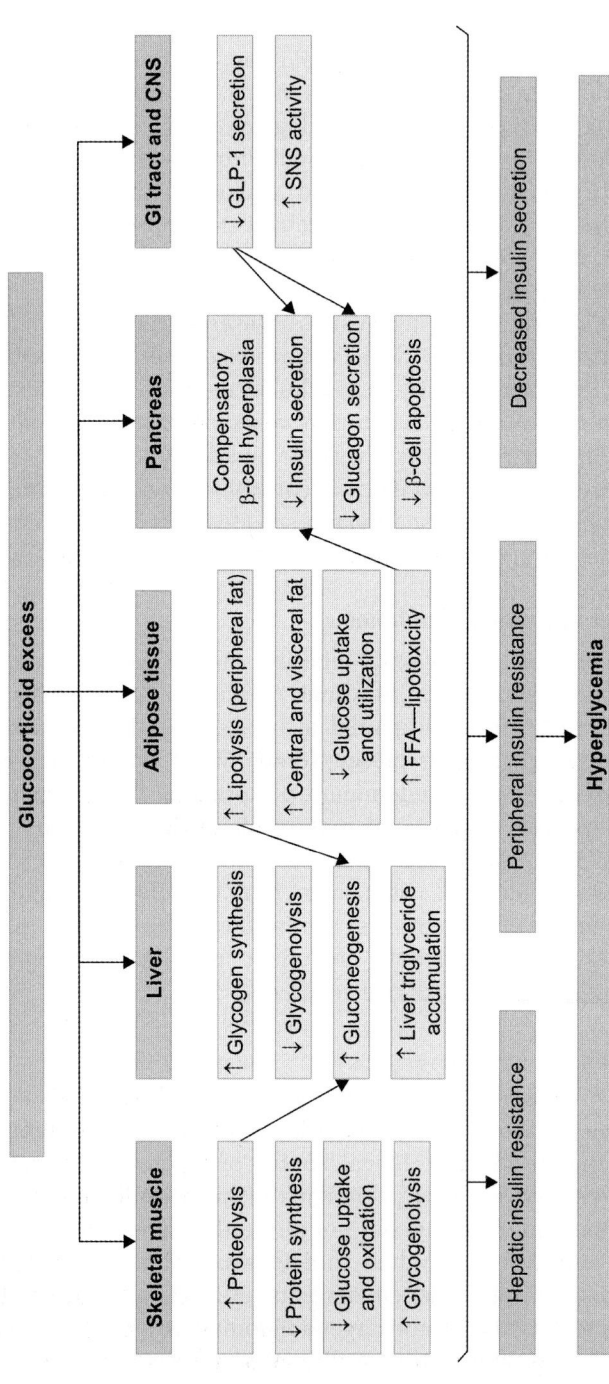

**FLOWCHART 1:** Pathogenesis of hyperglycemia due to glucocorticoid excess. Glucocorticoid excess contributes to hyperglycemia via multiple mechanisms. Glucocorticoids increase liver gluconeogenesis, both directly by upregulating several gluconeogenic enzymes and via increased availability of gluconeogenic precursors. While liver glycogen synthesis is increased, the net effect is an increase in hepatic glucose output. They also reduce peripheral glucose uptake and oxidation in skeletal muscle and adipose tissue, and increase glycogenolysis in skeletal muscle. Glucocorticoids increase the activity of hormone-sensitive lipase and lipolysis in subcutaneous adipose tissue by impairing insulin signaling in these tissues, but increase lipoprotein lipase activity and lipogenesis in visceral and upper body fat depots. In addition, increased free fatty acid flux results in ectopic fat deposition, including increased hepatic fat and skeletal muscle fat content. Proteolysis is increased and along with a net increase in free fatty acids and glycerol, and this results in increased availability of gluconeogenic precursors. The resultant lipotoxicity further contributes to insulin resistance and impaired insulin secretion. Glucocorticoids inhibit pancreatic insulin secretion and increase glucagon secretion, both directly and via inhibition of glucagon-like peptide-1 secretion.

(CNS: central nervous system; GI: gastrointestinal; GLP-1: glucagon-like peptide-1; FFA: free fatty acid; SNS: sympathetic nervous system) diabetes cannot be established at present. Therefore, the indications for laparoscopic adrenalectomy are not clearly defined and many patients can be followed closely with optimal management of metabolic abnormalities.

## Glucovigilance in Cushing's Syndrome: Screening for Hyperglycemia

Glucovigilance is important in individuals with Cushing's syndrome. They should be screened for hyperglycemia at diagnosis and periodically thereafter. Oral glucose tolerance test (OGTT) and hemoglobin A1c (HbA1c) measurement should be considered as fasting plasma glucose (FPG) may underestimate the prevalence of dysglycemia.[9] Periodic reassessment of glycemic status should be considered, though there are no guidelines on the frequency of such testing.

All individuals detected with adrenal incidentalomas, especially those who present with MS, should be evaluated for hyperglycemia and screening to detect subclinical Cushing's syndrome.

## Effect of Remission of Hypercortisolism on Glycemic Control

Resolution of hypercortisolism is associated with improvement in glycemic control and sometimes resolution of hyperglycemia. In patients who continue to require antidiabetic medications, antihyperglycemic treatment needs to be revised to avoid hypoglycemia due to improved insulin sensitivity. However, in many patients, insulin resistance, obesity, hyperglycemia, dyslipidemia and cardiovascular risk persists despite successful amelioration of cortisol excess.

## Effects of Therapeutic Strategy on Glycemic Control

- Surgical resection of pituitary microadenomas has remission rates ranging from 60% to 90%. Radiotherapy remains second option in patients with recurrent, persistent or inoperable disease. Hypopituitarism that may occur after surgery and/or radiotherapy, itself is associated with insulin resistance[9]
- In patients undergoing bilateral adrenalectomy, lifelong GC and MC treatment is needed. Any overdose of GCs may affect glycemic control
- For patients with adrenal tumors, adrenalectomy is usually associated with remission and does not require GC replacement
- Medical therapy for hypercortisolism may be considered preoperatively or in those in whom definitive treatment is not possible. Ketoconazole, metyrapone, mitotane, etomidate and LCI inhibit cortisol secretion from the adrenals. Ketoconazole, in doses of 200–1,200 mg/day, has been associated with significant improvements in insulin resistance, glycemic control, and lipids across several studies.[9] Similar benefits have been reported with metyrapone, in doses of 250–4,500 mg/day. Dopamine agonists, bromocriptine and cabergoline, also have a positive impact on glycemic control. However, somatostatin receptor (SSTR) agonists like octreotide, lanreotide and pasireotide also inhibit insulin and glucagon-like peptide-1 (GLP-1) secretion and worsen glycemic control despite reduction in cortisol levels. Individuals on pasireotide should be closely monitored for glycemic control.[9] Incretin-based antidiabetic drugs may be particularly useful to counter pasireotide-induced hyperglycemia.[11] Table 3 summarizes the effects of medical therapy on glucose homeostasis.

**TABLE 3** Effects of medical therapy for hypercortisolism on glucose homeostasis.

| | Dose | Mechanism of action | Mechanism of glycemic benefit | Trial evidence |
|---|---|---|---|---|
| **Adrenal-directed medical therapy** | | | | |
| Ketoconazole | 200–1,200 mg/day | Dose-dependent reversible inhibitors of adrenal steroidogenesis | Reduced cortisol levels | Improves glycemic control, lipids and insulin resistance |
| Metyrapone | 250–4,500 mg/day | | Reduced cortisol levels | Improved glycemic control |
| LCI699, Osilodrostat | – | | • Reduced cortisol levels<br>• Reduced aldosterone levels | Early evidence of glycemic benefit |
| Mitotane | 4,000 mg/day | Adrenolytic at dose >4 g/day | – | • Used in adrenal cancer<br>• Lack of long-term data |
| **Glucocorticoid receptor (GR) antagonist** | | | | |
| Mifepristone | 300–1,200 mg/day | • Progesterone receptor antagonist<br>• GR antagonist at higher concentrations | Block the effects of GCs mediated via GR | • Improved glycemic control<br>• Improved insulin sensitivity<br>• Weight reduction |
| **Pituitary-directed medical therapy** | | | | |
| D2-agonists Cabergoline Bromocriptine | 1–7 mg/day | Inhibit ACTH secretion mediated by D2 | • Reduced cortisol levels<br>• Reduced prolactin Regulation of biological clock<br>• Reduced appetite<br>• Reduced hepatic glucose output<br>• Increased splanchnic glucose uptake | • Improved glycemic control<br>• Quick-release bromocriptine approved for use in type 2 diabetes mellitus<br>• Good efficacy when combined with ketoconazole |
| Octreotide Lanreotide | Not recommended | Somatostatin receptor (SSTR) analogs | • Reduce cortisol levels<br>• Inhibit insulin secretion | May worsen glycemic control |
| Pasireotide | • 10–40 mg IM every 4 weeks<br>• 0.3–0.9 mg SC twice daily | • Multireceptor SST analog (SSTR1, 3 and 5)<br>• Potent SSTR5 agonists | • Reduced ACTH secretion and cortisol levels<br>• SSTR5 inhibits insulin secretion from pancreas<br>• Inhibits GLP-1 and GIP<br>• Inhibits GH/IGF-1 axis | • Can cause overt hyperglycemia or diabetes, reported in 73% patients in one study<br>• Can predispose patients to GHD—further contributes to insulin resistance |

(ACTH: adrenocorticotropic hormone; D2: dopamine; GH: growth hormone; GIP: gastric inhibitory polypeptide; GLP-1: glucagon-like peptide-1; IGF-1: insulin-like growth factor-1; IM: intramuscular; SC: subcutaneous; GC: glucocorticoid)

## Management of Hyperglycemia in Cushing's Syndrome

The optimal therapeutic approach for glycemic management in Cushing's syndrome has not been investigated in trials. Secondary diabetes due to Cushing's syndrome can be managed similar to type 2 diabetes mellitus (T2DM). Many patients will require insulin for glycemic control. Intravenous insulin infusion is required in those with acute hyperglycemic emergencies and intercurrent illness such as infections and for preoperative optimization. Others can be managed with basal-bolus insulin regimens with regular monitoring of blood glucose (BG). Optimal preoperative control reduces the risk of postoperative infections and complications. Many patients may show significant amelioration in hyperglycemia following surgical remission of hypercortisolism, necessitating down-titration of antidiabetic medications to avoid hypoglycemia.

In those patients who are not candidates for definitive treatment or have recurrent or persistent disease, long-term glycemic and metabolic control should be a priority. Insulin sensitizers can be used in conjunction with cortisol-lowering drugs. Incretin-based drugs may be promising agents, but need further evaluation. Many patients will require insulin for glycemic control. Close monitoring of BG is needed, especially since certain cortisol-lowering drugs (ketoconazole, metyrapone and cabergoline) can improve glycemic control while others (pasireotide) can worsen glycemic control.

## Exogenous Glucocorticoid-induced Diabetes

Glucocorticoids are used in physiological replacement doses in patients with primary or secondary adrenal insufficiency and congenital adrenal hyperplasia (CAH). In addition, GCs are used in a variety of acute and chronic conditions, including inflammatory, autoimmune and neurological disorders, and in chemotherapeutic and post-transplant regimens. However, they may worsen glycemic control in pre existing diabetes, cause transient hyperglycemia or new-onset diabetes. The incidence of new-onset hyperglycemia was 34–56% in individuals without pre-existing diabetes.[12] The odds ratio for new-onset diabetes with exogenous GCs was 1.5–2.5 in a recent meta-analysis.[13]

### Factors Increasing the Risk of Glucocorticoid-induced Hyperglycemia

The risk of GC-induced hyperglycemia has been variably reported due to several underlying factors.[14] Factors associated with increased risk of steroid-induced diabetes are listed in Table 4. The overall effect of GC depends on the dosage and duration of GC use and underlying susceptibility of the individual. More potent GCs such as dexamethasone and prednisolone are likely to result in greater degree of insulin resistance than hydrocortisone.

Glucocorticoid use is associated with predominantly postprandial hyperglycemia and BG elevations are typically seen in the afternoon and evening, for those taking the GC dose in the morning. Monitoring of FPG is often likely to miss the diagnosis.[15]

### Higher Risk of Complications

Diabetes may further contribute to the increased cardiovascular risk associated with chronic inflammatory conditions such as rheumatoid arthritis. It also increases the risk

| TABLE 4 | Factors associated with increased risk of glucocorticoid-induced diabetes. |
|---|---|
| Drug-associated factors | • Higher potency steroids<br>• Higher glucocorticoid dose<br>• Longer duration of exposure<br>• Higher cumulative dose<br>• Route of administration—less with topical, inhaled and ocular steroids than oral or parenteral steroids |
| Patient-specific factors | • Older age<br>• Family history of diabetes<br>• Higher BMI<br>• Abdominal obesity<br>• Pre-existing impaired glucose tolerance<br>• Previous history of gestational diabetes<br>• Concurrent drugs—immunosuppressants such as calcineurin inhibitors (especially tacrolimus), mycophenolate mofetil<br>• HCV positivity in post-transplant patients (NODAT)<br>• Hypomagnesemia (relation seen in post-transplant patients) |

(BMI: body mass index; HCV: hepatitis C virus; NODAT: new-onset diabetes after transplantation)

of microvascular complications. If left undetected and untreated, there is increased risk of acute hyperglycemic emergencies, including hyperglycemic hyperosmolar state or diabetic ketoacidosis. In hospitalized patients, GC-induced hyperglycemia increases the risk of infections, prolonged hospitalization, delayed would healing, readmission rates and overall mortality.[9] In addition, there is increased risk of graft failure in transplant recipients and reduced graft survival in patients with suboptimal glycemic control.[16]

## Management of Glucocorticoid-induced Hyperglycemia

There are no consensus guidelines for the management of GC-induced diabetes. All patients on GCs should be monitored regularly for BG levels. When GCs are used in hospitalized patients, regular BG monitoring should be done for at least 48 hours. If BG is less than 140 mg/day, subsequent monitoring frequency can be reduced. FPG estimation alone may miss many patients. Postprandial glucose after lunch and OGTT have more diagnostic sensitivity for the detection of GC-induced hyperglycemia.[9] HbA1c may fail to detect new-onset hyperglycemia seen due to recent initiation of GCs, but may be useful for monitoring of patients on long-term GC therapy. Therefore, OGTT or postprandial glucose (particularly postlunch) should be considered for monitoring patients on GCs in the short term with addition of HbA1c for screening patients on long-term steroids.

While an attempt should be made to keep the GC dose to minimal permissible, many patients will require long-term GC treatment and optimal metabolic control is required to minimize long-term risks. Management differs from standard treatment of diabetes in several aspects. Lifestyle modification should include adequate protein intake due to a negative protein balance caused by steroids. Regular physical activity with resistance training should be emphasized. Metformin remains the first-choice drug but may not be sufficient alone. Use of pioglitazone, however, may further worsen the risk of fluid retention, osteoporosis and fractures.[9]

Basal bolus insulin therapy is the cornerstone for glycemic management due to its greater efficacy and flexibility and ability to target individual BG values. Prandial and correction dose requirements are higher (approximately 70% of total insulin dose) with particularly higher doses needed around the mid-day and evening meals. Basal insulin requirements are usually lower (approximately 30%) and a higher dose of basal insulin, such as that used for type 1 diabetes mellitus (T1DM) or T2DM, can result in nocturnal hypoglycemia.[9] Intermediate-acting insulin neutral protamine Hagedorn (NPH) once in the morning can be considered in place of basal insulin analogs, especially when using intermediate-acting steroids since its peak coincides with the action of GCs.[16] However, the doses should be individually titrated based on 3-6 time point self-monitoring of blood glucose (SMBG) records.

Long-acting sulfonylureas do not specifically target postprandial hyperglycemia and may be associated with nocturnal hypoglycemia. If hyperglycemia is mild, a short-acting secretagogue such as repaglinide may be tried before meals. Incretin mimetics are promising agents as they reduce postprandial hyperglycemia. Short-acting GLP-1 analog exenatide was shown to be useful in patients on intermediate-acting GCs. Sodium-glucose cotransporter-2 (SGLT-2) inhibitors may increase the risk of genitourinary infections.[15]

When GC therapy is withdrawn or tapered down, there may be an increased risk of hypoglycemia due to steroid withdrawal. This calls for regular BG monitoring with appropriate down-titration of antihyperglycemic medications.

### Minimizing Glucocorticoid-induced Hyperglycemia

An attempt should be made to minimize the dose and duration of GC exposure, with the consideration of steroid-sparing regimens. However, even with physiological replacement regimens, such as those used in adrenal insufficiency, these regimens do not mimic endogenous rhythm of cortisol production and carry a risk of mild GC excess.[17] Factors that should be taken into consideration when initiating GCs include personal and family history of diabetes, obesity, hypertension, dyslipidemia and other cardiovascular risk factors. Individuals with a higher risk of steroid-induced hyperglycemia should be more closely monitored.

## Adrenal Insufficiency

Adrenal insufficiency, whether primary or secondary, is associated with a greater risk of hypoglycemia, but these individuals are also at risk of long-term mild GC excess related to GC replacement. In addition, autoimmune adrenal insufficiency may be related to T1DM.

### Increased Risk of Hypoglycemia

Deficient cortisol production is associated with reduced hepatic glucose output and increased risk of hypoglycemia. Individuals with adrenal insufficiency may present with unexplained hypoglycemia as an initial presentation. The risk of spontaneous hypoglycemia is more in those with secondary adrenal insufficiency who may have associated growth hormone deficiency or secondary hypothyroidism.[18]

## Long-term Exogenous Glucocorticoid Exposure

Adrenal insufficiency is managed with long-term GCs. Patients on long-term GC replacement may often be overtreated with GCs, thereby increasing the risk of exogenous GC-induced hyperglycemia, obesity and hypertension.[17] More physiological replacement regimens that mimic circadian rhythm are associated with less glucose intolerance.

In adrenal insufficiency, short-acting GCs administered in divided doses to mimic normal circadian rhythm are associated with less glycemic effects. Hydrocortisone has a half-life of 90 minutes, and can be used in doses of 15–20 mg/day, administered in two to three divided doses, with higher doses given on waking up, lower dose in early afternoon and lowest dose in late afternoon. Doses adjusted by weight (0.12 mg/kg/day) are more physiological.[17] On the other hand, longer acting and more potent GCs such as dexamethasone and prednisone should be avoided for GC replacement therapy. Newer formulations of hydrocortisone such as dual release hydrocortisone (with an immediate release outer coat and extended-release inner core) and Chronocort may mimic normal circadian rhythm with once and twice daily dosing, respectively, but are not currently available.[17] In addition, MC replacement with fludrocortisone in primary but not secondary adrenal insufficiency helps reduce the dose of GCs required. Patients should be monitored for features of GC excess.

## Coexistent Type 1 Diabetes Mellitus

About 10–15% of patients with primary adrenal insufficiency may develop T1DM. Some of these patients may have autoimmune polyglandular syndrome type 1 or 2. A high index of clinical suspicion can help in early detection of associated autoimmune disorders and optimal management. Optimal glycemic management would also require optimized GC replacement, as undertreatment may increase the risk of insulin-induced hypoglycemia and overtreatment may increase the risk of GC-induced metabolic side effects.

## Primary Hyperaldosteronism

Primary hyperaldosteronism (HA) can occur due to aldosterone-producing adenomas (APAs) or unilateral or bilateral adrenal hyperplasia. Secondary hyperreninemic hyperaldosteronism is more common, resulting from heart failure, chronic kidney disease or chronic liver disease.

Hyperaldosteronism is associated with sodium and water retention, hypokalemia and hypertension, and cardiovascular disease. In addition, these individuals also have reduced insulin sensitivity and impaired insulin secretion, both due to direct effects of MC excess and due to concomitant hypokalemia. Hypokalemia is associated with a high risk of incident diabetes as it impairs insulin secretion. Serum potassium concentration negatively correlated with 2-hour OGTT glucose concentration in patients with primary HA.[19] But potassium supplementation only partially improved glucose tolerance. HA also contributes to oxidative stress, chronic inflammation and endothelial dysfunction.

Primary HA is associated with insulin resistance, impaired glucose metabolism, MS and secondary diabetes.[20] Many studies report a higher prevalence of diabetes and MS in individuals with primary HA than hypertensive controls.[21] Surgical treatment of primary HA with normalization of aldosterone levels was associated with improvement in insulin sensitivity and glucose tolerance at 6–12 months.[22] However, the effects of MR antagonists on glycemic status are variable. While spironolactone has a negative impact on glycemic status, eplerenone is neutral.

## Congenital Adrenal Hyperplasia

The 21-hydroxylase deficiency is the most common cause of CAH. Long-term GC replacement remains the cornerstone of classic CAH, with the aim of replacement of cortisol and prevention of ACTH-induced androgen excess. However, this carries the risk of excess GC exposure, reversed circadian rhythm of cortisol, and adverse metabolic effects. Risk is higher with use of higher doses of more potent and long-acting synthetic GCs. Studies have reported CAH patients to have higher body mass index (BMI), insulin resistance, lipid abnormalities, diabetes and hypertension.[23]

The relative risk of diabetes in CAH has been reported to be higher than in primary adrenal insufficiency due to hyperandrogenism. Therefore, all patients with CAH should be monitored for weight, central obesity, blood pressure, glycemic status and lipids. Metformin and pioglitazone may be useful in patients with IGT as they also reduce androgen levels.[24]

# ADRENOVIGILANCE IN DIABETES

## Changes in Adrenal Cortical Physiology in Diabetes

Uncontrolled diabetes is associated with increased activation of hypothalamic–pituitary–adrenal (HPA) axis with higher levels of basal ACTH. However, by negative feedback, basal CRH secretion is reduced suggesting that HPA activation results from other factors such as insulin resistance. Individuals with T2DM have higher morning and nocturnal cortisol, but more significantly, the circadian rhythm of ACTH and cortisol is altered.[25] Suppression of cortisol in response to dexamethasone may also be diminished. Individuals with T1DM also exhibit increased 24-hour urinary-free cortisol, especially with longer disease duration and in those with microvascular and macrovascular complications. Too intensive glycemic control with recurrent hypoglycemia may lead to reduced response of ACTH and cortisol to hypoglycemia.

The enzyme 11βHSD1 increases local production of cortisol from cortisone in liver and adipose tissue. 11βHSD1 has been implicated in the pathogenesis of obesity. While circulating cortisol levels are not elevated in obesity and MS, adipose tissue and skeletal muscle have been shown to be hyperresponsive to GCs and increased expression of GRα and 11βHSD1 has been observed.

Obesity is associated with increased aldosterone levels, low adiponectin and high leptin levels, while weight reduction is associated with reduced aldosterone levels. Even in subjects without primary HA, increased levels of aldosterone are associated with greater insulin resistance and glucose intolerance.[5] Adipose tissue secretes several factors that promote excess aldosterone production that in turn worsens insulin resistance, oxidative stress, inflammation, and sodium retention. These maladaptive responses contribute to the development of hypertension in MS. Aldosterone, in turn, stimulates adipocyte expansion and increased leptin and reduced adiponectin expression.[5]

Aldosterone and angiotensin II are involved in vascular and cardiac remodeling and play an important role in mediating vascular complications in diabetes, including cardiovascular disease and diabetic kidney disease. Further, aldosterone may promote fibrosis and target organ damage. However, plasma levels of renin, angiotensin II, and aldosterone were not found to be high in animal models of diabetes. Therefore, local renin–angiotensin system (RAS) overactivity seems to be mediating vasculopathy.[25] Inhibitors of RAS are associated with reduced risk of the development and progression of vascular complications.

Dehydroepiandrosterone levels decrease with aging, with greater decline in women. DHEA and DHEAS levels are also reduced in men with T2DM and an association has been demonstrated between lower DHEAS levels and atherosclerosis in men.[25] Hyperglycemia has been implicated in this decline of DHEA and DHEAS, though the exact significance is unknown. On the other hand, DHEAS levels were normal or increased in women. No difference has been found in DHEAS or androstenedione levels in individuals with T1DM and their nondiabetic siblings.[25] In prospective studies, low DHEAS levels were linked to insulin resistance, cardiovascular disease and frailty.[26]

## Screening for Cushing's Syndrome in Individuals with Diabetes

Cushing's syndrome can cause "diabetes secondary to endocrinopathy". Previously undetected Cushing's syndrome was reported in 0.7% of individuals with T2DM in a large study.[27] While regular screening of all diabetics for Cushing's syndrome is not justified, a case-finding approach with evaluation for cortisol excess should be considered in any diabetic individual with a clinical phenotype suggestive of hypercortisolism.

In addition, when there is sudden worsening of glycemic control or there are significant fluctuations between hyperglycemia and hypoglycemia, one must be vigilant of the possible prescribed or surreptitious use of GCs, especially from indigenous medications. Off-label use of GCs is quite common in developing countries and a cause of worsened glycemic control.

## Screening for Adrenal Insufficiency in Individuals with Diabetes Mellitus with Unexplained Hypoglycemia

Individuals with T1DM may have increased prevalence of other autoimmune diseases, including primary adrenal insufficiency. Patients with secondary adrenal insufficiency with concomitant deficiencies in other anterior pituitary hormones are at higher risk of dyslipidemia, hypertension and cardiovascular disease. In previously controlled diabetic individuals, a history of recurrent hypoglycemia should prompt evaluation for adrenal insufficiency among other causes. GC replacement should preferably be done by hydrocortisone given in pattern that mimics circadian rhythm to minimize glycemic variability.

## Hyperaldosteronism in T2DM and Metabolic Syndrome

It is increasingly understood that MCs play an important role in the pathogenesis of MS, hypertension and cardiovascular and chronic kidney diseases.[28] The multiple ways in which aldosterone affects the pathophysiology of diabetes and its vascular complications are depicted in Flowchart 2. About 13% Asian type 2 diabetics subjects with difficult-to-control hypertension were detected to have primary HA. Therefore, systemic screening should be considered in those diabetic individuals with resistant hypertension.[29] MR blockade is particularly useful in the management of resistant hypertension and reduces cardiovascular and renal risk in diabetics.

Aldosterone blockade, in addition to RAS blockade, may have a role in preventing progression of chronic kidney disease, as suggested by Randomized Aldactone Evaluation Study (RALES) (spironolactone) and EPHESUS (eplerenone) trials.[30] Spironolactone reduced cardiovascular events and improved morbidity and mortality in heart failure in addition to RAS blockers. In EPHESUS trial, benefits with eplerenone were more pronounced in diabetic than nondiabetic subjects and were independent of reduction in blood pressure.

## Effects of Mineralocorticoid Antagonists on Glucose Homeostasis

Spironolactone, a nonselective MR antagonist, was associated with a negative effect on glucose homeostasis in heart failure patients with diabetes. In subjects with diabetes, spironolactone was associated with a slight rise in HbA1c (0.16–0.6%). This could be because while it blocks MR, aldosterone and cortisol levels are increased.[31] These effects are not seen with eplerenone. In fact, eplerenone did not seem to influence glycemic status.[32]

## NEW THERAPEUTIC AVENUES IN GLUCOCRINOLOGY OF ADRENALS

An improved understanding of the glucocrinology of adrenal cortex offers the potential to develop new therapeutic targets in diabetes and metabolic diseases. Some of these include:

- *11βHSD1 inhibitors*: Deficient activity of this enzyme has been associated with low risk of obesity and insulin resistance and lower triglycerides and low-density lipoprotein (LDL) cholesterol in mice.[33] The 11βHSD1 inhibitors selectively reduce GC activity in adipose tissue and muscle and are under investigation as a novel therapeutic option in T2DM. INCB13739 was found to reduce insulin resistance, HbA1c and weight along with improvement in lipid parameters in a phase 2 study
- *Selective GR modulators*: Selective GR modulators that block the metabolic effects of GCs but not their anti-inflammatory effects may be useful in patients using exogenous GCs. PF04171327 or the dissociated agonists of glucocorticoid receptor (DAGR) are under investigation and have been tested in animal models. However, long-term GR antagonism carries the risk of adrenal insufficiency, rebound activation of HPA axis, adrenal hyperplasia and increased cortisol secretion[34]

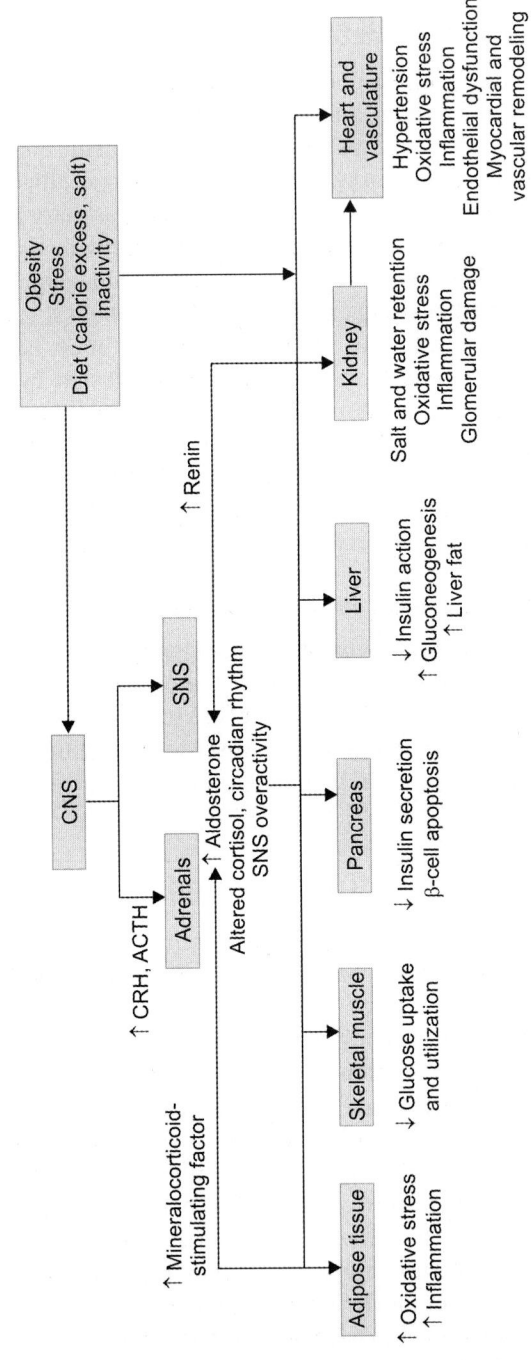

**FLOWCHART 2:** Role of aldosterone in the pathogenesis of type 2 diabetes mellitus and its complications.

(ACTH: adrenocorticotropic hormone; CRH: corticotropin-releasing hormone; CNS: central nervous system; SNS: sympathetic nervous system)

- *Dehydroepiandrosterone sulfate replacement*: While DHEA replacement has been considered in female infertility, menopause, osteoporosis, and depression, some animal studies suggested that DHEA replacement may be useful in diabetes and cardiovascular disease. DHEA may have positive effects on insulin resistance and secretion. Some studies report improvements in muscle strength, body composition, and physical performance. However, no benefit of DHEA on glycemic control, lipids, weight or BMI was found in postmenopausal women.[35]

## CONCLUSION

Glucocorticoids are important regulators of glucose and energy metabolism and act as counterregulatory hormones. GC excess or Cushing's syndrome, whether exogenous or endogenous, can lead to significant hyperglycemia due to reduced peripheral glucose uptake, increased hepatic glucose output and reduced insulin secretion. FPG may not be sufficient for detection of hyperglycemia as BG elevations are more marked in the postprandial period. Monitoring of BG, especially in postlunch period and OGTT, is recommended. While insulin sensitizers remain the first-line agents, many patients require insulin for the management of GC-induced hyperglycemia. Down-titration of antihyperglycemic therapy is required when tapering GC dose or after resolution of endogenous hypercortisolism. Primary HA and CAH are also associated with increased risk of hyperglycemia. On the other hand, patients with adrenal insufficiency may have an increased risk of hypoglycemia. An understanding of the glucocrinology of adrenal cortex will improve glucovigilance in adrenal cortical disorders and adrenovigilance in the diabetes care.

## REFERENCES

1. Kuo T, McQueen A, Chen TC, et al. Regulation of Glucose Homeostasis by Glucocorticoids. Adv Exp Med Biol. 2015;872:99-126.
2. Suh S, Park MK. Glucocorticoid-induced diabetes mellitus: an important but overlooked problem. Endocrinol Metab. 2017;32:180-9.
3. Fichna M, Fichna P. Glucocorticoids and beta-cell function. Endokrynol Pol. 2017;68(5):568-73.
4. Rafacho A, Ortsäter H, Nadal A, et al. Glucocorticoid treatment and endocrine pancreas function: implications for glucose homeostasis, insulin resistance and diabetes. J Endocrinol. 2014;223(3):R49-62.
5. Grossmann C, Gekle M. New aspects of rapid aldosterone signaling. Mol Cell Endocrinol. 2009;308(1-2):53-62.
6. Hayden MR, Sowers JR. Pancreatic renin-angiotensin-aldosterone system in the cardiometabolic syndrome and type 2 diabetes mellitus. J Cardiometab Syndr. 2008;3(3):129-31.
7. Baulieu E, Thomas G, Legrain S, et al. Dehydroepiandrosterone (DHEA), DHEA sulfate, and aging: contribution of the DHEAge study to a sociobiomedical issue. Proc Natl Acad Natl Sci U S A. 2000;97(8):4279-84.
8. Pasieka AM, Rafacho A. Impact of Glucocorticoid Excess on Glucose Tolerance: Clinical and Preclinical Evidence. Metabolites. 2016;6(3):E24.
9. Scaroni C, Zilio M, Foti M, et al. Glucose Metabolism Abnormalities in Cushing Syndrome: From Molecular Basis to Clinical Management. Endocr Rev. 2017;38(3):189-219.
10. Zografos GN, Perysinakis I, Vassilatou E. Subclinical Cushing's syndrome: current concepts and trends. Hormones (Athens). 2014;13(3):323-37.
11. Colao A, De Block C, Gaztambide MS, et al. Managing hyperglycemia in patients with Cushing's disease treated with pasireotide: medical expert recommendations. Pituitary. 2014;17(2):180-6.

12. Gonzalez-Gonzalez JG, Mireles-Zavala LG, Rodriguez-Gutierrez R, et al. Hyperglycemia related to high-dose GC use in noncritically ill patients. Diabetol Metab Syndr. 2013;5:18.
13. Clore JN, Thurby-Hay L. Glucocorticoid-induced hyperglycemia. Endocr Pract. 2009;15(5):469-74.
14. Gurwitz JH, Bohn RL, Glynn RJ, et al. Glucocorticoids and the risk for initiation of hypoglycemic therapy. Arch Intern Med. 1994;154(1):97-101.
15. Tamez-Pérez HE, Quintanilla-Flores DL, Rodríguez-Gutiérrez R, et al. Steroid hyperglycemia: Prevalence, early detection and therapeutic recommendations: A narrative review. World J Diabetes. 2015;6(8):1073-81.
16. Mazziotti G, Formenti AM, Frara S, et al. Diabetes in Cushing Disease. Curr Diab Rep. 2017;17(5):32.
17. Mazziotti G, Formenti AM, Frara S, et al. Management of endocrine disease: Risk of overtreatment in patients with adrenal insufficiency: current and emerging aspects. Eur J Endocrinol. 2017; 177(5):R231-48.
18. Bornstein SR, Allolio B, Arlt W, et al. Diagnosis and Treatment of Primary Adrenal Insufficiency: An Endocrine Society Clinical Practice Guideline. J Clin Endocrinol Metab. 2016;101(2):364-89.
19. Hanslik G, Wallaschofski H, Dietz A, et al. Increased prevalence of diabetes mellitus and the metabolic syndrome in patients with primary aldosteronism of the German Conn's Registry. Eur J Endocrinol. 2015;173(5):665-75.
20. Fallo F, Veglio F, Bertello C, et al. Prevalence and characteristics of the metabolic syndrome in primary aldosteronism. J Clin Endocrinol Metab. 2006;91(2):454-9.
21. Reincke M, Meisinger C, Holle R, et al. Is primary aldosteronism associated with diabetes mellitus? Results of the German Conn's Registry. Horm Metab Res. 2010;42(6):435-9.
22. Sindelka G, Widimský J, Haas T, et al. Insulin action in primary hyperaldosteronism before and after surgical or pharmacological treatment. Exp Clin Endocrinol Diabetes. 2000;108(1):21-5.
23. Mooij CF, Korese JM, Claahsen-van der Grinten HL, et al. Unfavourable trends in cardiovascular and metabolic risk in paediatric and adult patients with congenital adrenal hyperplasia? Clin Endocrinol (Oxf). 2010;73(2):137-46.
24. Krysiak R, Okopien B. The effect of metformin on androgen production in diabetic women with non-classic congenital adrenal hyperplasia. Exp Clin Endocrinol Diabetes. 2014;122(10):568-71.
25. Alrefai H, Allababidi H, Levy S, et al. The endocrine system in diabetes mellitus. Endocrine. 2002;18(2):105-19.
26. Aoki K, Terauchi Y. Effect of Dehydroepiandrosterone (DHEA) on Diabetes Mellitus and Obesity. Vitam Horm. 2018;108:355-65.
27. Ciccarelli E, Limone P, Crivellaro C, et al. Screening of Cushing's syndrome in outpatients with type 2 diabetes: results of a prospective multicentric study in Italy. J Clin Endocrinol Metab. 2012;97(10):3467-75.
28. Williams JS, Williams GH. 50th anniversary of aldosterone. J Clin Endocrinol Metab. 2003;88(6):2364-72.
29. Mukherjee JJ, Khoo CM, Thai AC, et al. Type 2 diabetic patients with resistant hypertension should be screened for primary aldosteronism. Diab Vasc Dis Res. 2010;7(1):6-13.
30. Epstein M. Aldosterone blockade: an emerging strategy for abrogating progressive renal disease. Am J Med. 2006;119(11):912-9.
31. Korol S, Mottet F, Perreault S, et al. A systematic review and meta-analysis of the impact of mineralocorticoid receptor antagonists on glucose homeostasis. Medicine (Baltimore). 2017;96(48):e8719.
32. Preiss D, van Veldhuisen DJ, Sattar N, et al. Eplerenone and new-onset diabetes in patients with mild heart failure: results from the Eplerenone in Mild Patients Hospitalization and Survival Study in Heart Failure (EMPHASIS-HF). Eur J Heart Fail. 2012;14(8):909-15.
33. Dube S, Norby BJ, Pattan V, et al. 11β-hydroxysteroid dehydrogenase types 1 and 2 activity in subcutaneous adipose tissue in humans: implications in obesity and diabetes. J Clin Endocrinol Metab. 2015;100(1):E70-6.
34. Tan H, Wang W, Yin X, et al. Identification of a selective glucocorticoid receptor ligand for the treatment of chronic inflammation in type 2 diabetes mellitus. Exp Ther Med. 2014;8(4):1111-4.
35. Elraiyah T, Sonbol MB, Wang Z, et al. The benefits and harms of systemic dehydroepiandrosterone (DHEA) in postmenopausal women with normal adrenal function: a systematic review and meta-analysis. Clin Endocrinol Metab. 2014;99(10):3536-42.

# Glucocrinology of Adrenal Medulla

*Ganesh HK, Kirtida Sandeep Acharya*

## INTRODUCTION

Adrenal medulla constitutes the inner most part of the adrenal glands and secretes catecholamines, namely adrenaline and noradrenaline. The adrenal medullary cells are, in fact, modified postganglionic neurons of the sympathetic autonomic nervous system (SNS) and are under regulation of the central nervous system. Adrenal medulla is capable of producing adrenaline, as it has the necessary enzyme phenylethanolamine N-methyltransferase (PNMT), which converts noradrenaline to adrenaline. Hence, adrenal medulla secretes both adrenaline and noradrenaline whereas rest of the sympathetic nerve endings can secrete only noradrenaline.

Catecholamines produced by adrenal medulla and sympathetic nervous system are popularly known as "fight and flight hormones". The effects of catecholamines are mediated via adrenergic receptors. There are mainly two types of adrenergic receptors $\alpha$ and $\beta$, which are again subdivided into $\alpha 1$, $\alpha 2$, $\beta 1$, $\beta 2$ and $\beta 3$.

Catecholamines are one of the key mediators of the fight-or-flight response to acute stress, characterized by a rise in heart rate and blood pressure, dilatation of bronchial smooth muscles and capillaries, peripheral vasoconstriction and increased fuel availability. While adrenaline and noradrenaline are recognized for their significant effects on cardiovascular system, it is increasingly understood that they have important metabolic effects as well. They help mobilize the body's energy stores to increase the availability of glucose and free fatty acids (FFAs) during periods of stress, including hypoglycemia.

In this chapter, we discuss the effect of adrenal medulla on glucose and energy homeostasis in both health and disease.

## GLUCOSE PHYSIOLOGY IN RELATION TO ADRENAL MEDULLA

Adrenaline or noradrenaline are receptor ligands to either $\alpha_1$, $\alpha_2$ or $\beta$-adrenoreceptors. Table 1 enlists the primary effects mediated via adrenergic receptors. The $\alpha_1$ adrenoreceptor couples to $G_q$, which results in increased intracellular $Ca^{2+}$ and subsequent smooth muscle contraction. The $\alpha_2$ adrenoreceptor, on the other hand, couples to $G_i$, which causes a decrease in neurotransmitter release, as well as a decrease of cyclic adenosine monophosphate (cAMP) activity resulting in smooth muscle contraction. The β-receptors couple to $G_s$, and increase intracellular cAMP activity, resulting in heart muscle contraction, smooth muscle relaxation and glycogenolysis.

Catecholamines increase heart rate (chronotropic), cardiac muscle excitability (bathmotropic), contractility (inotropic) and conduction velocity (dromotropic). Despite its profound effects on cardiovascular function, the contribution of adrenaline to normal cardiovascular regulation or to the development of essential hypertension is probably minimal. While they cause vasoconstriction in liver, kidney, intestine and skin through an effect on α-adrenergic receptors, catecholamines cause vasodilation in skeletal muscle through β-adrenergic receptors. Basal metabolic rate is increased with increase in thermogenesis.

Catecholamines regulate glucose and energy homeostasis in several ways (Table 2). The primary metabolic action of catecholamines is to mobilize and increase the availability of fuel during acute stress response. Therefore, they increase

**TABLE 1** Adrenergic receptors, mechanisms and effects.

| Ligand | Adrenoceptor | Mechanism (pathway involved) | Effects |
|---|---|---|---|
| Epinephrine, norepinephrine | $\alpha_1$ | Phospholipase C | Smooth muscle contraction |
| | $\alpha_2$ | Adenylyl cyclase | Inhibition of transmitter release |
| | β | Adenylyl cyclase | Cardiac muscle contraction, smooth muscle contraction and glycogenolysis |

**TABLE 2** Adrenoceptors and their effects on energy homeostasis.

| Target | Effects | Adrenoceptors |
|---|---|---|
| Endocrine pancreas | Decreased insulin secretion (predominant effect) | α2 |
| | Increased insulin secretion | β |
| | Increased glucagon secretion | β, α2 |
| Skeletal muscle | Increased release of gluconeogenic precursors (in response to adrenaline) | β |
| Adipose tissue | Increased lipolysis (predominant effect) | α1, β |
| | Decreased lipolysis | α2 |
| Liver | Increased gluconeogenesis (an indirect effect resulting from the increased availability of lactate and alanine from skeletal muscle and nonesterified fatty acids and glycerol from adipose tissue) | α1, β |
| | Decreased glycogenesis, increased glycogenolysis | α1, β |

glycogenolysis and lipolysis, inhibit insulin-mediated glycogenesis, and increase gluconeogenesis. Catecholamines also increase the rate of aerobic glycolysis, resulting in greater adenosine triphosphate (ATP) production. Adrenaline further stimulates adipose tissue lipase to increase lipolysis, resulting in increased FFA secretion, which can either undergo β-oxidation or provide substrate for gluconeogenesis. It reduces lipogenesis at the same time.

Han and Bonen studied the effect of epinephrine on glucose transport in muscles in rodents. Both insulin and epinephrine individually increase the presence of glucose transporter type 4 (GLUT4) on the plasma membrane. However, when both epinephrine and insulin are present together, the glucose transportation effect of GLUT4 was decreased. The transportation capacity of insulin-stimulated GLUT4 is potentially reduced or altered in the presence of high concentrations of epinephrine.[1] Thus, catecholamines reduce insulin-mediated peripheral glucose uptake.

In the liver, when adrenergic receptors are stimulated, they both act to increase gluconeogenesis and glycogenolysis.[2] Epinephrine increases glucagon secretion and hepatic glucose output. Saccà et al. evaluated the effect of epinephrine on glucose uptake by the liver.[3] When radiolabeled glucose was infused to healthy males, hepatic glucose production was found to shut down completely and insulin levels increased four-fold, with increase in splanchnic glucose uptake. However, this was not seen when radiolabeled glucose was administered along with epinephrine. With epinephrine infusion, hepatic glucose production failed to decrease despite an increase in insulin levels. Further addition of propranolol led to normalization of glucose metabolism with reduced hepatic glucose output.[4] This indicates that epinephrine-mediated hyperglycemia can be more-or-less reversed by blocking β-adrenergic receptors probably through decreasing glucagon secretion, as well as decreasing hepatic glucose production.

The noradrenergic system provides fine tuning to the endocrine pancreas activity through the function of α- and β-adrenergic receptors.[5] Stimulation of α2-adrenergic receptors predominantly inhibits insulin secretion from the β-cells of the pancreas. Stimulating β2- and α2-adrenergic receptors on the pancreatic α-cells will result in an increase in glucagon secretion.[2] Studies have shown that β2-adrenergic receptors on the pancreatic β-cells have a role in regulating insulin secretion.[6]

To summarize, adrenaline and noradrenaline have a net hyperglycemic effect by several mechanisms:
- Stimulating glycogenolysis and gluconeogenesis in liver
- Inhibiting insulin-mediated glucose uptake in skeletal muscle and adipose tissue
- Increasing glucagon secretion from pancreas
- Inhibiting insulin secretion from pancreas.

## Epinephrine versus Norepinephrine

Epinephrine infusion had a more significant effect on blood glucose elevation than norepinephrine infusion.[7] Norepinephrine infusion in the setting of moderate exercise caused an increase in glucose production but with a proportionate increase in glucose uptake, thus not causing significant hyperglycemia.[8]

## Pathophysiological Considerations

Animal models suggest that α-adrenergic receptors play an important role in glucose homeostasis. Studies in mice that lack postsynaptic α2-adrenergic receptors demonstrate that these mice have hyperinsulinemia and lower glucose levels. Genetic studies have revealed that human subjects with a certain α2-adrenergic receptor gene polymorphism (*ADRA2A* gene) have higher susceptibility to develop type 2 diabetes mellitus (T2DM).[9]

Increased α2-adrenoceptor signaling may result in β-cell dysfunction and increased risk of T2DM. Studies carried out with transgenic mice have nonetheless supported the notion that pancreatic β-cell α2-adrenoceptors tonically inhibit insulin secretion and have suggested that α2-adrenoceptor antagonists stimulate insulin secretion.[2]

More recent evidence shows that mice with simultaneous deletion of the three known genes encoding the β-adrenergic receptors (β1, β2 and β3) present a phenotype characterized by impaired glucose tolerance.[10] Studies with β2-adrenergic receptor agonists further suggest that the β2-adrenergic receptors may play an important role in regulating insulin secretion.[6] The β2-adrenergic receptors physiologically regulate pancreatic β-cell insulin secretion by modulating peroxisome proliferator-activated receptor gamma (PPAR-γ)/PDX-1/GLUT2 function.

## GLUCOVIGILANCE IN DISORDERS OF ADRENAL MEDULLA

Pheochromocytomas are rare catecholamine-secreting tumors often originating from the adrenal medulla (90%) but may arise from extra-adrenal chromaffin cells.

### Pheochromocytomas

High catecholamine secretion can result in reduced insulin secretion, increased glucagon secretion, increased glycogenolysis and gluconeogenesis. In addition, increased adipose tissue lipolysis and muscle glycolysis further increases the availability for gluconeogenic precursors. Peripheral glucose utilization is also reduced. The resultant insulin resistance and impaired insulin secretion are associated with an increased risk of glucose intolerance in patients with pheochromocytoma.

First phase of insulin secretion was selectively attenuated in patients with pheochromocytoma or paraganglioma (during a hyperglycemic clamp).[11] Overexpression of the α2-adrenergic receptor in mice or the presence of a variant of the receptor gene in humans has also been shown to result in suppression of the acute insulin secretory response.[12] The mechanism by which the adrenergic stimulus selectively attenuates the early phase of insulin secretion is not fully understood. The Epac2A-Rap1 pathway, which is activated by cAMP-dependent signaling, has been shown to play an important role in the acute insulin secretory response.[13] It is possible that an alternation in this signaling pathway contributes to the pathological effects of the adrenergic stimulus on insulin secretion in pancreatic β-cells.

## Clinical Presentation

Glucose intolerance has been reported in approximately 25–75% of pheochromocytoma patients. In fact, in some cases, pheochromocytoma may present with new-onset diabetes or worsening of pre-existing diabetes. There are case reports of pheochromocytomas presenting with acute hyperglycemic emergencies, such as diabetic ketoacidosis or hyperglycemic hyperosmolar state.

Most adrenal pheochromocytomas and especially large extra-adrenal tumors predominantly secrete norepinephrine. However, the adrenaline-dominant type tumors have a greater propensity to cause hyperglycemia due to higher affinity of adrenaline for β-receptor. Reduction in urinary metanephrine levels led to improvement in homeostatic model assessment (HOMA)-β and no effect on HOMA-insulin resistance, suggesting that adrenaline affects glucose intolerance mainly by impaired secretion of insulin.

## Management of Hyperglycemia

Many patients may have only impaired glucose tolerance or mild hyperglycemia and can be managed with medical nutrition therapy and oral antidiabetic medications. For patients requiring insulin, subcutaneous regular or rapid-acting insulin along with basal insulin would remain an optimal choice until definitive treatment of pheochromocytoma. In rare patients presenting with an acute hyperglycemic emergency, aggressive hydration along with insulin infusion should be instituted.

While α-blockers and β-blockers are important to manage the cardiovascular symptoms and preoperative preparation of the patient, there is no evidence that they improve glycemic control. Insulin remains the drug of choice for perioperative glycemic control with close monitoring of capillary blood glucose levels. One-hourly blood glucose monitoring with intravenous insulin infusion should be considered till the patient is hemodynamically stable. Later, patients may be switched to basal-bolus regimen, depending on insulin requirements.

Surgical treatment of pheochromocytoma has been shown to improve insulin sensitivity as evaluated by hyperinsulinemic-euglycemic clamp analysis.[14] With resection of pheochromocytomas and sudden decrease in α-adrenergic activity, hypoglycemia is a distinct possibility requiring careful titration of insulin doses.

In majority of the cases, hyperglycemia due to adrenal medullary tumors resolves completely after surgical resection of the tumor, unlike hypertension which may remain persistent. According to a study by Beninato T et al., removal of pheochromocytoma improved diabetes in over 90% of patients, with resolution in 79%.[15] Patients with other risk factors for developing T2DM, such as elevated body mass index (BMI), are more likely to continue to require medication for diabetes postoperatively.

## Paragangliomas

Most paragangliomas are nonfunctioning; however, a small percentage of them can secrete catecholamines. The main catecholamine that is produced by these tumors is norepinephrine because they lack PNMT, an enzyme that converts norepinephrine to epinephrine in the adrenal tissue. While epinephrine has greater hyperglycemic effect, norepinephrine has more effect on α-adrenergic receptors. However, there is insufficient data support any difference in glucose homeostasis between adrenal pheochromocytomas and paragangliomas.

### Glucovigilance with the Pharmacological Use of Catecholamines

Epinephrine is an emergency drug used in acute cardiac arrest, ventricular fibrillation, anaphylactic shock and angioedema, while norepinephrine infusion is often used for its inotropic properties in hypotensive states. These drugs may contribute to stress hyperglycemia or worsening of hyperglycemia in pre-existing diabetes. Epinephrine infusion had a more significant effect on blood glucose elevation than norepinephrine infusion.[7]

## ADRENOVIGILANCE IN DIABETES

### Vigilance for Adrenal Disorders in Diabetes

Pheochromocytomas may cause worsening of glycemic control in individuals with diabetes or new-onset hyperglycemia. Presence of classical symptoms suggesting catecholamine excess (sustained or paroxysmal hypertension, palpitations, headache, chest pain, anxiety, excess sweating, etc.) in an individual with newly diagnosed diabetes or pre-existing diabetes with sudden worsening of glycemic control should prompt evaluation for catecholamines. A high index of suspicion may be required in individuals with acute hyperglycemic emergencies, since osmotic and catabolic symptoms may mask the symptoms of catecholamine excess. Incidental detection of adrenal neoplasms in a diabetic individual should also prompt evaluation to exclude pheochromocytomas.

A 24-hour urinary free catecholamines and fractionated metanephrines and/or plasma metanephrines should be estimated to establish a biochemical diagnosis. Localization of the tumor can be done with contrast-enhanced CT scan or MRI and $I^{123}$ metaiodobenzylguanidine (MIBG) scan.

### Impaired Counter-regulation to Hypoglycemia

Catecholamine secretion is one of the major defense mechanisms against hypoglycemia. In fact, majority of the hypoglycemic symptoms (palpitations, sweating, tremors and anxiety) are adrenergic in nature. Adrenergic symptoms are the first to appear, easily recognized, and the individual is prompted to eat as soon as he/she starts developing these symptoms.

In fact, in a normal person, the adrenal medulla and sympathetic nervous system play a major role in mounting a response against hypoglycemia. Glucagon, catecholamines, cortisol, and growth hormone are classically recognized as the counterregulatory hormones that are activated in response to hypoglycemia.

Depriving the brain of glucose (neuroglucoprivation) activates the glucose counter-regulatory response to restore normoglycemia. In humans, the glucose counter-regulatory response consists of release into the circulation of the rapid-acting hormones: glucagon from the pancreatic α-cells and adrenaline from the adrenal medulla.[16] Growth hormone and cortisol are slow-acting counter-regulatory hormones (few hours). Glucagon acts exclusively by stimulating glucose production in the liver, whereas, adrenaline acts by suppressing endogenous insulin secretion, stimulation of hepatic glucose production, stimulation of lipolysis (β3-adrenoceptor-mediated activation of lipase in adipose tissue) and reduction of glucose utilization. In addition, α2-adrenoceptors seem to be critically important for the counterregulatory response to sulfonylurea-induced hypoglycemia in mice. The barosensitive receptors in rostral ventromedial medulla (RVM) that are activated by glucoprivation are most probably C1 neurons.

In diabetic individuals, a reduction in insulin secretion by the β-cell and increased glucagon secretion by α-cell are the first two defense mechanisms to hypoglycemia. However, in type 1 diabetes mellitus and advanced T2DM, adrenaline is the predominant counter-regulatory hormone as the first two defense mechanisms are lost.[17] Repeated bouts of hypoglycemia can also lead to reduced catecholamine secretion and "hypoglycemia unawareness". This is seen more often in patients with long-standing diabetes with autonomic neuropathy, where adrenaline secretion is reduced. With such hypoglycemia unawareness, classic warning symptoms of hypoglycemia fail to develop, and the patient is at risk of progressing to neuroglycopenia and coma.

Whenever a diabetic patient starts developing hypoglycemia without any plausible etiology, adrenal insufficiency should be ruled out. Both primary and secondary adrenal insufficiency can cause hypoglycemia. Basal and, if required, stimulated cortisol should be a part of the work-up in all patients with unexplained hypoglycemia.

## CONCLUSION

Catecholamines secreted by the adrenal medulla and sympathetic nervous system play an important role in the glucose/energy homeostasis in humans. They form an important defense mechanism against hypoglycemia. On the other hand, excessive production of these hormones from tumors like pheochromocytoma can cause hyperglycemia/diabetes. Resection of pheochromocytoma leads to normoglycemia in majority.

## REFERENCES

1. Han XX, Bonen A. Epinephrine translocates GLUT-4 but inhibits insulin-stimulated glucose transport in rat muscle. Am J Physiol. 1998;274:E700-7.
2. Fagerholm V, Haaparanta M, Scheinin M. α2-adrenoceptor regulation of blood glucose homeostasis. Basic Clin Pharmacol Toxicol. 2011;108:365-70.
3. Saccá L, Morrone G, Cicala M, et al. Influence of epinephrine, norepinephrine, and isoproterenol on glucose homeostasis in normal man. J Clin Endocrinol Metab. 1980;50:680-4.
4. Deibert DC, Defronzo RA. Epinephrine-induced insulin resistance in man. J Clin Invest. 1980;65:717-21.
5. Abe I, Fujii H, Ohishi H, et al. Differences in the actions of adrenaline and noradrenaline with regard to glucose intolerance in patients with pheochromocytoma. Endocr J. 2019;66:187-192.
6. Santulli G, Lombardi A, Sorriento D, et al. Age-Related Impairment in Insulin Release, The Essential Role of β2-Adrenergic Receptor. Diabetes. 2012;61:692-701.

7. DiSalvo RJ, Bloom WL, Brust A, et al. A comparison of the metabolic and circulatory effects of epinephrine, norepinephrine and insulin hypoglycemia with observations on the influence of autonomic blocking agents. J Clin Invest. 1956;35:568-77.
8. Kreisman SH, Ah Mew N, Halter JB, et al. Norepinephrine infusion during moderate-intensity exercise increases glucose production and uptake. J Clin Endocrinol Metab. 2001;86:2118-24.
9. Chen X, Liu L, He W, et al. Association of the ADRA2A polymorphisms with the risk of type 2 diabetes: a meta-analysis. Clin Biochem. 2013;46:722-6.
10. Sieg A, Su J, Muñoz A, et al. Epinephrine-induced hyperpolarization of islet cells without KATP channels. Am J Physiol Endocrinol Metab. 2004;286:E463-71.
11. Komada H, Hirota Y, So A, et al. Insulin secretion and insulin sensitivity before and after surgical treatment of pheochromocytoma or paraganglioma. J Clin Endocrinol Metab. 2017;102:3400-5.
12. Rosengren AH, Jokubka R, Tojjar D, et al. Overexpression of alpha2A-adrenergic receptors contributes to type 2 diabetes. Science. 2010;327:217-20.
13. Zhang CL, Katoh M, Shibasaki T, et al. The cAMP sensor Epac2 is a direct target of antidiabetic sulfonylurea drugs. Science. 2009;325:607-10.
14. Wiesner TD, Bluher M, Windgassen M, et al. Improvement of insulin sensitivity after adrenalectomy in patients with pheochromocytoma. J Clin Endocrinol Metab. 2003;88:3632-6.
15. Beninato T, Kluijfhout W, Drake F, et al. Resection of Pheochromocytoma Improves Diabetes Mellitus in the Majority of Patients. Ann Surg Oncol. 2017;24:1208-13.
16. Bolli GB, Fanelli CG. Physiology of glucose counterregulation to hypoglycemia. Endocrinol Metab Clin North Am. 1999;28:467-93.
17. Verberne AJ, Korim WS, Sabetghadam A. Adrenaline: insights into its metabolic roles in hypoglycaemia and diabetes. Br J Pharmacol. 2016;173:1425-37.

# CHAPTER 7

# Glucocrinology of Pancreas

Sakthivel Sivasubramanian, Partha Pratim Chakraborthy, Senthil Senniappan

## INTRODUCTION

Pancreas is a complex exocrine/endocrine organ that plays a key role in the regulation of macronutrient digestion and glucose, protein and lipid metabolism and energy homeostasis through secretion of various digestive enzymes into the gastrointestinal tract and pancreatic hormones (insulin and glucagon) into the circulation. The key pancreatic hormones, insulin and glucagon, maintain blood glucose concentrations within a very narrow range.

Diabetes is classically understood to be a disease of the endocrine pancreas; resulting from impaired insulin secretion and/or impaired insulin action in the liver and peripheral tissues, that formed the initial triumvirate of diabetes pathogenesis. Disorders of pancreas, whether they involve the endocrine or exocrine component, are in fact, associated with significant alterations in glucose homeostasis. Secretory defects in insulin include both undersecretion and oversecretion; impaired insulin secretion manifests as hyperglycemia and unregulated excess secretion results in hypoglycemia.

While pancreatic diseases manifest as dysglycemia on the one hand, diabetes itself is associated with changes in both endocrine as well as exocrine pancreas. Hyperglycemia and resultant glucotoxicity as well as lipotoxicity have been implicated in the progressive decline of β-cell function in type 2 diabetes mellitus (T2DM). In addition, diabetes is associated with increased risk of pancreatitis and pancreatic cancer.

## GLUCOCRINOLOGY OF PANCREAS: HISTORICAL PERSPECTIVES

The connection between pancreas and diabetes was suggested in 1788 when Cawley reported a shriveled pancreas in an autopsy of a person with diabetes. However, Lancereaux related pancreas to diabetes with certainty much later in 1877.[1] Mering and Minkowski demonstrated that extirpation of pancreas in a dog caused diabetes.[1]

The endocrine component of pancreas was discovered by Paul Langerhans in 1869, but its role in the pathogenesis of diabetes was not identified until Eugene Opie demonstrated hyaline changes in the islets in patients with diabetes.[1] In 1910, Sharpey-Schafer postulated that diabetes resulted from deficiency of a secretory substance from pancreas, that he named "insulin".[1] While the discovery of insulin is credited to the team of Frederick Banting, Charles Best, John Macleod and Bertram Collip in 1921, Nicolae Paulescu had also developed an extract of pancreas in 1916 that was found to lower blood glucose in dogs.[1] Glucagon was later identified from pancreatic extracts by Kimball and Murlin in 1923.[1]

Initial experiments suggested that ligation of pancreatic duct with destruction of exocrine pancreas did not result in diabetes. But by latter half of 18th century, glycosuria was documented in patients with acute pancreatitis by several authors.[1] Before that, Cawley had described pancreatic calcification in an obese man with diabetes in 1788 but he thought the kidney was the cause of diabetes. Later, association between pancreatic cancer and diabetes was also reported.[1]

This chapter focuses on the role of pancreas (endocrine and exocrine) in glucose homeostasis in health and disease, and discusses the need for glucovigilance in pancreatic disorders and pancreatic vigilance in diabetes.

## GLUCOSE PHYSIOLOGY IN RELATION TO PANCREAS

The bulk of the gland is composed of acinar or exocrine cells that secrete pancreatic juices containing digestive enzymes, such as amylase, pancreatic lipase and trypsinogen, into the pancreatic ducts. The endocrine component includes clusters of endocrine cells that form islets of Langerhans within the exocrine pancreatic tissue and constitute only 1–2% of the organ. The islets are composed of five different cell types releasing various hormones that have endocrine, paracrine and autocrine effects and regulate energy homeostasis. These are enlisted in Table 1.

Pancreatic hormones, particularly glucagon and insulin, maintain blood glucose levels within a very narrow range of 72–108 mg/dL (4–6 mmol/L).[2] Glucose homeostasis is achieved by the opposing and balanced actions of glucagon and insulin. Blood glucose levels are low during sleep or in between meals. Glucagon is a catabolic

**TABLE 1** Cell types of islets of Langerhans and their predominant secretion.

| Cell type | Percentage population of the total islet cells | Hormone secretion | Physiological role |
|---|---|---|---|
| α-cells | 15–20% | Glucagon | Increases glucose concentration |
| β-cells | 65–80% | Insulin, C-peptide and amylin | Reduces glucose concentration |
| γ-cells | 3–5% | Pancreatic polypeptide | Regulate the exocrine and endocrine secretion of pancreas |
| δ-cells | 3–10% | Somatostatin | Inhibits glucagon and insulin secretion |
| ε-cells | 1% | Ghrelin | Increases appetite |

hormone that is released from α-cells to promote hepatic glycogenolysis. Additional glucagon drives hepatic and renal gluconeogenesis to increase endogenous blood glucose levels during prolonged fasting.

Insulin, an anabolic hormone, is secreted from β-cells in response to elevated exogenous glucose levels, such as those occurring after a meal. After combining with its suitable receptor on muscle and adipose tissue, insulin enables the insulin-dependent uptake of glucose into these tissues and hence lowers blood glucose levels by removing the exogenous glucose from the bloodstream.[2] Furthermore, insulin promotes glycogenesis, lipogenesis and the incorporation of amino acids into proteins.

## Glucose Sensing by Pancreas

Pancreatic β-cells closely regulate insulin secretion in response to circulating blood glucose concentrations. Glucose sensing and glucose-responsive insulin secretion is mediated via uptake of glucose into pancreatic β-cells.[2] The main stimulus for insulin release in β-cells is elevated blood glucose levels. The circulating blood glucose is taken up by the facilitative glucose transporter-2 (GLUT-2), which is located on the surface of the β-cells. Upon entry inside the cell, glucose undergoes glycolysis, thereby generating adenosine triphosphate (ATP), resulting in an increased ATP/ADP ratio. This increased ratio then leads to the closure of ATP-sensitive potassium (KATP) channels.[2]

## Kinetics of Insulin Secretion

In nonstimulated conditions, the KATP channels are open to ensure the maintenance of a resting potential by transporting positively charged $K^+$ ions down their concentration gradient out of the cell. Upon closure, the subsequent decrease in the magnitude of the outwardly directed $K^+$ current elicits the depolarization of the membrane, followed by the opening of voltage-dependent $Ca^{2+}$ channels (VDCCs).[3] Insulin is stored in large dense-core vesicles that are recruited to the proximity of the plasma membrane following stimulation such that insulin is readily available. The increase in intracellular calcium concentrations eventually triggers the fusion of insulin-containing granules with the membrane and the subsequent release of their content, as depicted in Figure 1.

In this biphasic secretory process, the first phase peaks around 5 minutes after the glucose stimulus with the majority of insulin being released during this first phase. The second phase, somewhat slower, is when the remaining insulin is secreted.[3] Figure 2 depicts the biphasic secretion of insulin. The insulin secretion occurs in an oscillatory pattern with "fast oscillations" ranging from 5–15 minutes and slow "ultradian oscillations" that occur over 80–180 minutes.[3]

## Role of Insulin and Glucagon in Glucose Homeostasis

Plasma glucose concentration is a function of the rate of glucose entering the circulation (glucose appearance) balanced by the rate of glucose removal from the circulation (glucose disappearance). In the bihormonal model of glucose homeostasis,

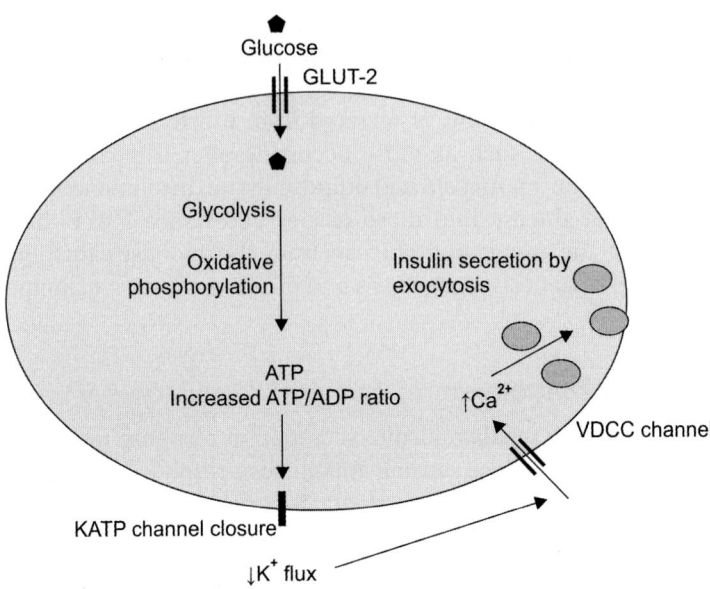

**FIG. 1:** Mechanism of insulin secretion from the pancreatic β-cells. Glucose is taken by pancreatic β-cells through glucose transporter-2 (GLUT2); following glycolysis, there is increased ATP production and increase in ATP/ADP ratio. This results in closure of the ATP-sensitive potassium (KATP) channels and subsequent membrane depolarization. Subsequently, there is activation of voltage-dependent calcium channels (VDCC), resulting in calcium influx that triggers secretion of insulin from stored granules by exocytosis.

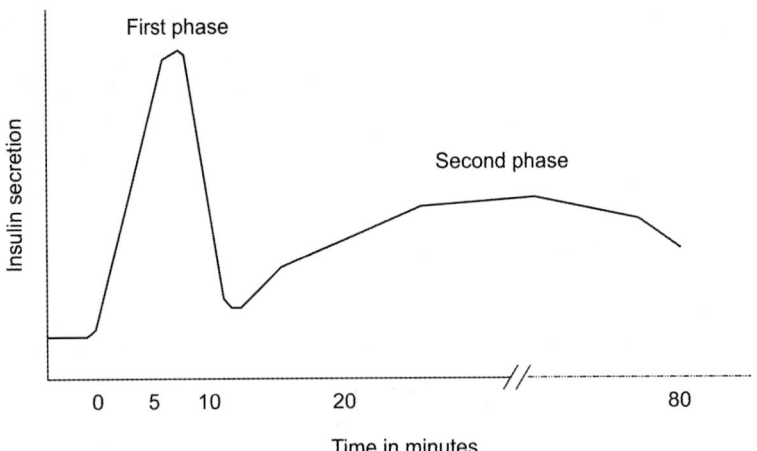

**FIG. 2:** Biphasic insulin secretion. In response to a rise in blood glucose concentration, there is an initial rapid release of insulin prestored in the secretory granules by exocytosis. This results in an immediate peak of insulin secretion, followed by later rise in insulin secretion that results from increased insulin synthesis within the pancreatic β-cells.

insulin is the key regulatory hormone of glucose disappearance, and glucagon is a major regulator of glucose appearance. Glucoregulatory hormones include insulin, glucagon, amylin, glucagon-like polypeptide-1 (GLP-1), glucose-dependent insulinotropic peptide (GIP), epinephrine, cortisol and growth hormone.[2] Of these, insulin and amylin are derived from the β-cells, glucagon from the α-cells of the pancreas and GLP-1 and GIP from the L-cells and K-cells of the intestine. The glucoregulatory hormones of the body work in close harmony to maintain circulating glucose concentrations in a relatively narrow range.

Circulating glucose is derived from three sources:
1. Intestinal absorption during the fed state,
2. Glycogenolysis or the breakdown of glycogen which is the polymerized storage form of glucose during the fasting state, and
3. Gluconeogenesis or the formation of glucose primarily from lactate and amino acids during the fasting state.

Glycogenolysis and gluconeogenesis are partly under the control of glucagon, a hormone produced in the α-cells of the pancreas.[2] During the first 8-12 hours of fasting, glycogenolysis is the primary mechanism by which glucose is made available. Glucagon facilitates this process and thus promotes glucose appearance in the circulation. Over longer periods of fasting, glucose, produced by gluconeogenesis, is released from the liver.

In the fasting state, glucose leaves the circulation at a constant rate. To keep pace with glucose disappearance, endogenous glucose production is necessary. For all practical purposes, the sole source of endogenous glucose production is the liver. Renal gluconeogenesis contributes substantially to the systemic glucose pool only during periods of extreme starvation. Although most tissues have the ability to hydrolyze glycogen, only the liver and kidneys contain glucose-6-phosphatase, the enzyme necessary for the release of glucose into the circulation.[2]

Following ingestion of a meal, glucose levels rise to reach a post-meal peak; and then decrease during the next several hours, eventually returning to fasting levels. In the immediate post-feeding state, glucose removal into skeletal muscle and adipose tissue is driven mainly by insulin. At the same time, endogenous glucose production is suppressed by:
- The direct action of insulin, delivered via the portal vein, in the liver; and
- The paracrine effect or direct communication within the pancreas between the α- and β-cells, which results in glucagon suppression.

In the endocrine pancreas, α- and β-cells, in the islets of Langerhans, regulate each other reciprocally by paracrine effects and thereby systemic glucose levels are maintained within narrow range. Pancreatic α-cells also serve as guardians or protectors of β-cells to preserve the capacity for the islets to produce insulin. In normal physiological conditions, these cells produce glucagon but in conditions of β-cell injury, they also produce GLP-1, a growth and survival factor for β-cells.[4] In euglycemic individuals, insulin levels go up postprandially which in turn suppresses glucagon secretion. Patients with T2DM, however, have a subnormal insulin response and a paradoxical rise in glucagon.

## Pancreatic Defects in Pathogenesis of Type 1 Diabetes Mellitus

Type 1 diabetes mellitus (T1DM) results from the destruction of insulin-producing pancreatic β-cells by a β-cell-specific autoimmune process.[5] Several factors mediate this autoimmune destruction of islet cells. β-cell autoantigens are thought to be released from β-cells by cellular turnover or damage and are processed and presented to T-helper cells by antigen-presenting cells. Macrophages and dendritic cells are the first cell types to infiltrate the pancreatic islets. Naive CD4+ T-cells that circulate in the blood and lymphoid organs, including the pancreatic lymph nodes, may recognize major histocompatibility complex (MHC) and β-cell peptides presented by dendritic cells and macrophages in the islets.[6] These CD4+ T cells can be activated by interleukin-2 (IL-2) released from macrophages and dendritic cells.

While this process takes place, β-cell antigen-specific CD8+ T-cells are activated by IL-2 produced by the activated TH1 CD4+ T-cells, differentiate into cytotoxic T-cells and are recruited into the pancreatic islets. These activated TH1 CD4+ T-cells and CD8+ cytotoxic T-cells are involved in the destruction of β-cells.[6]

In addition, β-cells can also be damaged by granzymes and perforin released from CD8+ cytotoxic T-cells and by soluble mediators such as cytokines and reactive oxygen molecules released from activated macrophages in the islets. Thus, activated macrophages, TH1 CD4+ T-cells and β-cell-cytotoxic CD8+ T-cells act synergistically to destroy β-cells, resulting in autoimmune T1DM.[6]

## Pancreatic Defects in Pathogenesis of Type 2 Diabetes Mellitus

The pathogenesis of T2DM is multifactorial and yet to be crystallized. Insulin insensitivity is an early phenomenon partly related to obesity and adipose tissue dysfunction. While there is initial compensatory rise in insulin secretion, over time pancreas β-cell function fails to compensate for insulin resistance and declines gradually over time before the onset of clinical hyperglycemia.[7] Several mechanisms have been proposed to explain the pathogenesis of insulin resistance in T2DM including increased nonesterified fatty acids, lipotoxicity, mitochondrial dysfunction, inflammatory cytokines, adipokines, mitochondrial dysfunction and glucotoxicity. Over time, several factors mediate β-cell dysfunction including glucotoxicity, lipotoxicity, endoplasmic reticulum stress, mitochondrial dysfunction, inflammation and amyloid formation.[7]

A reduction in β-cell mass and impaired β-cell function have both been demonstrated in T2DM. There is a loss of the pulsatile pattern of insulin secretion in early stages of the disease, even before the appearance of glucose intolerance.[8] Early loss of first phase of insulin secretion has been regarded as a key abnormality since long. In addition, individuals with T2DM have shorter and very irregular "fast oscillations." In addition, alterations in ultradian oscillations have also been reported with reduced amplitude and greater irregularity of ultradian pulses.[8] Pulsatile secretion is required to maintain the metabolic effects of insulin, especially the suppression of hepatic glucose production.

Over time, as the duration of diabetes increases, there occurs progressive decline in β-cell mass. At the time of diagnosis of overt diabetes, β-cell function decline of 50% has been reported based on homeostasis model assessment (HOMA) models.[9] The decline in β-cell function and mass progresses over time and has been attributed to several factors including glucotoxicity and lipotoxicity. This was believed to be due to β-cell apoptosis and death.

Recently β-cell dedifferentiation, rather than death, has been proposed as the underlying mechanism responsible for β-cell failure in T2DM.[10] Dedifferentiation involves gained expression of embryonic progenitor-cell markers such as Ngn3 that results in secretion of non-β cell hormones such as somatostatin and glucagon. β-cell expression of a key transcription factor Foxo1 is markedly decreased during stress.[10] These stressed β-cells also lose expression of β-cell specific genes such as those including insulin, GLUT-2, glucokinase, the proinsulin processing enzyme PCSK1 (proprotein convertase subtilisin/kexin type 1) and major transcription factors (such as MafA). Therefore, early insulin secretory defects in T2DM are partially reversible.[10]

To summarize, β-cell function in T2DM progresses through distinct stages of initial compensatory response to insulin resistance, followed by stable adaptation manifesting as prediabetes, early transient and then stable decompensation manifesting as overt diabetes, followed by severe decompensation when there is a near-absolute insulin deficiency.[9] These stages are enlisted in Table 2.

However, T2DM is characterized by not just β-cell dysfunction, but also α-cell dysfunction. A number of postulates have been put forward and hyperglucagonemia (both fasting and post-prandial), as a result of α-cell dysfunction, is a well-established abnormality in T2DM.[11] Loss of insulin mediated intra-islet paracrine inhibition of glucagon secondary to loss of pulsatile insulin secretion and desensitization of α-cells to the suppressive effect of glucose following prolonged hyperglycemia play a role in inappropriate hyperglucagonemia.[11,12] Interestingly, impaired glucagon secretory response of α-cells to low glucose levels is also a manifestation of α-cell dysfunction in T2DM.[13]

The histological appearance of islets in T2DM is characterized by relative/absolute deficiency of β-cells and relative preponderance of α-cells that equals or exceeds the loss of β-cell mass.[13] Compared to β-cells, α-cells are better equipped to adapt to and survive metabolic and inflammatory stress by expressing higher levels of survival factors like Bcl-xL (BCL2L1) and superoxide dismutase 2, a major scavenging enzyme, respectively.[11] This may partly explain the preserved α-cell mass in T2DM.

Moreover, the disease has a strong genetic component, but only a handful of genes have been identified so far—genes for calpain 10, potassium inward-rectifier 6.2, peroxisome proliferator-activated receptor γ and insulin receptor substrate-1.

## GLUCOVIGILANCE IN PANCREATIC DISORDERS

Acute and chronic pancreatitis are primarily considered as disorders of the exocrine pancreas. However, they may be associated with secondary pancreatic diabetes. Several names have been proposed for secondary diabetes due to exocrine pancreatic disorders including diabetes of the exocrine pancreas (DEP), pancreatogenic diabetes or type 3c diabetes mellitus (T3cDM).[14] It may result from a wide range of pancreatic disorders including acute, recurrent or chronic pancreatitis, pancreatic injury, postpancreatectomy, pancreatic carcinoma, fibrocalculous pancreatopathy, hemochromatosis and cystic fibrosis. The various causes are enlisted in Table 3.

**TABLE 2** Stages of beta-cell insufficiency.

| Stage | Description | β-cell mass | β-cell function | Glycemic status | Proposed taxonomy | Treatment strategy |
|---|---|---|---|---|---|---|
| 1 | Compensation | Insulin resistance and/or decreasing β-cell mass | Maintenance of differentiated function; normal GSIS | Normoglycemia | β-cell sufficiency | Lifestyle |
| 2 | Stable state of β-cell adaptation | Changes in β-cell phenotype (gene and protein expression) Loss of β-cell mass or β-cell hypertrophy (glucose-driven response stopping short of replication) | Diminished first phase GSIS Second phase GSIS partially preserved Acute insulin responses to non-glucose secretagogues (isoproterenol, arginine) largely intact | Prediabetes | Partial/reversible β-cell insufficiency | Lifestyle; insulin sensitizers |
|  | Transient unstable period of early decompensation | Critical decline of β-cell mass and/or increase in insulin resistance | Insulin mRNA/function falls rapidly | Glucose levels rise relatively rapidly |  | Lifestyle; insulin sensitizers |
|  | Stable decompensation | More severe β-cell dedifferentiation β-cell mass reduced to ~50% of normal | Reduced efficiency Loss in insulin production | Frank diabetes |  | As per clinical situation secretagogues may be used insulin, if required, will be short term |
| 3 | Severe decompensation | Profound reduction in β-cell mass | Absent insulin production | Progression to ketosis | Complete/irreversible β-cell insufficiency | Long-term insulin |

Source: Adapted with permission from Kalra S, Gupta Y. Beta-cell Insufficiency. Eur Endocrinol. 2017;13(2):51-3.
(GSIS: glucose-stimulated insulin secretion)

**TABLE 3** Causes of pancreatogenic or type 3c diabetes mellitus.

|  | Etiology |
|---|---|
| Congenital | Agenesis of the pancreas |
|  | Cystic fibrosis-related pancreatitis |
|  | Hemochromatosis |
| Pancreatitis | Severe acute pancreatitis |
|  | Chronic pancreatitis |
|  | Chronic calcific pancreatitis |
|  | Fibrocalculous pancreatopathy |
| Postsurgical | Total pancreatectomy |
|  | Partial pancreatectomy |
| Malignant | Ductal adenocarcinoma of the pancreas |

Therefore, glucovigilance is required in the gastroenterology and internal medicine practice, when treating individuals with pancreatitis. In this section, authors discuss the need for glucose monitoring and management issues related to diabetes associated with exocrine pancreatic disorders.

## Acute Pancreatitis

Acute pancreatitis may often be associated with early transient hyperglycemia, but may also reveal underlying pre-existing diabetes. The pathophysiological mechanisms leading to hyperglycemia in acute pancreatitis are not completely understood. Transient hyperglycemia may be the result of stress hyperglycemia in critically ill patients but may also be associated with necrosis and damage to the pancreatic β-cells.

Most cases of acute pancreatitis present with mild disease, but 10–20% individuals may develop varying degree of necrosis of the gland and multiorgan involvement.[15] The multisystem involvement in acute pancreatitis is a reflection of the pancreatic gland's capacity to produce a number of potent vasoactive peptides, hormones and enzymes. The various prognostic criteria are early evaluations of these metabolic derangements. The pathogenesis of hypocalcemia, long recognized as an indicator of severity of acute pancreatitis, is multifactorial. Imbalances of parathyroid hormone (PTH)-calcitonin, the interactions of glucagon, gastrin and other pancreatic hormones with PTH-calcitonin, the role of free fatty acids in binding serum calcium with albumin, and the translocation of calcium ion in muscles and liver, have been recently described but remain conflicting theories.

Blood glucose values should be regularly monitored during hospitalization for acute pancreatitis; in addition, glycated hemoglobin (HbA1c) measurement may inform pre-existing diabetes or new-onset hyperglycemia. Management of hyperglycemia would require intensive fluid replacement and intravenous insulin infusion. Once oral intake is sufficient, patient should be transitioned to multiple subcutaneous insulin injections. In some cases, hyperglycemia may resolve over the period of recovery while in others, persistent hyperglycemia requires long-term insulin therapy.

Both transient hyperglycemia and pre-existing diabetes are associated with more severe pancreatitis, greater risk of multiorgan failure and greater morbidity and mortality related to acute pancreatitis. Furthermore, individuals with acute pancreatitis are also at short-term as well as long-term risk of developing diabetes.[16] In a series of 113 patients hospitalized for acute pancreatitis, 30.1% had persistent diabetes and 29.2% had impaired glucose tolerance on follow-up after discharge.[15] Occurrence of hyperglycemia during the acute episode, presence of pancreatic necrosis as well as the presence of other metabolic abnormalities such as hypertension, nonalcoholic fatty liver disease, dyslipidemia and obesity predicted greater risk of overt diabetes.[16] Therefore, while regular glucose monitoring is needed during the acute phase of hospitalization for acute pancreatitis, long-term glucovigilance is also required. Monitoring of fasting plasma glucose (FPG) or HbA1c alone may not detect early abnormalities of glucose tolerance; oral glucose tolerance test (OGTT) is more sensitive for detection of hyperglycemia in such individuals.

## Chronic Pancreatitis

Most cases of pancreatogenic diabetes occur due to chronic pancreatitis. The pathogenesis of diabetes in the setting of chronic pancreatitis is not completely understood, but damage to pancreas is associated with disruption of insulin and glucagon secretion, impaired incretin secretion and nutrient malabsorption. This is usually accompanied by varying degrees of exocrine pancreatic insufficiency.

The pathogenesis of diabetes related to chronic pancreatitis involves impaired insulin secretion resulting from inflammation and later fibrosis; individuals with chronic calcific pancreatitis are more susceptible. The decline in endocrine function parallels the decline in exocrine function. In early stages, this may manifest as impaired glucose tolerance rather than overt diabetes. With progressive fibrosis, there is loss of islet mass and more marked hyperglycemia with glycemic variability.[17]

In patients with insulin-dependent diabetes secondary to chronic pancreatitis, β-cell function is preserved to a greater extent and glucoregulation is better than in individuals with T1DM due to relatively slower destruction of the β-cells. Individuals with secondary pancreatogenic diabetes have significant glycemic variability due to several factors—(1) loss of glucagon secretion; (2) blunted epinephrine response to insulin-induced hypoglycemia; and (3) malabsorption.[17] A fraction of chronic pancreatitis patients may show glucagon secretion from residual α-cell function during intravenous arginine and meal stimulation but not with insulin-induced hypoglycemia or insulin withdrawal despite complete absence of endogenous insulin production. Peripheral insulin sensitivity does not seem to be significantly affected but there may be some degree of hepatic insulin resistance due to reduced secretion of pancreatic polypeptide (PP).[17]

Diabetes mellitus caused by pancreatic exocrine disease is a unique clinical and metabolic form of diabetes. These individuals have increased levels of circulating gluconeogenic amino acids, lower insulin requirements, low risk of development of ketosis, low cholesterol levels, an increased risk of medication-induced hypoglycemia and the clinical impression of brittle diabetes. In addition, they may have pancreatic calcification or clinically demonstrable pancreatic exocrine dysfunction.

Ewald and Bretzel[18] proposed the following diagnostic criteria for T3cDM:
- Presence of exocrine pancreatic insufficiency,
- Abnormal features of imaging of pancreas, and
- Absence of autoantibodies that characterize T1DM.

However, T3cDM may be misclassified using these stringent criteria as chronic pancreatitis is relatively painless and may not be accompanied by evident exocrine pancreatic insufficiency if a high index of suspicion is not maintained. In addition, individuals with diseases of the exocrine pancreas should be periodically screened for hyperglycemia. Since FPG test may underestimate the prevalence of hyperglycemia in these individuals, OGTT is a better strategy.[19]

Management of pancreatogenic diabetes requires a multidisciplinary team approach with collaboration between gastroenterologists, endocrinologists, gastrointestinal surgeons and nutritionist. Pancreatic imaging using ultrasound, computed tomography (CT), magnetic resonance cholangiopancreatography (MRCP) and endoscopic retrograde cholangiopancreatography (ERCP) is indicated in chronic pancreatitis to assess for pancreatic morphology, calculi, duct dilatation, obstruction and cyst formation. Assessment of exocrine pancreatic function is cumbersome and includes measurement of serum trypsin, stool fat content, fecal elastase-1 (FE-1), fecal chymotrypsin and secretin-pancreozymin test.

General lifestyle modification should focus on the maintenance of adequate nutrition in addition to physical activity. Greater intake of soluble fiber and reduced fat intake along with oral pancreatic enzyme supplements are useful to prevent malabsorption, malnutrition, micronutrient deficiencies and steatorrhea, especially in the setting of exocrine pancreatic insufficiency. Cessation of smoking and abstinence from alcohol should be encouraged as smoking and alcohol can further pancreatic damage.

Oral hypoglycemic agents may be appropriate for milder hyperglycemia. Metformin may reduce the risk of pancreatic cancer but may cause troublesome weight loss and gastrointestinal side effects. Insulin secretagogues can be used. However, incretin-based drugs are not recommended as they are associated with increased risk of pancreatitis. Insulin is required for most individuals with pancreatogenic diabetes. While there are no guidelines for pharmacological management of pancreatogenic diabetes, multiple subcutaneous insulin injections with regular self-monitoring of blood glucose is the most optimal regimen. Since these individuals may have "brittle diabetes", avoiding hypoglycemia is a key concern.

Pancreatic enzyme replacement therapy may be used for the management of abdominal pain and exocrine pancreatic insufficiency, but it also improves incretin response by improvement of nutrient absorption.[17] Therefore, it may improve glycemic control as well. Select patients with recurrent attacks of pancreatitis may benefit from surgical intervention. Novel therapies such as PP are under evaluation for management of chronic pancreatitis-associated diabetes.

The risk for microvascular and macrovascular complications also seems to be similar to that seen with T1DM and T2DM. There is an increased risk of vitamin D deficiency and osteoporosis. The incidence of pancreatic cancer is significantly higher; some studies report incidence rates as high as 30% for pancreatic cancer.

## Fibrocalculous Pancreatic Diabetes

Fibrocalculous pancreatic diabetes (FCPD) is a unique form of diabetes secondary to tropical chronic calcific pancreatitis. The pathogenesis is not understood, but genetic susceptibility, malnutrition, cassava toxicity, dietary toxins, trace element deficiencies and oxidative stress have been implicated. FCPD usually affects the poorer strata of society and patients are lean and often frankly malnourished. The hallmarks of the disease are the occurrence of pain in abdomen in childhood and pancreatic calculi associated with dilatation of the pancreatic duct and fibrosis of the gland in adolescence.[20]

Diabetes sets in by early adulthood, is severe and brittle. Individuals are usually lean built and present with history of recurrent abdominal pain, malabsorption and steatorrhea. Plain radiographs, ultrasound or CT of the abdomen may reveal multiple large intraductal pancreatic calculi.

Individuals with FCPD usually require insulin for management of diabetes though ketosis is rare. Patients of FCPD are at greater risk of hypoglycemia due to deficiency of glucagon. Pancreatic enzyme supplements reduce the risk of malabsorption. Recurrent pain not responding to pharmacological measures may require surgical intervention.[21]

While microvascular complications occur at increased rates, the risk of macrovascular complications is not significantly elevated. The risk of pancreatic cancer is particularly high in FCPD and a high index of suspicion is required for early detection.

## Pancreatic Cancer

Diabetes may develop in individuals with pancreatic ductal adenocarcinoma, especially in elderly individuals. In a population-based study, almost 1% of individuals with new-onset diabetes at age ≥50 years were found to have secondary diabetes due to pancreatic cancer.[22] There seems to be a temporal relationship between diagnosis of diabetes and pancreatic cancer, with diabetes preceding cancer by almost 1-2 years. The prevalence of dysglycemia is very high in pancreatic cancer with impaired fasting glucose, impaired glucose tolerance or diabetes reported in over 80% of cancer patients.[17]

However, unlike other forms of T3cDM, dysglycemia does not seem to result from islet destruction resulting in insulinopenia. Rather, most of these individuals exhibit insulin resistance.[17] While the exact pathogenesis of diabetes remains unclear, it has been hypothesized that diabetes may be a paraneoplastic effect of pancreatic cancer that results in both β-cell toxicity and insulin resistance. Candidate molecules for this paraneoplastic effect include PP, adrenomedullin and the adipokine lipocalin 2.[17]

In fact, treatment of underlying malignancy has been reported to result in improvement in glycemic status. There may occur resolution of hyperglycemia in those with recent history of diabetes following surgical resection of the tumor; on the other hand, those with long-standing diabetes do not show improved glycemic status.

The primary goal of management is amelioration of symptomatic hyperglycemia with the use of oral antidiabetic agents as well as insulin. Metformin has antineoplastic properties and may have a protective effect. On the other hand, incretin-based therapies have been linked to increased risk of pancreatic cancer, albeit controversially. Coexistent diabetes in individuals with pancreatic cancer has a worse prognosis with greater risk of postoperative complications, infection and mortality.

## Insulinoma

The classic example of hypoglycemia due to a pancreatic disorder is insulinoma. Individuals with an insulinoma typically have fasting hypoglycemia but may occasionally also experience postprandial hypoglycemia.[23] Diagnosis requires documentation of hyperinsulinemia during a hypoglycemic episode. It is usually not possible to obtain laboratory data during a spontaneous event, and for that reason a 72-hour monitored fast is often required to make the diagnosis. Most, but not all, patients with the disease experience hypoglycemia within 72 hours. Hypoglycemia occurs in less than 24 hours in about two-thirds of cases, and in less than 48 hours of fasting in the great majority of affected patients.

By the time an insulinoma comes to clinical attention, hypoglycemic events are typically characterized by episodes of neuroglycopenia. Often patients are given other diagnoses such as seizure disorder, before hypoglycemia due to an insulinoma is considered. Common neuroglycopenic symptoms include confusion and personality changes or bizarre behavior that may not be recognized as metabolic in origin. Patients may have amnesia for the hypoglycemic events. Once diagnosis is established, treatment remains surgical excision of the tumor. Pharmacological agents that may be used include diazoxide, somatostatin receptor analogs and mTOR inhibitors (everolimus).[23] Endogenous hyperinsulinemic hypoglycemia has been discussed in the chapter "Hypoglycemia in Endocrinopathy".

## Glucagonoma

Rare glucagon-producing tumors of the pancreatic α-cells can also result in hyperglycemia. Glucagonoma syndrome is typically characterized by a triad of glucagon-secreting tumors, diabetes and necrolytic migratory erythema. The typical skin rash is often the initial clinical presentation of glucagonomas. Glucagon levels are significantly elevated. Treatment is primarily surgical removal of the tumor, but somatostatin analogs and radionuclide therapy have also been used.[24]

## PANCREATIC VIGILANCE IN DIABETES

Both T1DM and T2DM are associated with functional and morphological changes in endocrine pancreas that are both a cause and consequence of hyperglycemia, as discussed in the section "Glucose Physiology in Relation to Pancreas".

While diabetes is classically considered a disease of the endocrine pancreas, significant alterations have been reported in exocrine pancreatic health as well. On the one hand, primary pancreatic disorders are a recognized cause of secondary or T3cDM, the prevalence of such disorders is comparatively low. T2DM remains the most common disorder, followed by T1DM and both are themselves associated with altered health of exocrine pancreas. Individuals with diabetes are at increased risk of acute pancreatitis, chronic pancreatitis, exocrine pancreatic insufficiency and pancreatic cancer. Therefore, there is a clear need for pancreatic vigilance in the diabetes clinic.

## Risk of Acute Pancreatitis in Diabetes

As discussed in the earlier section, individuals with T2DM have a greater risk of developing acute pancreatitis. In fact, a meta-analysis of observational studies reported an increased risk (relative risk 1.92; 95% CI 1.50–2.47) of acute pancreatitis in individuals with T2DM, even after correction for other risk factors such as alcohol intake, gallstone disease and hypertriglyceridemia.[25]

How diabetes increases the risk of acute pancreatitis remains unknown. Multiple factors may contribute including hyperglycemia, inflammation, oxidative stress and amyloid deposition. Other confounding risk factors including obesity, gallstone disease, hypertriglyceridemia, alcohol intake and chronic pancreatitis may also be present. In addition, incretin-based drugs have been reported to be associated with increased risk of pancreatitis and should be avoided in individuals with current or previous history of pancreatitis.[26]

## Risk of Chronic Pancreatitis in Diabetes

While a significant proportion of patients with chronic pancreatitis develop secondary diabetes over time, there is a significant overlap between pancreatitis and T2DM. The prevalence of pancreatitis in a cohort of individuals with diabetes was estimated at 9.2% (172 or 1,868 individuals).[17] The association between chronic pancreatitis and diabetes has been discussed in the previous section.

## Risk of Exocrine Pancreatic Insufficiency in Diabetes

Exocrine pancreatic insufficiency is observed in about 26–74% patients of T1DM and 28–36% patients of T2DM using either direct (secretin-pancreozymin test) or indirect (FE-1 concentrations) tests of pancreatic function.[27-29]

Exocrine insufficiency probably is more prevalent in poorly controlled diabetes of long duration as serum amylase, serum trypsin and fecal elastase concentration were shown to be inversely correlated with diabetes duration, FPG and HbA1c levels and positively correlated with C-peptide levels in different studies.[28,29] On the contrary, exocrine pancreatic insufficiency as evidenced by low FE-1 concentration in a mixed cohort of T1DM, insulin treated T2DM, and noninsulin-treated T2DM was as low as 5.4%.[30] Pancreatic exocrine insufficiency is seen some varieties of maturity onset diabetes in young (MODY) like MODY 3 (mutation in HNF 1α), MODY 5 (mutation in HNF 1β) and MODY 8 (defect in cholesterol ester lipase). Prevalence of exocrine pancreatic insufficiency was seen in 12.7% of 63 adults with MODY 3.

Various hypotheses have been put forward to explain exocrine pancreatic insufficiency in nonpancreatic diabetes. Acinar cells situated in close vicinity of the nearby islets are comparatively bigger and produce more enzymes than those located at a distance. Insulin is considered a trophic factor for the nearby exocrine tissue and this may explain relatively higher prevalence of low FE-1 concentration in T1DM and longstanding T2DM. Islet hormones other than insulin may also play a role. Hyperglucagonemia and elevated somatostatin (absolute/relative), seen in both T1DM and T2DM, have been suggested to contribute to exocrine damage and dysfunction.

Autoimmune destruction of both endocrine and exocrine pancreas can explain exocrine insufficiency in autoimmune diabetes. Antibodies directed against different exocrine antigens [pancreatic cytokeratin, bile salt-dependent lipase (BSDL), lactoferrin or carbonic anhydrase] have been detected in about two-third of patients of T1DM.[31]

Exocrine pancreatic insufficiency may also arise as a result of autonomic neuropathy and microangiopathy. The enteropancreatic reflexes, which play a dominant role in pancreatic response after a meal, are impaired in autonomic neuropathy and may result in exocrine insufficiency. Moreover, gastroparesis secondary to autonomic neuropathy culminates in reduced cholecystokinin (CCK) secretion and subsequent impaired exocrine pancreatic secretion. This is supported by positive correlation of exocrine insufficiency with duration of diabetes. The other probable mechanisms are direct hyperglycemic injury to the pancreas, abnormal secretion of CCK, acinar cell insensitivity to CCK and simultaneous damage of exocrine and endocrine tissues by viral infections.

The consequences of exocrine insufficiency can be manifold. It may result in clinically significant steatorrhoea and possible deficiency of fat-soluble vitamins. More importantly perhaps is the possible alteration in incretin axis that in turn may result in deterioration in glycemic control.

## Risk of Pancreatic Cancer in Diabetes

Diabetes is associated with increased risk of chronic ductal adenocarcinoma of the pancreas, especially in individuals with concurrent diabetes and chronic pancreatitis. Individuals with long-standing diabetes are at almost 1.5–2 times increased risk of pancreatic ductal adenocarcinoma.[17] The risk is higher in those with diabetes duration of greater than 5 years. Several factors have been implicated in this increased risk including insulin resistance with increased insulin concentrations within the pancreas that may promote tumor formation, oxidative stress and obesity which is an independent risk factor for pancreatic cancer.[32] A high index of suspicion for pancreatic cancer should be maintained in individuals with T2DM—clinical indicators could include unexplained weight loss, jaundice and abdominal pain. At present, there are no biomarkers that can assist in screening for pancreatic cancer. Diagnosis can be established by endoscopic ultrasound, CT or MR imaging.

## Risk of Pancreatitis with Antidiabetic Drugs

Various oral and injectable antidiabetics may contribute to the risk of pancreatitis in diabetes. This requires pancreatic vigilance with the use of these medications in patients at risk of or with a previous history of pancreatitis.[33]

*Metformin*: Metformin was linked to pancreatitis, secondary to overdose or in case of impaired renal function. While the underlying mechanisms are not known, metformin toxicity could result in acinar cell injury with subsequent intercellular leakage of digestive enzymes from the ductules. Metformin should be discontinued during an episode of acute pancreatitis, but at present a strong association between pancreatitis risk and metformin does not exist. In individuals with T2DM, metformin was associated with 60% risk reduction for pancreatic carcinoma; however, this evidence came from only case-control studies.[17] More recent meta-analysis did not demonstrate such a benefit.[34]

*Sulfonylureas*: Acute and chronic administration of sulfonylurea drugs act on KATP channels to increase insulin secretion and also enhance β-cell sensitivity to the potentiating effect of glucose. In cohort studies, sulfonylureas have been linked to increased risk of pancreatitis.

*Meglitinides*: No association with risk of pancreatitis has been reported.

*Alpha-glucosidase inhibitors*: Acarbose, voglibose or miglitol do not seem to increase pancreatitis risk.

*Thiazolidinediones*: Thiazolidinediones have been reported to have a protective effect on the pancreas in animal studies and found to attenuate pancreatic damage.[33]

*Sodium-glucose cotransporter 2 inhibitors*: This class of drugs also seems to be neutral in terms of pancreatitis risk.

*Dipeptidylpeptidase-4 inhibitors*: There have been a series of case reports of acute pancreatitis and pancreatic cancer related to the use of gliptins and therefore, caution has been recommended. But most randomized controlled trials including the large cardiovascular outcome trials and retrospective analysis of outpatient databases have not demonstrated such an association.[35]

*GLP-1 receptor agonists*: GLP-1 receptor agonists have also been linked to an increased risk of pancreatitis and pancreatic cancers. However, large cardiovascular outcome trials of GLP-1 receptor agonists failed to demonstrate such risk, though an increased risk of cholelithiasis was detected, possibly related to weight loss.[36]

Caution is needed when using incretin-based drugs such as dipeptidyl peptidase 4 (DPP4) inhibitors and GLP-1 receptor agonists in individuals at risk of pancreatitis. In addition, these drugs should be avoided in individuals with previous history of acute or chronic pancreatitis and discontinued if pancreatitis develops. Both DPP4 inhibitors and GLP-1 receptor agonists may be associated with modest increase in serum amylase and lipase levels; however, routine measurement of amylase and lipase is not recommended in the pharmacovigilance for these drugs.

## CONCLUSION

Patients with various endogenous pancreatic disorders including acute or chronic pancreatitis are at increased risk of developing diabetes; hence, they should be screened for diabetes at diagnosis and periodically thereafter. In addition, diabetes is associated with significant changes in both endocrine and exocrine pancreatic function and antidiabetic drugs may have variable effects on pancreatic health. There exists a bidirectional association between acute pancreatitis, chronic pancreatitis and pancreatic cancer and diabetes. Presence of chronic pancreatitis and diabetes together poses significant management challenges due to high glycemic variability and carries an increased risk of pancreatic cancer.

The Consortium for the Study of Chronic Pancreatitis, Diabetes, and Pancreatic Cancer (CPDPC) aims to evaluate the complex pathophysiological relationship between diabetes and pancreatic disorders. Research should focus on understanding the mechanisms behind these associations, appropriate classification of various forms of pancreatogenic diabetes and optimal approach to management.

## REFERENCES

1. Menon S, Rajesh G, Balakrishnan V. Pancreas and diabetes mellitus: the relationship between the organ and the disease. J Assoc Physicians India. 2015;63(10):51-8.
2. Röder PV, Wu B, Liu Y, et al. Pancreatic regulation of glucose homeostasis. Exp Mol Med. 2016; 48:e219.
3. Tengholm A, Gylfe E. Oscillatory control of insulin secretion. Mol Cell Endocrinol. 2009;297(1-2):58-72.
4. Habener JF, Stanojevic V. Alpha cells come of age. Trends Endocrinol Metab. 2013;24(3):153-63.
5. Faideau B, Larger E, Lepault F, et al. Role of beta-cells in type 1 diabetes pathogenesis. Diabetes. 2005;54(Suppl 2):S87-96.
6. Pino SC, Kruger AJ, Bortell R. The role of innate immune pathways in type 1 diabetes pathogenesis. Curr Opin Endocrinol Diabetes Obes. 2010;17(2):126-30.
7. White MG, Shaw JA, Taylor R. Type 2 diabetes: the pathologic basis of reversible β-Cell dysfunction. Diabetes Care. 2016;39(11):2080-8.
8. Satin LS, Butler PC, Ha J, et al. Pulsatile insulin secretion, impaired glucose tolerance and type 2 diabetes. Mol Aspects Med. 2015;42:61-77.
9. Kalra S, Gupta Y. Beta-cell Insufficiency. Eur Endocrinol. 2017;13(2):51-3.
10. Talchai C, Xuan S, Lin HV, et al. Pancreatic beta cell dedifferentiation as a mechanism of diabetic beta cell failure. Cell. 2012;150(6):1223-34.
11. Wali JA, Thomas HE. Pancreatic alpha cells hold the key to survival. EBioMedicine. 2015;2(5):368-9.
12. Meier JJ, Kjems LL, Veldhuis JD, et al. Postprandial suppression of glucagon secretion depends on intact pulsatile insulin secretion: further evidence for the intraislet insulin hypothesis. Diabetes. 2006;55(4):1051-6.
13. Menge BA, Grüber L, Jørgensen SM, et al. Loss of inverse relationship between pulsatile insulin and glucagon secretion in patients with type 2 diabetes. Diabetes. 2011;60(8):2160-8.
14. Makuc J. Management of pancreatogenic diabetes: challenges and solutions. Diabetes Metab Syndr Obes. 2016;9:311-5.
15. Tu J, Zhang J, Ke L, et al. Endocrine and exocrine pancreatic insufficiency after acute pancreatitis: long-term follow-up study. BMC Gastroenterol. 2017;17(1):114.
16. Yuan L, Tang M, Huang L, et al. Risk Factors of Hyperglycemia in Patients After a First Episode of Acute Pancreatitis: A Retrospective Cohort. Pancreas. 2017;46(2):209-18.
17. Hart PA, Bellin MD, Andersen DK, et al. Consortium for the Study of Chronic Pancreatitis, Diabetes, and Pancreatic Cancer (CPDPC). Type 3c (pancreatogenic) diabetes mellitus secondary to chronic pancreatitis and pancreatic cancer. Lancet Gastroenterol Hepatol. 2016;1(3):226-37.
18. Ewald N, Bretzel RG. Diabetes mellitus secondary to pancreatic diseases (type 3c)—are we neglecting an important disease? Eur J Intern Med. 2013;24(3):203-6.
19. Meier JJ, Giese A. Diabetes associated with pancreatic diseases. Curr Opin Gastroenterol. 2015;31(5):400-6.
20. Unnikrishnan R, Mohan V. Fibrocalculous pancreatic diabetes (FCPD). Acta Diabetol. 2015;52(1):1-9.
21. Barman KK, Premalatha G, Mohan V. Tropical chronic pancreatitis. Postgrad Med J. 2003;79(937):606-15.
22. Chari ST, Leibson CL, Rabe KG, et al. Probability of pancreatic cancer following diabetes: a population-based study. Gastroenterology. 2005;129:504-11.
23. Matej A, Bujwid H, Wroński J. Glycemic control in patients with insulinoma. Hormones (Athens). 2016;15(4):489-99.
24. John AM, Schwartz RA. Glucagonoma syndrome: a review and update on treatment. J Eur Acad Dermatol Venereol. 2016;30(12):2016-22.

25. Xue Y, Sheng Y, Dai H, et al. Risk of development of acute pancreatitis with pre-existing diabetes: a meta-analysis. Eur J Gastroenterol Hepatol. 2012;24:1092-8.
26. Kikuta K, Masamune A, Shimosegawa T. Impaired glucose tolerance in acute pancreatitis. World J Gastroenterol. 2015;21(24):7367-74.
27. Hardt PD. High prevalence of exocrine pancreatic insufficiency in diabetes mellitus. A multicenter study screening fecal elastase 1 concentrations in 1,021 diabetic patients. Pancreatology. 2003; 3(5):395-402.
28. Ewald N, Raspe A, Kaufmann C, et al. Determinants of Exocrine Pancreatic Function as Measured by Fecal Elastase-1 Concentrations (FEC) in Patients with Diabetes mellitus. Eur J Med Res. 2009;14(3):118-22.
29. Terzin V, Várkonyi T, Szabolcs A, et al. Prevalence of exocrine pancreatic insufficiency in type 2 diabetes mellitus with poor glycemic control. Pancreatology. 2014;14(5):356-60.
30. Vujasinovic M, Zaletel J, Tepes B, et al. Low prevalence of exocrine pancreatic insufficiency in patients with diabetes mellitus. Pancreatology. 2013;13(4):343-6.
31. Taniguchi T, Okazaki K, Okamoto M, et al. High prevalence of autoantibodies against carbonic anhydrase II and lactoferrin in type 1 diabetes: concept of autoimmune exocrinopathy and endocrinopathy of the pancreas. Pancreas. 2003;27(1):26-30.
32. De Souza A, Irfan K, Masud F, et al. Diabetes Type 2 and Pancreatic Cancer: A History Unfolding. JOP. 2016;17(2):144-8.
33. Giorda CB, Nada E, Tartaglino B, et al. A systematic review of acute pancreatitis as an adverse event of type 2 diabetes drugs: from hard facts to a balanced position. Diabetes Obes Metab. 2014;16(11):1041-7.
34. Singh S, Singh PP, Singh AG, et al. Anti-diabetic medications and risk of pancreatic cancer in patients with diabetes mellitus: a systematic review and meta-analysis. Am J Gastroenterol. 2013;108(4):510-9.
35. Azoulay L, Filion KB, Platt RW, et al. Association between incretin-based drugs and the risk of acute pancreatitis. JAMA Intern Med. 2016;176(10):1464-73.
36. Monami M, Nreu B, Scatena A, et al. Safety issues with glucagon-like peptide-1 receptor agonists (pancreatitis, pancreatic cancer and cholelithiasis): data from randomized controlled trials. Diabetes Obes Metab. 2017;19(9):1233-41.

# CHAPTER 8

# Glucocrinology of Reproductive System: Male

*Om J Lakhani, Khalid Sheikh*

## INTRODUCTION

The field of male reproductive medicine primarily pertains to the endocrinology of reproductive and sexual health of boys and men. Any aberration along the hypothalamic–pituitary–gonadal axis can cause abnormalities in testosterone production or action and spermatogenesis. Traditionally, testosterone is considered important in the development of the male phenotype. However, the role of testis in the maintenance of vigor, muscle strength, and vitality has been understood since the times of ancient Roman and Chinese civilizations, when animal testicular extracts were used for this purpose. Modern research clearly suggests that testosterone has significant impact on metabolic health in addition to the maintenance of reproductive functions. The incidence of diabetes and metabolic syndrome (MetS) has been reported to be higher in men with hypogonadism.

In addition, more than one-third of men with diabetes mellitus have low testosterone levels. Both the total testosterone and free testosterone levels are reduced in patients with type 2 diabetes mellitus (T2DM) and MetS.[1] Testosterone supplementation is associated with metabolic benefits in hypogonadal men. However, an age-old chicken or egg question that emerges is whether deficiency of testosterone leads to insulin resistance and hence MetS and T2DM or does MetS and T2DM lead to low testosterone levels?

In this chapter, we have explored the interesting bilateral relationship between glucose physiology and testosterone and glucocrinology in relation to the male reproductive system. We have also discussed the clinical implications and suggestions for screening and treatment in appropriate scenarios.

# GLUCOSE PHYSIOLOGY IN RELATION TO MALE REPRODUCTIVE SYSTEM

## Relationship of Testosterone with Glucose Metabolism and Insulin Resistance

It is well-known that testosterone therapy, in otherwise healthy hypogonadal men, is associated with an increase of muscle mass and reduction of fat-free mass. This is because testosterone promotes the conversion of pluripotent stem cells to myocytes in preference of adipocytes. This has been proven in experimental studies on mouse models.[2] The favorable change in body composition with an increase in myocytes and reduction of adipocytes leads to improved insulin sensitivity.

The effects of testosterone on insulin sensitivity are further mediated via both genomic and nongenomic actions. Glucose transporter type 4 (GLUT4) is an insulin-regulated glucose transporter found mainly on adipocytes, skeletal muscle cells and cardiac myocytes. Testosterone increases the expression and translocation of GLUT4 via both nongenomic and genomic effects, thereby, promoting glucose uptake by these cells.[3] It has been shown to increase the expression of GLUT4, GLUT3 and GLUT1, increase membrane translocation of GLUT4, and positively modulate insulin signaling via PI3K/AKT/mammalian target of rapamycin (mTOR) and RAS/ERK pathways. Testosterone has also been shown to protect murine pancreatic β-cells from apoptosis by reducing the expression of angiotensin II type 1 receptor (AGTR1) and decreasing glucotoxicity-induced oxidative stress.[4]

Additionally, the impact of testosterone on insulin resistance may be indirect. Studies have shown that hypogonadal mice have reduced physical activity which can contribute to poor metabolic health (Flowchart 1).[5] Testosterone may also have central hypothalamic effects via androgen receptors as well as estrogen receptors and facilitates the effects of leptin to increase energy expenditure and reduce whole body fat mass particularly white adipose tissue.

Apart from testosterone, studies have also shown a link between increased prolactin levels and insulin resistance.[6] It was initially thought that supraphysiological prolactin levels, as seen in hyperprolactinemia due to prolactinoma or antipsychotic drugs, is associated with increased insulin resistance and prolactin levels within physiological limits have little impact on insulin sensitivity. Treatment of prolactinoma with a dopamine agonist was associated with improvement in metabolic parameters in men.[6] However, Daimon et al. showed that among nondiabetic men with serum prolactin within normal physiological range, a positive association was found between higher prolactin values and HOMA-IR.[7]

Hyperprolactinemia induces hypogonadism in both sexes.[8] Interestingly, hyperprolactinemia reduces testosterone levels in men leading to hypogonadism, while in women it is associated with increased testosterone levels leading to clinical symptoms which masquerade as polycystic ovary syndrome (PCOS). It is well-known that reduced testosterone levels in men and increased testosterone levels in women have a significant association with insulin resistance and the risk of T2DM.[9] Whether the impact of prolactin on insulin resistance is mediated via its impact on testosterone needs further assessment; however, it is certainly deemed to be plausible.

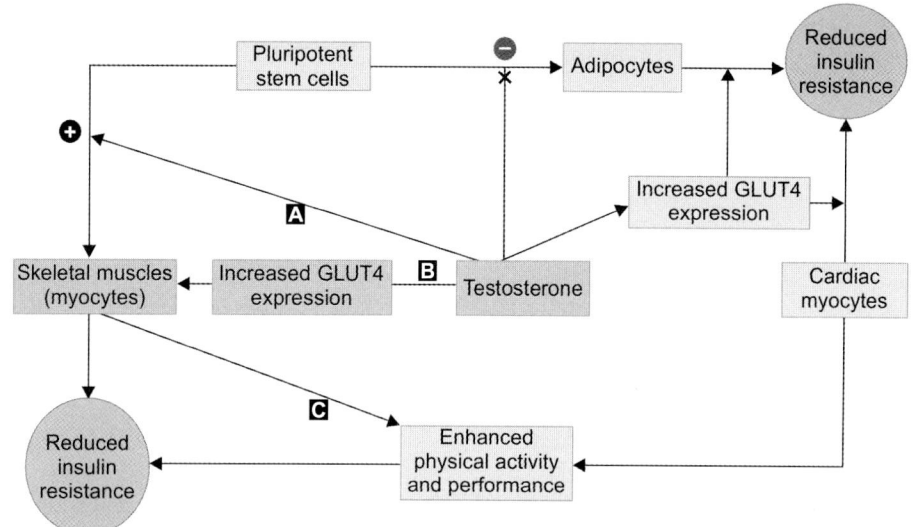

**FLOWCHART 1:** Relationship of testosterone with glucose metabolism and insulin resistance. (a) Testosterone increases the differentiation of pluripotent stem cells to myocytes in preference over adipocytes. This leads to reduced insulin resistance; (b) Testosterone increases the glucose transporter type 4 (GLUT4) expression on skeletal myocytes, cardiac myocytes and adipose cells leading to enhanced insulin sensitivity; and (c) Testosterone enhances physical activity and performance leading to reduced insulin resistance.

Hence, reduced testosterone level in males is associated with insulin resistance and increased risk and incidence of T2DM (Flowchart 1).

## Impact of Obesity, Metabolic Syndrome and Type 2 Diabetes Mellitus on Testosterone Levels

The other obvious question is whether obesity and metabolic abnormalities lead to low testosterone levels seen more frequently in men with obesity, MetS and T2DM. Insulin resistance is associated with a reduction in sex hormone-binding globulin (SHBG) levels.[1] Hence, total testosterone levels are lower in men with features of insulin resistance. On the other hand, women with PCOS have hyperinsulinemia which results in reduced SHBG and higher free testosterone levels, leading to hyperandrogenic symptoms.[10] Studies have clearly shown that both MetS and T2DM have a significant association with lower total as well as free testosterone levels (Flowchart 2).[11,12]

Hypogonadism and androgen deficiency in males can be broadly divided into two categories. One is organic androgen deficiency (OAD) which is secondary to a pathological cause, including hypogonadotropic hypogonadism, androgen deprivation therapy (ADT) in prostate cancer, or Klinefelter syndrome (KS). On the other hand, a condition which is much more common, yet much less understood is functional androgen deficiency (FAD) which is secondary to obesity and aging.[13]

An interesting cross-sectional study conducted by Tajar et al. in more than 3,000 European men between ages of 40–79 years evaluated the impact of aging and obesity

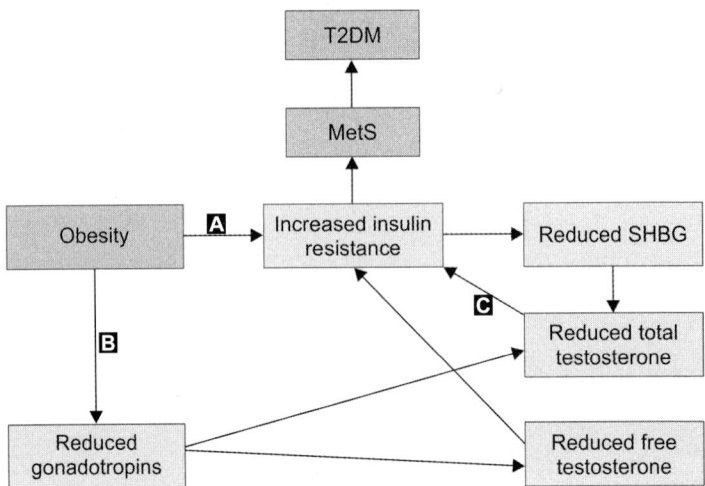

**FLOWCHART 2:** Summary of the bidirectional relationship between testosterone and metabolic syndrome (MetS) and type 2 diabetes mellitus (T2DM). (a) Obesity is associated with increased insulin resistance which leads to reduction in sex hormone-binding globulin (SHBG) levels; (b) Obesity also results in reduced gonadotropin levels that are associated with reduction in both total and free testosterone levels in males; and (c) Reduced testosterone levels in males are associated with increased insulin resistance leading to MetS and T2DM.

on testosterone levels. The study population was divided into four groups based on testosterone and luteinizing hormone (LH) levels. Aging was associated with primary hypogonadism (low testosterone with elevated LH) and compensated hypogonadism (normal testosterone and elevated LH). While on the other hand, obesity was associated with secondary hypogonadism (low testosterone and normal or low LH). What is interesting to note, however, was that testosterone levels were 30% lower in men with obesity even after adjusting for age. This suggests that obesity has an impact on androgen deficiency which is independent of aging especially when dealing with late-onset hypogonadism.[14] In fact, another observational study by Sartorius et al. showed that healthy aging was not associated with androgen deficiency and late-onset hypogonadism was predominantly associated with obesity and smoking. Therefore, late-onset hypogonadism may be a consequence of the battle scars of unhealthy aging rather than true deficiency associated purely with age.[15]

An interesting prospective study conducted in Finland showed that those with MetS were 2.6 times more likely to have hypogonadism a decade later.[16] A recent meta-analysis has shown that higher total and free testosterone is associated with reduced risk of T2DM by as much as 30–40%.[17]

## Lower Testosterone as a Predictor of Poor Health in Patients with Type 2 Diabetes Mellitus

Men with T2DM and lower testosterone levels are more likely to be obese and have more adverse cardiometabolic profile than those with normal testosterone levels.[13] A cross-sectional study in diabetic men showed that lower total and free testosterone levels were associated with higher C-reactive protein levels and carotid intima-media thickness and were more likely to have endothelial dysfunction.[18] A meta-analysis by Corona et al. showed that patients with lower testosterone and higher estradiol (E2) had higher cardiovascular mortality. The findings were independent of diabetes status.[12] However, replacement of testosterone to reduce cardiovascular risk, especially in patients with FAD, remains controversial.[19]

It seems that testosterone may be a biomarker of poor metabolic health and higher cardiovascular mortality rather than the cause. However, this is an area of active research in the field of andrology.

## GLUCOVIGILANCE IN MALE REPRODUCTIVE DISORDERS

Since it is clear that the risk of T2DM is higher in men with hypogonadism, it is important to monitor the glycemic and metabolic status of men suffering from OAD.

### Glucovigilance in Men with Congenital Hypogonadotropic Hypogonadism

Congenital hypogonadotropic hypogonadism (CHH), also known as idiopathic or isolated hypogonadotropic hypogonadism, is an important cause of secondary hypogonadism.[20] Few studies have specifically looked at the risk of T2DM in patients with CHH. Two small studies in about 20 men each with CHH showed that testosterone therapy in men with CHH was associated with improvement in HOMA-IR, QUICKI, and fasting insulin levels.[21,22] An interesting study showed that short-term (2 weeks) withdrawal of androgen therapy in patients with CHH was associated with significant elevation of fasting blood glucose and fasting insulin levels without any appreciable change in body composition.[23] This shows that compliance with therapy in case of CHH may have importance not only from androgenization point of view but also from a metabolic perspective.

At present, there are no clear guidelines for screening men with CHH for diabetes. In the absence of any specific guidelines on the same, we suggest the following:

- Compliance of androgen replacement therapy (either testosterone or gonadotropins) in men with CHH must be ensured to reduce the risk of the adverse metabolic consequences of hypogonadism. Studies have shown that correction of androgen deficiency provides protection from adverse metabolic disturbances. Additionally, even short-term withdrawal of testosterone in these patients is associated with worsening of insulin resistance
- In patients with CHH who are treated with adequate androgen replacement, the screening for T2DM may be as per the current recommendations for the general population. There is no evidence to suggest enhanced glucovigilance in patients with CHH who are treated and compliance of treatment is ensured.

### Glucovigilance in Men on Androgen Deprivation Therapy for Prostate Cancer

Androgen deprivation therapy for prostate cancer is in the form of either surgical orchiectomy which leads to hypergonadotropic hypogonadism or the use of gonadotropin-releasing hormone (GnRH) agonist which leads to hypogonadotropic hypogonadism.[24] Grossman et al. provide an excellent review of the metabolic effects of ADT.[25] Within 3 months of the commencement of ADT, there is increased visceral fat associated with an increase in insulin resistance. Continued therapy for a period greater than 1 year is associated with an increased risk of diabetes. The number needed to harm is one confirmed case of diabetes per 100 patients on ADT.[13]

In the light of available evidence, the following are suggested for glucovigilance:
- Men on ADT are undoubtedly at increased risk of worsening of metabolic health. Hence, lifestyle measures should be initiated or enhanced in these patients to prevent adverse metabolic consequences. Diet, exercise and smoking cessation should be encouraged
- Increased vigilance and, if necessary, intensification of therapy for pre-existing diabetes, hypertension and dyslipidemia must be considered
- Screening for diabetes, hypertension and dyslipidemia must be considered at baseline and every 3–6 months after commencement of ADT, at least for the first few years after commencement of therapy.

## Glucovigilance in Men with Acquired Hypogonadotropic Hypogonadism as Part of Hypopituitarism

Acquired hypogonadotropic hypogonadism may result from any intervention or disease that impacts pituitary and hypothalamic function. Surgery of the pituitary gland and/or associated radiotherapy may induce hypopituitarism.[26]

Multiple factors affect insulin sensitivity in hypopituitarism. On one hand, uncorrected central adrenal insufficiency may increase insulin sensitivity and may cause fasting hypoglycemia, hypogonadotropic hypogonadism may lead to insulin resistance. Additionally, treatment with exogenous glucocorticoids and growth hormone (GH) may have an impact on the risk of developing diabetes. Glucovigilance among these groups of patients is summarized as follows:
- The Endocrine Society guidelines recommend checking blood glucose levels every 6 months in patients on GH therapy for hypopituitarism
- Even in patients not on GH replacement, enhanced glucovigilance is advisable as glucocorticoid and androgen replacement is seldom optimal. However, because of the heterogeneity of the situation, monitoring should be individualized.

## Glucovigilance in Men with Klinefelter Syndrome

Klinefelter syndrome is the classical prototype for a man with hypergonadotropic hypogonadism. Increased insulin resistance in men with KS is very well-known. In fact, studies have shown that changes in body composition predate pubertal onset and hence, may be multifactorial and not limited to just hypogonadism.[13]

Almost one-third of patients with KS have abnormal oral glucose tolerance test (OGTT). In fact, the prevalence of abnormal OGTT in KS is so high that Salzano et al. suggested that KS should be considered a prediabetic condition. Additionally, patients with KS also have an increased risk of autoimmune disease.[27] Hence, the prevalence of type 1 diabetes mellitus is also 2.5 times higher in patients with KS compared to the general population.[28] While obesity is more common in KS as reported from a Korean registry, the prevalence of diabetes is high in even nonobese patients.[29]

There are also some characteristic differences between diabetes associated with KS compared to the general population. T2DM tends to occur almost a decade earlier, with the mean age of onset of diabetes around 30 years.[27] These patients also have increased mortality attributable to diabetes. Additionally, as described earlier, diabetes is associated with both obese and nonobese men with KS. Interestingly, testosterone replacement in these patients prevents the development of diabetes but has little impact on its course. Therefore, other factors beyond hypogonadism clearly play a role in the pathogenesis of diabetes.[27] Another interesting aspect of diabetes management in KS is that insulin does not seem to be very effective in the management of T2DM associated with KS.[30]

Considering the unique nature of diabetes in KS, we have summarized some suggestions for glucovigilance in KS:

- The screening for diabetes and dyslipidemia in KS should start earlier than the general population. Groth et al. have suggested that the screening must start at baseline at the time of diagnosis and then repeated every 3 months initially and then annually after the first few years[31]
- Presence of "categories of increased risk" (prediabetes) among patients with KS must be looked at seriously. Serious attempts must be made to delay the progression of diabetes using lifestyle measures. The threshold for the use of pharmacological therapy starting with metformin for prevention of diabetes should be lower
- Testosterone replacement in patients with KS may not prevent the development of diabetes in these patients unlike other patients with hypogonadism. Hence, the screening and preventive measures for diabetes must continue even with androgen replacement
- Once diagnosed to have diabetes, consideration must be given for medications like metformin and glucagon-like peptide-1 (GLP-1) receptor agonists which reduce fat and improve body composition in these patients in preference to sulfonylurea or insulin.[32] The role of sodium-glucose cotransporter-2 (SGLT-2) inhibitors merits exploration.

## Glucovigilance in Men with Hyperprolactinemia

Hyperprolactinemia in men may be due to medications which disturb the dopamine pathway or prolactin-producing pituitary adenomas. Hyperprolactinemia is associated with insulin resistance and increased risk of diabetes. It has also been observed that the treatment of hyperprolactinemia with dopamine agonists in patients with prolactinoma improves glucose metabolism.[6]

We have summarized the suggestions for glucovigilance in men with hyperprolactinemia:

- It is prudent to screen patients with hyperprolactinemia for diabetes at baseline considering the association between prolactin and T2DM
- Dopamine agonist therapy in patients with prolactinoma is shown to reduce the risk of diabetes. In fact, bromocriptine is used as a novel antidiabetic agent in T2DM patients. Hence, strong consideration should be given to appropriately treat these patients with a dopamine agonist.

# GONADAL VIGILANCE IN DIABETES MELLITUS AND METABOLIC SYNDROME

So far in this chapter, we have explored the need for glucovigilance in patients with hypogonadism. The corollary to the same is to screen for hypogonadism in patients with diabetes and MetS. However, when we discuss FAD, we have to understand that benefits of treatment with testosterone in these patients are less clear and hence screening must be looked at from a perspective of risk versus benefits derived from treatment. The evidence so far suggests that testosterone replacement is beneficial in patients with clear evidence of hypogonadism associated with MetS, while the risk of treatment outweigh the benefits in case of patients with MetS but no clear evidence of hypogonadism.[1]

## Screening for Hypogonadism in Patients with Diabetes and Metabolic Syndrome

Should all men with diabetes and MetS be screened for hypogonadism? This is a contentious question and the current Endocrine Society guidelines do not recommend screening for hypogonadism in patients with diabetes. Screening for testosterone deficiency is definitely indicated in patients if they have osteoporosis, infertility, erectile dysfunction, decreased libido or have a pituitary lesion, or are taking medications known to cause hypogonadism. However, diabetes is not listed as a condition in which active case finding should be considered.[1] Testing for hypogonadism in patients with T2DM must be considered in patients who present to the clinician with symptoms of hypogonadism such as reduced libido and erectile dysfunction. This is also consistent with the recommendations of the American Diabetes Association.[33]

There is limited information about sensitivity and specificity of various screening instruments like Androgen Deficiency in Aging Males, the Aging Males' Symptoms Rating Scale, the Massachusetts Male Aging Study Questionnaire, the Hypogonadism Impact of Symptoms Questionnaire, and the Sexual Arousal, Interest and Drive Scale. The Endocrine Society does not give a broad recommendation about the use of these instruments in screening men for hypogonadism.[1] ANDROTEST© (a structured interview for the screening of hypogonadism in patients with sexual dysfunction) is useful for screening male patients for hypogonadism and the score more than eight in this questionnaire correlates with lower calculated free testosterone levels.[34]

## Testing for Hypogonadism in Patients with Diabetes

Screening for androgen deficiency starts with the measurement of morning fasting total testosterone concentration. Since SHBG levels are typically reduced in patients with hypogonadism, measurement of SHBG and albumin to calculate free testosterone concentration must be considered in individuals with diabetes. If free testosterone assay with equilibrium dialysis is available, it may be the preferred initial test.[1] Low values must be reconfirmed by repeat test with evaluation of follicle-stimulating hormone (FSH) and LH to distinguish primary from secondary hypogonadism.

If a patient is found to have primary hypogonadism, a karyotype must be sent to rule out KS. As discussed earlier, diabetes is found in as much as 30–40% of patients with KS. Additionally, FAD in T2DM is mainly secondary (i.e. hypogonadotropic) and hence elevated FSH and LH levels are more likely to suggest an OAD in this population.

Secondary hypogonadism in patients with T2DM may be either organic or functional. Grossman et al. have suggested that total testosterone levels less than 140 ng/dL in patients with diabetes must be considered a red flag for screening for OAD.[13] To rule out other causes of secondary hypogonadism, prolactin levels must be assessed in most patients. Tests for iron saturation are useful in a population having a high genetic risk of hereditary hemochromatosis. Additionally, exogenous use of androgens and glucocorticoids or any other medications which can potentially cause hypogonadism, must be ruled out by taking a good clinical history.

An MRI of the pituitary is indicated in the following subset of patients with secondary hypogonadism:[1]
- Total testosterone levels less than 150 ng/dL
- Elevated prolactin (especially prolactin levels >100 pg/mL)
- Evidence of anterior pituitary hormone dysfunction
- Symptoms of tumor mass effect:
  - Visual field defect
  - A new-onset headache
  - Visual impairment.

## Treatment of Hypogonadism in Males with Type 2 Diabetes Mellitus

The first important step when treating males with hypogonadism in association with T2DM and MetS is to differentiate organic versus FAD. OAD must be treated in all cases (barring absolute noted contraindications to testosterone therapy). Some organic causes of hypogonadism like hyperprolactinemia may be corrected by treating the underlying cause rather than replacing testosterone. In most of the organic causes, treatment of hypogonadism is associated with improvement in body composition, reduction in hemoglobin A1c (HbA1c) and improvement in markers of atherosclerosis, and reduced risk of cardiovascular disease.[13]

Treating FAD associated with T2DM and MetS is controversial. The current Endocrine Society guidelines unambiguously recommend against treating asymptomatic men with low testosterone levels with T2DM as a means of improving glycemic control or reducing complications. Men with symptoms of hypogonadism and low testosterone levels and in whom organic causes of hypogonadism have been ruled out may be treated to improve the symptoms of erectile dysfunction, reduced libido, increase of muscle mass and improved well-being. Whether this leads to improved glycemic control and reduced risk of complications is unclear.[1]

## CONCLUSION

Obesity, MetS and T2DM have a bidirectional association with testosterone levels in men (Flowchart 2). Testosterone enhances the conversion of pluripotent stem cells to develop myocytes in preference to adipocytes leading to improved insulin sensitivity.

Hypogonadal men have increased risk of diabetes and MetS. Therefore, glucovigilance in patients diagnosed to have OAD is essential. Among the various organic causes of hypogonadism in males, specific recommendations for screening for diabetes can be given for ADT in men with prostate cancer and men having KS.

Metabolic syndrome and T2DM predate the development of functional hypogonadism though the mechanism for the same is unclear. Routine screening for hypogonadism in men with T2DM and MetS is not recommended. Those having symptoms of hypogonadism may be screened. Calculated or directly measured free testosterone is more useful in comparison to total testosterone because insulin resistance reduces SHBG levels. Treatment of OAD and symptomatic FAD in men with T2DM is suggested; however, treatment of asymptomatic men with low testosterone and FAD in T2DM is not recommended.

## REFERENCES

1. Bhasin S, Brito JP, Cunningham GR, et al. Testosterone Therapy in Men with Hypogonadism: An Endocrine Society. J Clin Endocrinol Metab. 2018;103(5):1715-44.
2. Singh R, Artaza JN, Taylor WE, et al. Androgens stimulate myogenic differentiation and inhibit adipogenesis in C3H 10T1/2 pluripotent cells through an androgen receptor-mediated pathway. Endocrinology. 2003;144(11):5081-8.
3. Mitsuhashi K, Senmaru T, Fukuda T, et al. Testosterone stimulates glucose uptake and GLUT4 translocation through LKB1/AMPK signaling in 3T3-L1 adipocytes. Endocrine. 2016;51(1):174-84.
4. Hanchang W, Semprasert N, Limjindaporn T, et al. Testosterone Protects Against Glucotoxicity-Induced Apoptosis of Pancreatic β-Cells (INS-1) and Male Mouse Pancreatic Islets. Endocrinology. 2013;154(11):4058-67.
5. Rana K, Fam BC, Clarke MV, et al. Increased adiposity in DNA binding-dependent androgen receptor knockout male mice associated with decreased voluntary activity and not insulin resistance. Am J Physiol Metab. 2011;301(5):E767-78.
6. Serri O, Li L, Mamputu JC, et al. The influences of hyperprolactinemia and obesity on cardiovascular risk markers: Effects of cabergoline therapy. Clin Endocrinol (Oxf). 2006;64(4):366-70.
7. Daimon M, Kamba A, Murakami H, et al. Association between serum prolactin levels and insulin resistance in non-diabetic men. PLoS One. 2017;12(4):e0175204.
8. Melmed S, Casanueva FF, Hoffman AR, et al. Diagnosis and treatment of hyperprolactinemia: An endocrine society clinical practice guideline. J Clin Endocrinol Metab. 2011;96(2):273-88.
9. Ding EL, Song Y, Malik VS, et al. Sex differences of endogenous sex hormones and risk of type 2 diabetes: a systematic review and meta-analysis. JAMA. 2006;295(11):1288-99.
10. Facchinetti F, Bizzarri M, Benvenga S, et al. Results from the International Consensus Conference on Myo-inositol and d-chiro-inositol in Obstetrics and Gynecology : the link between metabolic syndrome and PCOS. Eur J Obstet Gynecol Reprod Biol. 2015;195:72-6.
11. Corona G, Monami M, Rastrelli G, et al. Testosterone and metabolic syndrome: a meta-analysis study. J Sex Med. 2011;8(1):272-83.
12. Corona G, Rastrelli G, Monami M, et al. Hypogonadism as a risk factor for cardiovascular mortality in men: a meta-analytic study. Eur J Endocrinol. 2011;165(5):687-701.
13. Grossmann M. Testosterone and glucose metabolism in men: current concepts and controversies. J Endocrinol. 2014;220(3):R37-55.
14. Tajar A, Forti G, O'Neill TW, et al. Characteristics of secondary, primary, and compensated hypogonadism in aging men: evidence from the European Male Ageing Study. J Clin Endocrinol Metab. 2010;95(4):1810-8.
15. Sartorius G, Spasevska S, Idan A, et al. Serum testosterone, dihydrotestosterone and estradiol concentrations in older men self-reporting very good health: the healthy man study. Clin Endocrinol (Oxf). 2012;77(5):755-63.

16. Laaksonen DE, Niskanen L, Punnonen K, et al. The MetS and Smoking in Relation to Hypogonadism in Middle-Aged Men: A Prospective Cohort Study. J Clin Endocrinol Metab. 2005;90(2):712-9.
17. Yao QM, Wang B, An XF, et al. Testosterone level and risk of T2D in men: a systematic review and meta-analysis. Endocr Connect. 2018;7(1):220-31.
18. Farias JM, Tinetti M, Khoury M, et al. Low Testosterone Concentration and Atherosclerotic Disease Markers in Male Patients With T2D. J Clin Endocrinol Metab. 2014;99(12):4698-703.
19. Anawalt BD, Yeap BB. Conclusions about testosterone therapy and cardiovascular risk. Asian J Androl. 2018;20(2):152-3.
20. Boehm U, Bouloux PM, Dattani MT, et al. Expert consensus document: European Consensus Statement on congenital hypogonadotropic hypogonadism-pathogenesis, diagnosis and treatment. Nat Rev Endocrinol. 2015;11(9):547-64.
21. Wu X, Mao J, Lu S, et al. Testosterone replacement therapy improves insulin sensitivity and decreases high sensitivity C-reactive protein levels in hypogonadotropic hypogonadal young male patients. Chin Med J (Engl). 2009;122(23):2846-50.
22. Naharci M, Pinar M, Bolu E, et al. Effect of Testosterone on Insulin Sensitivity in Men with Idiopathic Hypogonadotropic Hypogonadism. Endocr Pract. 2007;13(6):629-35.
23. Yialamas MA, Dwyer AA, Hanley E, et al. Acute Sex Steroid Withdrawal Reduces Insulin Sensitivity in Healthy Men with Idiopathic Hypogonadotropic Hypogonadism. J Clin Endocrinol Metab. 2007;92(11):4254-9.
24. Golabek T, Belsey J, Drewa T, et al. Evidence-based recommendations on androgen deprivation therapy for localized and advanced prostate cancer. Cent Eur J Urol. 2016;69(2):131-8.
25. Grossmann M, Zajac JD. Androgen deprivation therapy in men with prostate cancer: How should the side effects be monitored and treated? Clin Endocrinol (Oxf). 2011;74(3):289-93.
26. Fleseriu M, Hashim IA, Karavitaki N, et al. Hormonal replacement in hypopituitarism in adults: An endocrine society clinical practice guideline. J Clin Endocrinol Metab. 2016;101(11):3888-921.
27. Salzano A, D'Assante R, Heaney LM, et al. Klinefelter syndrome, insulin resistance, MetS, and diabetes: review of literature and clinical perspectives. Endocrine. 2018;61(2):194-203.
28. Bojesen A, Birkebæk NH, Juul S, et al. Morbidity in Klinefelter Syndrome: A Danish Register Study Based on Hospital Discharge Diagnoses. J Clin Endocrinol Metab. 2006;91(4):1254-60.
29. Han SJ, Kim KS, Kim W, et al. Obesity and Hyperglycemia in Korean Men with Klinefelter Syndrome: The Korean Endocrine Society Registry. Endocrinol Metab (Seoul). 2016;31(4):598-603.
30. Nielsen J, Johansen K, Yde H. Frequency of diabetes mellitus in patients with Klinefelter's syndrome of different chromosome constitutions and the XYY syndrome. Plasma insulin and growth hormone level after a glucose load. J Clin Endocrinol Metab. 1969;29(8):1062-73.
31. Groth KA, Skakkebæk A, Høst C, et al. Klinefelter syndrome—A clinical update. J Clin Endocrinol Metab. 2013;98(1):20-30.
32. Giagulli VA, Carbone MD, Ramunni MI, et al. Adding liraglutide to lifestyle changes, metformin and testosterone therapy boosts erectile function in diabetic obese men with overt hypogonadism. Andrology. 2015;3(6):1094-103.
33. American Diabetes Association. Diabetes Care: Standards of Medical Care in Diabetes—2018. Diabetes Care. 2018;41(Suppl 1):S3-159.
34. Corona G, Mannucci E, Petrone L, et al. ANDROTEST©: A structured interview for the screening of hypogonadism in patients with sexual dysfunction. J Sex Med. 2006;3(4):706-15.

# CHAPTER 9

# Glucocrinology of Reproductive System: Female

*Lakshmana Perumal Nandhini, Dayakshi DK Abeyaratne, Gagan Priya*

## INTRODUCTION

The subject of female reproductive endocrinology deals with a study of reproductive health and sexual function in women. The primary function of the reproductive system is procreation and maintenance of progeny. What is often overlooked is that the hypothalamic–pituitary–ovarian (HPO) axis is a complex endocrine axis that works in close harmony with other endocrine and metabolic pathways in a bidirectional manner. In fact, female reproductive hormones play an important role in the regulation of feeding behavior, maintenance of body weight and metabolism. The physiological changes across the lifespan of a woman impact her metabolic status. Pregnancy is associated with a physiological increase in insulin resistance (IR) that may lead to gestational diabetes in at-risk women. Following menopause, the protective effects of estrogen are lost with a resultant rise in the incidence of diabetes and cardiovascular disease.

Several female reproductive disorders are often associated with increased risk of diabetes and metabolic syndrome (MS). Likewise, diabetes itself alters the hormonal milieu and impacts reproductive and sexual health of women. In this chapter, we discuss the reciprocal interaction between female reproductive physiology and glucose and energy homeostasis in health and disease.

## GLUCOSE PHYSIOLOGY IN RELATION TO FEMALE REPRODUCTIVE SYSTEM

### Effects of Estrogen on Metabolism

The predominant circulating form of estrogen in women, 17β-estradiol, is synthesized by the ovaries. In men and postmenopausal women, estradiol is largely synthesized in extragonadal sites like adipose tissue, breast, muscle and bone through aromatization of androgens and exerts its actions in a paracrine or intracrine manner. The actions of

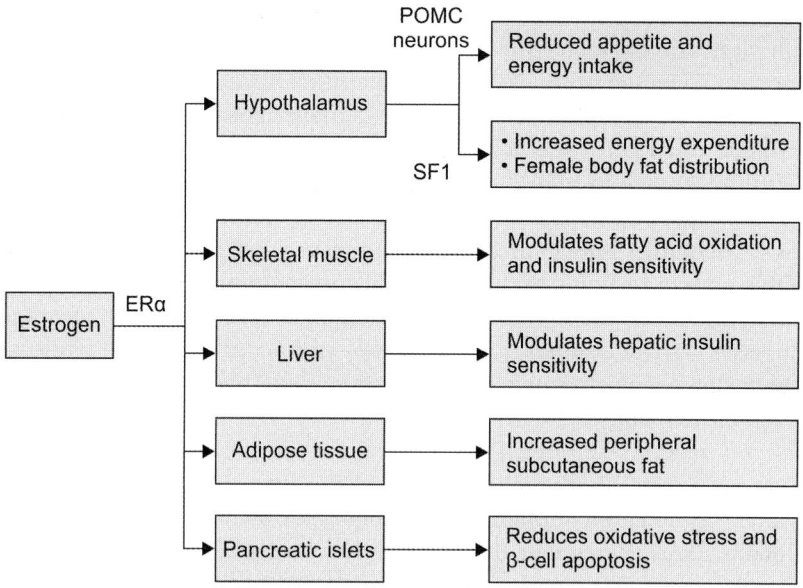

**FLOWCHART 1:** Effects of estrogen on energy homeostasis and metabolism.

(ERα: estrogen receptor alpha; POMC: pro-opiomelanocortin; SF1: steroidogenic factor-1)

estrogens are mediated through two isoforms of estrogen receptors (ERs)—(1) ERα and (2) ERβ. Majority of the metabolic actions are mediated through the ERα isoform.[1]

The effects of estrogen on metabolism and energy homeostasis can be summarized as here and are delineated in Flowchart 1:

- *Central actions to regulate food intake and energy balance*: Estrogens play a major role in regulating food intake and energy expenditure. Among mammals, feeding behavior varies with the ovarian cycle. Food intake is reduced during peri-ovulatory period, when plasma estrogen level peaks.[1]

  Estrogen receptors are abundantly expressed in various hypothalamic nuclei involved in energy balance, namely, ventromedial (VMN) nucleus, arcuate nucleus, medial preoptic and paraventricular nuclei.[1] Stimulation of ERs results in a surge in excitatory impulse to the pro-opiomelanocortin (POMC) neurons in the arcuate nucleus, that secrete alpha-melanocyte-stimulating hormone (α-MSH) causing marked reduction in appetite and food intake and an increase in energy expenditure. ERα expressed in VMH neurons mediates thermogenesis, physical activity and body fat distribution without affecting food intake. Estradiol also suppresses food intake by enhancing the actions of cholecystokinin on satiety.

  Estrogens increase the sensitivity of target nuclei to the actions of leptin, an adipokine secreted by adipose tissue.[2] Leptin reduces food intake and promotes energy expenditure. Supplementation of estrogen also suppressed ghrelin, a gut-derived orexigenic hormone and reduced food intake and body weight in ovariectomized rats. The anorexigenic action of estrogen is further mediated by attenuating the expression of neuropeptide Y (NPY) and agouti-related peptide (AgRP) in the arcuate nucleus[1]

- *Regulation of body fat distribution*: Estrogen influences body fat distribution resulting in the characteristic sex-specific deposition of adipose tissue. In premenopausal women, adipose tissue is predominantly distributed in subcutaneous and gluteofemoral region. In men and postmenopausal women, there is greater intra-abdominal and visceral fat.[3] Intra-abdominal fat depots probably provided survival advantage to men during early evolution, where rapid mobilization of adipose tissue was crucial for providing energy during hunting and protection against predators. Subcutaneous adipose tissue, on the other hand, provides a stable source of lipids and fuel which ensures maintenance of reproductive capacity and meets the increased energy demands during lactation.[3] Estrogen also suppresses fatty acid uptake, adipogenesis and accumulation of white adipose tissue by down regulating enzymes like fatty acid synthase, acetyl-CoA carboxylase and lipoprotein lipase
- *Effects on insulin sensitivity*: Physiological concentrations of estrogens promote insulin sensitivity in both men and women. The estrogen action on muscle insulin sensitivity is mediated through ERα.[1] Though the exact mechanism is still a matter of debate, ERα may regulate downstream insulin signaling, AKt phosphorylation and p38 mitogen-activated protein kinase (MAPK) pathways. It may improve hepatic insulin sensitivity by suppressing hepatic lipogenesis, lipid accumulation and lipotoxicity. Deficiency of ERα is associated with hepatic IR
- *Effects on pancreatic beta-cell function*: Animal models offer insight into the β-cell protective actions of estrogen. Treatment of nonobese diabetic mouse with estrogen prevented insulitis and development of type 1 diabetes mellitus (T1DM) by restoring the immunomodulatory function of natural killer cells.[1] Estrogen reduced oxidative stress and β-cell apoptosis. In rodent models of type 2 diabetes mellitus (T2DM), estrogen suppressed lipogenesis and accumulation of fatty acid intermediates in β-cells and offered protection from lipotoxicity. Estrogens may also enhance insulin secretion and β-cell sensitivity to stimuli like glucose.[1] The insulinotropic action is particularly important in pregnancy to overcome IR and enhanced metabolic needs.

## Effects of Progestins on Metabolism

Progestins enhance basal as well as glucose-stimulated insulin secretion, but this effect is mediated at high progestin levels such as those seen during pregnancy.[4] This effect is potentiated by estrogen. On the other hand, 19-nortestosterone derivatives have been associated with impaired insulin sensitivity and glucose intolerance, an effect not seen with second- or third-generation progestins.[4] Medroxyprogesterone acetate (MPA) has glucocorticoid activity and may increase IR.

## Effects of Androgens on Female Metabolism

The effects of androgens on metabolism seem to be sex-specific. In men, testosterone deficiency is associated with visceral obesity and IR and testosterone replacement improves insulin sensitivity.[5] The effects of androgen receptor on metabolism in females are not well-understood, though it seems to be in contrast to men.

# CHAPTER 9: Glucocrinology of Reproductive System: Female

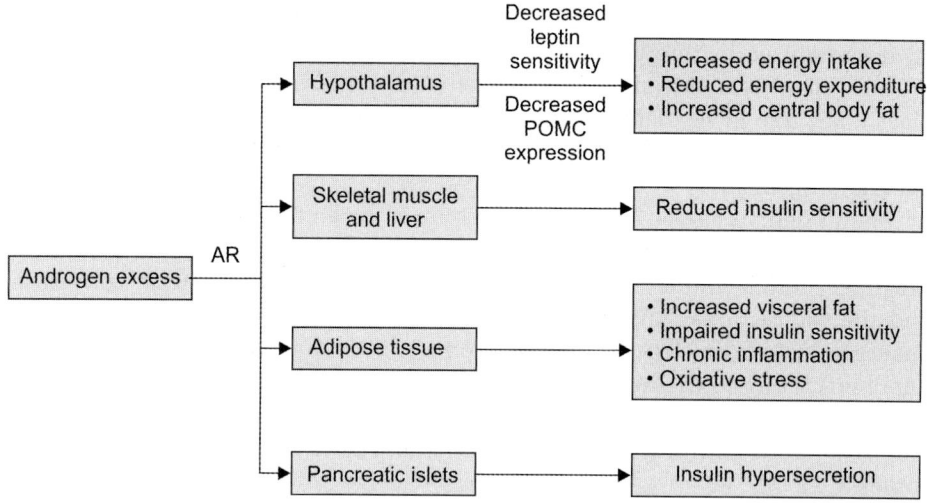

(AR: androgen receptor; POMC: pro-opiomelanocortin)

**FLOWCHART 2:** Metabolic effects of androgen excess in females.

Hyperandrogenism in women is associated with IR and increased risk of diabetes. Low sex hormone-binding globulin (SHBG) and high free testosterone levels have been associated with increased incidence of T2DM among women of reproductive age as well as postmenopausal women.[5]

Androgen excess in women increases skeletal muscle IR and visceral adiposity, both by reducing brown adipose tissue thermogenesis and by central action via melanocortin system. These improve partially with treatment of the hyperandrogenic state. Hyperandrogenic women also exhibit pancreatic β-cell dysfunction, though exact mechanism is not well-understood.[6] This may be due to oxidative stress, chronic inflammation, direct effect on β-cell, or a result of compensatory failure to IR. The metabolic effects of androgen excess in females are depicted in Flowchart 2.

## Effects of Metabolic Health on Reproductive Health

The relationship between female reproductive physiology and energy balance is not a one-way street. Adipose tissue and the gastrointestinal tract secrete several hormones (leptin, resistin, adiponectin, ghrelin, NPY and AgRP) that not only influence energy intake and expenditure, but also modulate HPO axis. Energy status modulates reproductive function at multiple levels:

- Hypothalamic gonadotropin-releasing hormone (GnRH) and pituitary gonadotropin secretion through the effect of several neuropeptides and hormones
- Regulation of ovarian steroidogenesis and folliculogenesis, by interaction with growth hormone-IGF-insulin system and local mediators.[7]

It is not surprising that the hypothalamic arcuate nucleus is involved in the regulation of both metabolism and reproductive function. Kisspeptin and GnRH neurons sense changes in glucose availability and glucose is involved in the hypothalamic regulation of luteinizing hormone (LH) secretion.[7] Glucose is also a major substrate for oocytes and embryo. In addition, the adipose tissue is an important endocrine gland, involved in the conversion of precursor steroids to estrogen by aromatization in both men and women. The insulin receptor also plays a key role in regulating fertility at the ovarian level. Hyperinsulinemia with increased signaling through IR is associated with ovulatory dysfunction and hyperandrogenism.

Energy deficits as well as energy excess are associated with altered reproductive physiology and affect steroidogenesis, folliculogenesis, fertilization, implantation, pregnancy and lactation.[7] All these reproductive functions are energy consuming and the bidirectional talk between metabolic health and reproductive system ensures adequate nutrient availability. A critical body mass is required for initiation of puberty. Long-term undernutrition can suppress female reproductive function, as seen in functional hypothalamic amenorrhea. On the other hand, obesity may also interfere with HPO axis function and lead to ovulatory dysfunction and subfertility.

## Glycemic Variability during Menstrual Cycle

Fluctuations in sex hormone levels during various phases of the menstrual cycle are known to affect insulin sensitivity, with an increase in IR noted prior to ovulation and a peak during luteal phase. While these changes may not be clinically significant in normal women, few women with brittle T1DM may experience clinically significant variability in glycemic control. Few studies have reported reduced incidence of hypoglycemic episodes and a greater incidence of hyperglycemia during luteal phase in women with T1DM.[8]

## Glucose Physiology during Pregnancy

Pregnancy is associated with significant and dynamic metabolic changes over the gestational period.[9] Early pregnancy is an anabolic state (a net increase in maternal triglycerides and fat accumulation) primarily due to an increase in insulin secretion, with little change in insulin sensitivity. This anabolic state is accompanied by increased energy intake.

There occurs a switch from anabolic to a net catabolic state in later gestation to meet the increased energy demands of both the mother and the fetus. The lipid deposits are a source of fuel for maternal requirements, while glucose is preferentially spared as fuel for the growing fetus. The catabolic phase is associated with an increase in liver gluconeogenesis, adipose tissue lipolysis and ketogenesis. This switch is mediated by a physiological rise in IR, attributed to the effect of placental hormones [placental lactogen (PL), human placental growth hormone] and adipose tissue cytokines (tumor necrosis factor-$\alpha$).[9] A compensatory rise in insulin secretion and an expansion of $\beta$-cell mass maintains the glucose concentration in a narrow range. In fact, this increase in insulin secretion occurs prior to the onset of IR and is postulated to be mediated by PL, prolactin, hepatic growth factor, progestins and estrogen.[10] Gestational diabetes mellitus (GDM) may result from an inability to compensate for the physiological impairment of insulin sensitivity. Following delivery, these metabolic changes revert rapidly with restoration of insulin sensitivity.

# GLUCOVIGILANCE IN DISORDERS OF FEMALE REPRODUCTIVE TRACT

Several female reproductive disorders are associated with abnormal metabolism with an increased risk of obesity, MS and diabetes. This calls for a need for glucovigilance and metabolic vigilance when managing these patients.

## Polycystic Ovary Syndrome

Polycystic ovary syndrome (PCOS) is the most common endocrine disorder in reproductive age women. The clinical presentation of PCOS spans a spectrum, ranging from menstrual irregularities, acne and hirsutism in adolescent girls and young women, to concerns over fertility. However, it is being increasingly recognized that the syndrome extends beyond reproductive health and has long-term cardiometabolic implications.

### Pathophysiological Links with Insulin Resistance

Polycystic ovary syndrome is a complex disorder resulting from an interaction between genetic, metabolic and environmental factors. Several pathophysiological mechanisms have been described to explain the development of this syndrome, including gonadotropin dysfunction with increased LH secretion and excess ovarian and adrenal androgen secretion.

Intrinsic IR, often compounded by extrinsic IR due to obesity and hyperinsulinemia, has been recognized as a key pathogenic factor in PCOS. A postreceptor defect in insulin sensitivity associated with hyperinsulinemia may independently contribute hyperandrogenism and ovulatory dysfunction through several mechanisms, as delineated in Flowchart 3. Hyperinsulinemia worsens hyperandrogenemia by directly stimulating ovarian androgen secretion, augmenting LH-mediated effects on androgen secretion, and reducing SHBG levels.[11] Also, it promotes proliferation of ovarian theca cells. Hyperandrogenism, in turn, can induce IR at the level of adipose tissue and skeletal muscle, promoting a vicious cycle.[11]

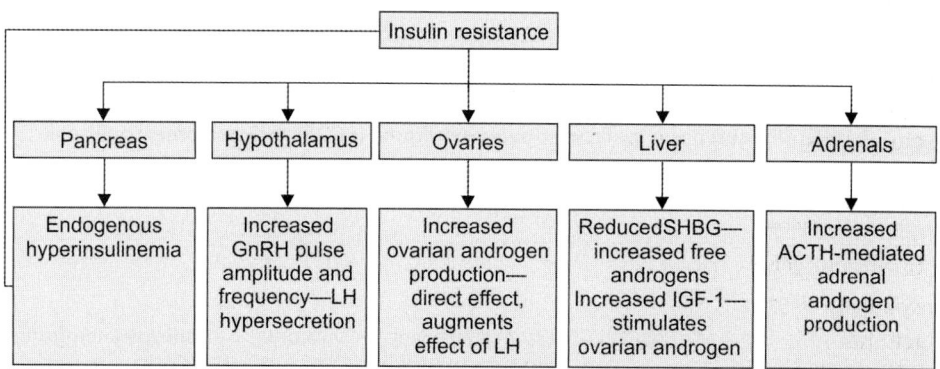

(ACTH: adrenocorticotropic hormone; GnRH: gonadotropin-releasing hormone; IGF-1: insulin-like growth factor-1; LH: luteinizing hormone; SHBG: sex hormone-binding globulin)

**FLOWCHART 3:** Insulin resistance in the pathogenesis of polycystic ovary syndrome.

A large percentage of women with PCOS are overweight or obese, with prevalence rates varying from 30% to 80%, depending on the population studied. IR is noted in 75% of lean and 95% of obese women with PCOS in clamp studies.[12] While obesity is not required for the development of PCOS, it may further compound the underlying pathophysiological defects and lead to a more severe clinical phenotype. In fact, IR is highest among women with hyperandrogenemia and obesity.[13] IR is accompanied by compensatory hyperinsulinemia but there may be subtle insulin secretory defects, primarily related to first-phase insulin release.[14]

## Risk of Diabetes and Metabolic Syndrome in Polycystic Ovary Syndrome

Understandably, PCOS is associated with abnormal glucose metabolism and an increased risk of diabetes. Approximately, 30–40% of reproductive age PCOS women may have impaired glucose tolerance (IGT) and 10% have been reported to have overt diabetes.[15] This risk has been described even in lean PCOS women.

Diabetes may manifest at a younger age and comparatively lower body mass index (BMI) in PCOS compared to non-PCOS women. The overall risk for diabetes is 2–3-fold, while obesity increases the risk up to 3–5-fold. The rate of progression from normal glucose tolerance (NGT) to IGT and T2DM is 5–15% within 5 years and over 50% within 10 years.[15] Increasing age, obesity and a family history of diabetes are associated with greater risk. Certain PCOS phenotypes, as depicted in Table 1 that are characterized by hyperandrogenism [phenotypes A and B or the National Institutes of Health (NIH) phenotypes], are associated with greater metabolic risk.[15] The risk of PCOS is also reported to be higher in girls with T1DM (12–19%), but this seems to be a consequence of treatment-related supraphysiological systemic insulin levels and weight gain.[16]

Women with PCOS are at a greater risk for developing MS [odds ratio (OR) 3.35; 95% confidence interval (CI) 2.44, 4.59].[17] The prevalence of MS was found to be greater among women with PCOS even after adjusting for BMI, emphasizing the role of intrinsic IR in the pathophysiology of PCOS and its complications. A recent meta-analysis of studies in women with PCOS and lean body habitus, however, found no increase in the risk of MS.[17]

**TABLE 1** Phenotypes of polycystic ovary syndrome (PCOS) and cardiometabolic risk.

| Diagnostic criteria | Phenotype A | Phenotype B | Phenotype C | Phenotype D |
|---|---|---|---|---|
| Oligoanovulation | + | + | – | + |
| Hyperandrogenism | + | + | + | – |
| PCO morphology | + | – | + | + |
| Alternate nomenclature | Classic PCOS | Essential National Institutes of Health criteria | Ovulatory PCOS | Nonhyperandrogenic PCOS |

*Note:* Phenotypes A and B are associated with more insulin resistance and greater cardiometabolic risk. Women with phenotypes C and D have normal insulin sensitivity or mild insulin resistance.

## Screening for Diabetes in Women with Polycystic Ovary Syndrome

All women with PCOS should be assessed for weight, BMI and waist circumference, clinical features of IR and blood pressure. The Androgen Excess Society guidelines recommend that all women with PCOS should be screened using a 75-g oral glucose tolerance test (OGTT).[18] Since postprandial hyperglycemia predominates in early stages, fasting plasma glucose (FPG) may not be sufficient. For those with normal OGTT, periodic testing is advised every 3–5 years. However, high-risk women (obese, age >40 years, previous GDM, or family history of diabetes) should be screened every 1–2 years.[18] Guidelines recommend against the measurement of serum insulin levels as they do not add to the therapeutic decision. Serum lipids should be monitored at least every 2 years.

## Glucocrinological Issues in Management of Polycystic Ovary Syndrome

The concomitant presence of PCOS and metabolic risk raises several dilemmas in management. Weight loss of 5–10% is associated with improvement in both reproductive and metabolic manifestations and therefore, lifestyle modification should be recommended.

- *Use of antidiabetic medications in PCOS*: Several antidiabetic drugs have been evaluated for their role in PCOS. Insulin sensitizers including metformin and pioglitazone lead to significant improvements in IR and may improve symptoms related to hyperandrogenism, menstrual irregularities and subfertility. Metformin use results in small but significant improvements in weight, menstrual cyclicity, ovulation rates and clinical pregnancy rates. Therefore, it should be considered as the first-line drug in women with PCOS and diabetes. It may also be used in women with IGT if they do not improve with lifestyle modification.[15] Pioglitazone carries the risk of teratogenicity and therefore, it may not be suitable in women of reproductive age.

    Small studies with glucagon-like peptide-1 (GLP-1) receptor agonists including exenatide and liraglutide have shown significant improvement in PCOS phenotype and can be considered, especially in obese PCOS women with diabetes. Sodium-glucose cotransporter-2 (SGLT-2) inhibitors are associated with significant weight reduction but, their role in PCOS is uncertain. However, in women planning pregnancy, caution must be used with antidiabetic medications, as the effects of fetal exposure have not been ascertained

- *Role of statins in PCOS*: PCOS is associated with increased prevalence of several cardiovascular risk factors, including obesity, diabetes or IGT, MS, hypertension, dyslipidemia, endothelial dysfunction and chronic inflammation. Statins lead to significant improvements in lipid parameters and have anti-inflammatory properties. In addition, they may ameliorate hyperandrogenic features to a small extent. But they may have a teratogenic effect and guidelines do not recommend the routine use of statins in PCOS[15]

- *Effect of PCOS therapy on metabolic risk*: Combined oral contraceptives (COCs) are often used as first-line drugs for the management of menstrual irregularity and hyperandrogenism in PCOS. COCs contain supraphysiological doses of estrogen and may be associated with weight gain, IR, an abnormal effect on glucose and lipid metabolism and increase in blood pressure. The adverse metabolic risk depends on the dose of estrogen and type of progestin. The effect of low-dose estrogen preparations (20–35 µg) on glucose metabolism seems to be minimal.[18] Androgenic progestins such as norethindrone have greater adverse metabolic effect, while antiandrogenic progestins (drospirenone, cyproterone acetate) seems to have minimal effect but greater thromboembolic risk. COCs are associated with an increased risk of venous thromboembolism that must be considered especially in women with cardiometabolic risk factors.[15]

On the other hand, progestogen-only contraceptives (POCs) have less metabolic impact. Antiandrogenic drugs such as spironolactone that have a neutral effect on metabolic milieu can be used in conjunction with POCs in high-risk women.[15]

- *Pregnancy planning and risk of GDM*: Prenatal counseling should include advice on weight reduction, lifestyle modification, assessment and optimization of glycemic and blood pressure control. However, potentially teratogenic drugs should be discontinued prior to conception. While metformin can be safely continued, many diabetic women with PCOS will require insulin initiation during pregnancy.[15] In addition, GDM has been observed in almost 50% of women with PCOS and is associated with increased risk of maternal and fetal complications. Therefore, screening for GDM should be universal and treatment should be initiated promptly.

## Glucovigilance in Turner Syndrome

About 10–34% of Turner syndrome (TS) patients have IGT and TS is associated with an increased risk of both T1DM and T2DM.[19] The underlying mechanisms for this risk are not entirely clear, but it may result for the deletion of specific genes on the X-chromosome (Xp haplotype insufficiency) that are involved in β-cell function. Thus, impaired insulin secretion seems to be the primary mechanism of dysglycemia in TS.[19] In addition, most studies have demonstrated that TS is also associated with increased IR. This may be due to concomitant central obesity, resulting from reduced physical fitness and sedentary lifestyle. TS is also associated with increased risk of autoimmune diseases due to X-chromosome haploinsufficiency, including T1DM.

### Screening for Diabetes in Turner Syndrome

The International Guidelines recommend that all girls with TS should undergo routine screening for glucose abnormalities with hemoglobin A1c (HbA1c) and FPG at least once a year, starting at 10 years age. Lipid profile should be monitored from 18 years onward, especially in those with cardiovascular risk factors.[20]

### Glucocrinological Considerations of Treatment in Turner Syndrome

Growth hormone is used in many girls with TS for optimization of height and there are concerns that it may exacerbate IR. However, prospective data does not suggest that GH therapy in TS girls is associated with increased risk of diabetes.[19,20]

Hormone replacement therapy (HRT) remains the cornerstone of management. Estrogen has a positive influence on insulin signaling and β-cell function, but some studies have raised the concern that estrogen replacement may aggravate IR. The studies of effect of HRT on metabolic health of TS have demonstrated mixed results, with some showing increased risk of IGT, while others showing no to beneficial effects on glucose metabolism.[19,20] Transdermal estradiol preparations that bypass liver have the least metabolic effects, but there is insufficient evidence for the same.

## Glucovigilance in Menopause

In addition to symptoms like mood disturbances, hot flashes and deterioration of bone health, menopause is associated with an increased risk of cardiometabolic diseases. This has been attributed to a dramatic and sudden reduction in estrogen levels. Given the metabolic effects of estrogens, menopause is characterized by changes in body composition, reduced energy expenditure, impairment of insulin sensitivity and reduced insulin secretion. The perimenopausal transition period is associated with increase in central adiposity, decreased basal metabolic rate and reduced lean body mass. The resultant IR along with aging increases the risk of diabetes. An early and/or surgical menopause has been associated with greater diabetes risk.[21]

### Prevalence of Metabolic Syndrome and Diabetes in Postmenopausal Women

In fact, menopause is an independent risk factor for MS, regardless of age. The prevalence of MS among postmenopausal women has been reported to be higher than that of the general population.[22] A recent meta-analysis of 31 studies reported a greater prevalence of MS components in postmenopausal women when compared to menstruating women. Serum triglyceride and low-density cholesterol levels were raised by a mean of 20.44 mg/dL and 20.77 mg/dL in postmenopausal women. It was also seen that surgical menopause was associated with greater odds of MS when compared to naturally attained menopause.[22]

Epidemiological studies assessing the impact of menopause on diabetes risk, however, have not found a significant association with menopausal status. However, diabetes prevalence has been reported to be higher in women with premature menopause and those with a shorter reproductive lifespan.[23] But at the same time, high endogenous estrogen levels in postmenopausal women have also been associated with increased diabetes risk, possibly attributed to obesity.[23] Most endogenous estrogen in postmenopausal women is derived from aromatization of androgens in adipose tissue. Such a risk has not been demonstrated with HRT.

The impact of diabetes mellitus on the age of menopause is controversial. The increased prevalence of premature ovarian insufficiency (POI) among women with T1DM, due to the shared risk of autoimmunity, is known. Few studies on women with T1DM have reported earlier onset of menopause while other studies (Ovarian Ageing in Type 1 Diabetes Mellitus and the Epidemiology of Diabetes Interventions and Complications) have not shown the same. However, advanced micro vascular complications are likely to be associated with an earlier menopause.[24]

### Glucocrinological Considerations of Hormone Replacement Therapy

Hormone replacement therapy can reverse the adverse metabolic effects associated with menopause. Redistribution of body fat, enhanced lipid oxidation, energy expenditure and improved insulin sensitivity have been demonstrated with HRT.[25,26] The beneficial effects of HRT are experienced by both women with and without diabetes. The Heart and Estrogen/Progestin Replacement Study (HERS) and the Women's Health Initiative (WHI) study reported a reduction in the incidence of T2DM in women receiving HRT by 35% and 21%, respectively.[27,28] However, HRT cannot be recommended for diabetes prevention.

Oral administration of estrogen has a stronger effect on reducing IR when compared to the transdermal route, which bypasses the hepatic first-pass metabolism. Ironically, the increased hepatic exposure to estrogen is also responsible for the increased synthesis of triglycerides, C-reactive protein and clotting factors, which contribute to adverse effects. The addition of progesterone to estrogen in HRT seems to offset the glycemic benefits in a dose-dependent manner. Natural and nonandrogenic progestogens like norethisterone and dydrogesterone are neutral in this regard and are preferred.

Among women with T2DM, menopausal hormonal therapy (MHT) may improve glycemic control and components of MS.[29] The increased risk of cardiovascular disease among patients with diabetes was perceived as a deterrent to HRT in the past. However, the benefits of HRT in carefully selected women, after a thorough assessment of cardiovascular risk factors, seem to outweigh the risks.

## GONADAL VIGILANCE IN DIABETES

Metabolic syndrome, obesity and T2DM are important risk factors for the development of type 1 endometrial cancer. The relative risk for endometrial cancer among patients with MS is 1.89 (95% CI 1.34–2.67).[30] MS also predisposes to more advanced and aggressive endometrial cancer. The hyperestrogenic state that results from increased conversion of androgens to estrogens in the adipose tissue and hyperinsulinemia are believed to be key factors that initiate endometrial hyperplasia. The risk for benign endometrial pathologies like endometrial polyps and hyperplasia, without atypia, is also increased.

Central obesity and IR can also increase the risk of uterine fibroids. IR results in the upregulation of serum insulin-like growth factor-1 and epidermal growth factor levels which contribute to the development of uterine fibroid through direct action on myometrium and by promoting ovarian hormone secretion.[31]

In addition, diabetes itself impacts the reproductive health of women including the age of menarche, ovulatory and endometrial functions, fertility and fecundity. Diabetes poses unique challenges during pregnancy and lactation. These are discussed in the Chapter "Reproductive Health in Diabetes".

## CONCLUSION

Estrogen is a key player in several processes that regulate metabolism and energy homeostasis. On the other hand, androgen excess in women is associated with IR.

Female reproductive disorders are often associated with increased risk of diabetes and MS. PCOS shares a common pathophysiological and bidirectional link with IR and diabetes. The risk of diabetes is also higher in women with TS and POI. Similarly, cardiometabolic risk rises steeply after menopause and may be reduced with HRT. Likewise, diabetes itself alters the hormonal milieu and impacts the reproductive and sexual health and fertility in women. An understanding of glucocrinology of female reproductive system is crucial to improving clinical care in both obstetrics and gynecology and endocrinology practices.

## REFERENCES

1. Mauvais-Jarvis F, Clegg DJ, Hevener AL. The role of estrogens in control of energy balance and glucose homeostasis. Endocr Rev. 2013;34(3):309-38.
2. Ainslie DA, Morris MJ, Wittert G, et al. Estrogen deficiency causes central leptin insensitivity and increased hypothalamic neuropeptide Y. Int J Obes Relat Metab Disord. 2001;25(11):1680-8.
3. Enzi G, Gasparo M, Biondetti PR, et al. Subcutaneous and visceral fat distribution according to sex, age, and overweight, evaluated by computed tomography. Am J Clin Nutr. 1986;44(6):739-46.
4. Beck P. Effect of progestins on glucose and lipid metabolism. Ann N Y Acad Sci. 1977;286:434-45.
5. Navarro G, Allard C, Xu W, et al. The role of androgens in metabolism, obesity, and diabetes in males and females. Obesity (Silver Spring). 2015;23(4):713-9.
6. Schiffer L, Kempegowda P, Arlt W, et al. Mechanisms in endocrinology: The sexually dimorphic role of androgens in human metabolic disease. Eur J Endocrinol. 2017;177(3):R125-43.
7. Garcia-Garcia RM. Integrative control of energy balance and reproduction in females. ISRN Vet Sci. 2012;2012:121389.
8. Barata DS, Adan LF, Netto EM, et al. The effect of the menstrual cycle on glucose control in women with type 1 diabetes evaluated using a continuous glucose monitoring system. Diabetes Care. 2013;36(5):e70.
9. Zeng Z, Liu F, Li S. Metabolic Adaptations in Pregnancy: A Review. Ann Nutr Metab. 2017;70(1):59-65.
10. Moyce BL, Dolinsky VW. Maternal β-Cell Adaptations in Pregnancy and Placental Signalling: Implications for Gestational Diabetes. Int J Mol Sci. 2018;19(11):E3467.
11. Dumesic DA, Oberfield SE, Stener-Victorin E, et al. Scientific Statement on the Diagnostic Criteria, Epidemiology, Pathophysiology, and Molecular Genetics of Polycystic Ovary Syndrome. Endocr Rev. 2015;36(5):487-525.
12. Stepto NK, Cassar S, Joham AE, et al. Women with polycystic ovary syndrome have intrinsic insulin resistance on euglycaemic-hyperinsulaemic clamp. Hum Reprod. 2013;28(3):777-84.
13. Barber TM, Wass JAH, McCarthy MI, et al. Metabolic characteristics of women with polycystic ovaries and oligo-amenorrhoea but normal androgen levels: implications for the management of polycystic ovary syndrome. Clin Endocrinol (Oxf). 2007;66(4):513-7.
14. Holte J. Disturbances in insulin secretion and sensitivity in women with the polycystic ovary syndrome. Baillieres Clin Endocrinol Metab. 1996;10(2):221-47.
15. Glintborg D, Andersen M. Management of endocrine disease: morbidity in polycystic ovary syndrome. Eur J Endocrinol. 2017;176(2):R53-65.
16. Codner E, Cassorla F. Puberty and ovarian function in girls with type 1 diabetes mellitus. Horm Res. 2009;71(1):12-21.
17. Lim SS, Kakoly NS, Tan JW, et al. Metabolic syndrome in polycystic ovary syndrome: a systematic review, meta-analysis and meta-regression. Obes Rev. 2019;20(2):339-52.
18. Goodman NF, Cobin RH, Futterweit W, et al. American Association of Clinical Endocrinologists, American College of Endocrinology, and Androgen Excess and PCOS Society Disease State Clinical Review: Guide to the Best Practices in the Evaluation and Treatment of Polycystic Ovary Syndrome - Part 2. Endocr Pract. 2015;21(12):1415-26.
19. Sun L, Wang Y, Zhou T, et al. Glucose Metabolism in Turner Syndrome. Front Endocrinol (Lausanne). 2019;10:49.

## SECTION 1: The Scope of Glucocrinology

20. Gravholt CH, Andersen NH, Conway GS, et al. Clinical practice guidelines for the care of girls and women with Turner syndrome: proceedings from the 2016 Cincinnati International Turner Syndrome Meeting. Eur J Endocrinol. 2017;177(3):G1-70.
21. Farahmand M, Ramezani Tehrani F, Simbar M, et al. Does metabolic syndrome or its components differ in naturally and surgically menopausal women? Climacteric. 2014;17(4):348-55.
22. Pu D, Tan R, Yu Q, et al. Metabolic syndrome in menopause and associated factors: a meta-analysis. Climacteric. 2017;20(6):583-91.
23. Brand JS, van der Schouw YT, Onland-Moret NC, et al. Age at menopause, reproductive life span, and type 2 diabetes risk: results from the EPIC-InterAct study. Diabetes Care. 2013;36(4):1012-9.
24. Sjöberg L, Pitkäniemi J, Harjutsalo V, et al. Menopause in women with type 1 diabetes. Menopause. 2011;18(2):158-63.
25. Aubertin-Leheudre M, Goulet ED, Dionne IJ. Enhanced rate of resting energy expenditure in women using hormone-replacement therapy: preliminary results. J Aging Phys Act. 2008;16(1):53-60.
26. Duncan AC, Lyall H, Roberts RN, et al. The effect of estradiol and a combined estradiol/progestagen preparation on insulin sensitivity in healthy postmenopausal women. J Clin Endocrinol Metab. 1999;84(7):2402-7.
27. Margolis KL, Bonds DE, Rodabough RJ, et al. Effect of oestrogen plus progestin on the incidence of diabetes in postmenopausal women: results from the Women's Health Initiative Hormone Trial. Diabetologia. 2004;47(7):1175-87.
28. Kanaya AM, Herrington D, Vittinghoff E, et al. Glycemic effects of postmenopausal hormone therapy: the Heart and Estrogen/progestin Replacement Study. A randomized, double-blind, placebo-controlled trial. Ann Intern Med. 2003;138(1):1-9.
29. Stuenkel CA. Menopause, hormone therapy and diabetes. Climacteric. 2017;20(1):11-21.
30. Esposito K, Chiodini P, Capuano A, et al. Metabolic syndrome and endometrial cancer: a meta-analysis. Endocrine. 2014;45(1):28-36.
31. Wise LA, Palmer JR, Spiegelman D, et al. Influence of body size and body fat distribution on risk of uterine leiomyomata in U.S. black women. Epidemiology. 2005;16(3):346-54.

# SECTION 2

# Glucovigilance in Endocrinology

# CHAPTER 10

# Metabolic Syndrome in Endocrinopathy

*Jubbin Jagan Jacob, Abraham Alex Kodiatte, Vishal Bhatia*

## INTRODUCTION

It is a well-known fact that metabolic syndrome (MetS) increases the risk for cardiovascular disease (CVD). There is growing evidence that MetS is not merely a lifestyle disorder, but results from a complex interplay of genetic and environmental influences. The endocrine system is a key regulator of glucose, protein and lipid metabolism, and disorders affecting endocrine health have far-reaching effects on metabolic health. Endocrinopathies are often associated with changes in body weight and body composition, dysglycemia, hypertension, dyslipidemia, endothelial dysfunction, and chronic inflammation in addition to the unique manifestations caused by hormone deficiency or excess. Therefore, the clinical profile of several endocrine disorders resembles MetS to a great extent which itself is associated with an increased risk of CVD. This chapter focuses on the endocrine disorders, both hormone excess and deficiency states, which contribute to the pathogenesis of MetS. Management of MetS associated with endocrine disorders requires a multipronged approach, including lifestyle modification, pharmacological management of components of MetS, and appropriate hormonal supplementation or ablation treatments. Such multifactorial approach is essential to slow or halt the drive toward CVD.

## DEFINING METABOLIC SYNDROME/ SYNDROME X/INSULIN-RESISTANCE SYNDROME

Metabolic syndrome encompasses a cluster of risk factors that contribute toward the development of CVD. It is a constellation of interconnected risk factors, the fundamental mechanisms of which are exacerbated by a convoluted chemistry between a deficient lifestyle and a calorie-surplus state. MetS was first described in 1923 by Kylin as a clinical association between hypertension and gout. However, the term was first coined by Reaven in 1988 to highlight insulin resistance as the

**TABLE 1** Diagnostic criteria for metabolic syndrome.

| International Diabetes Federation (IDF) definition of metabolic syndrome | | |
|---|---|---|
| **Must fulfill the two criteria** | | |
| 1. Central obesity (defined as waist circumference with ethnicity specific values) | | |
| Europids, Sub-Saharan Africans, Eastern Mediterranean and Middle East | Male | ≥94 cm |
| | Female | ≥80 cm |
| South Asians, Ethnic South and Central Americans, Chinese and Japanese | Male | ≥90 cm |
| | Female | ≥80 cm |
| 2. Any two of the following four factors: | | |
| Raised triglycerides | ≥150 mg/dL or on specific treatment | |
| Reduced HDL cholesterol | <40 mg/dL in males <50 mg/dL in females or on specific treatment | |
| Raised blood pressure | Systolic BP ≥130 mm Hg or diastolic BP ≥85 mm Hg or on specific treatment | |
| Raised FPG | FPG ≥100 mg/dL or on specific treatment | |

(BP: blood pressure; FPG: fasting plasma glucose; HDL: high-density lipoprotein)

shared nucleus for each of the risk factors, all of which contribute towards the CVD epidemic.

Individuals with this complex web of metabolic factors have the propensity to lure the treacherous duet of CVD and diabetes mellitus (DM). According to various studies, the prevalence of MetS in India was found to be ranging from 24.9% to 33.5%. The clinical heterogenicity of this syndrome can be explained by its significant impact on glucose, fat, and protein metabolism, cellular growth, inflammation and endothelial dysfunction.

The International Diabetes Federation (IDF) in 2005 put forward the definition of MetS which incorporated easily available yet critical parameters, as depicted in Table 1.[1] Apart from these factors, increased levels of markers denoting pro-inflammatory state (C-reactive protein) and prothrombotic state (plasminogen activator inhibitor-1, fibrinogen) may also be observed in MetS.

# ENDOCRINE SYSTEM—METABOLIC EFFECTS

## Effect of Thyroid Hormones on Metabolic Health

### Thyroid and Lipid Metabolism

Thyroid hormones have multiple effects on the regulation of lipid synthesis, absorption and metabolism. Thyroid hormones lead to mobilization of lipids from adipose tissue and reduce fat stores. They also increase the circulating levels of free fatty acid in the plasma and greatly accelerate the oxidation of free fatty acids by various cells. Elevated thyroid hormone reduces cholesterol and triglycerides.

One of the mechanisms by which thyroid hormone decreases plasma cholesterol concentration is to significantly increase the rate of cholesterol secretion in the bile and consequent loss in the feces. Thyroid hormones upregulate the expression of low-density lipoprotein (LDL) receptors on hepatocytes, thereby increasing the hepatic uptake and clearance of LDL particles.[2,3]

## Thyroid and Arterial Hypertension

Hypothyroidism is associated with diastolic hypertension whereas hyperthyroidism is associated with systolic hypertension.

## Thyroid and Obesity

Thyroid hormone excess or deficiency is associated with significant impact on body weight. Hypothyroidism contributes to weight gain primarily by accumulation of edema, but it is also associated with reduced basal metabolic rate and reduced energy expenditure. On the other hand, hyperthyroidism amplifies the catabolic effects of thyroid hormones on adipose and muscle tissue and often manifests with weight loss.

## Thyroid and Glucose Intolerance

The Health, Aging and Body Composition Study reported a positive correlation of hypothyroidism with elevated fasting glucose levels.[4,5] Hypothyroidism is associated with impaired insulin sensitivity and overt or subclinical hypothyroidism has been reported at a higher prevalence in individuals with diabetes (both type 1 and type 2 diabetes mellitus) than the general population. There is also an increased insulin response to an oral glucose tolerance test in patients with subclinical and overt hyperthyroidism.[6] The effects of thyroid hormones on individual components of MetS have been summarized in Flowchart 1.

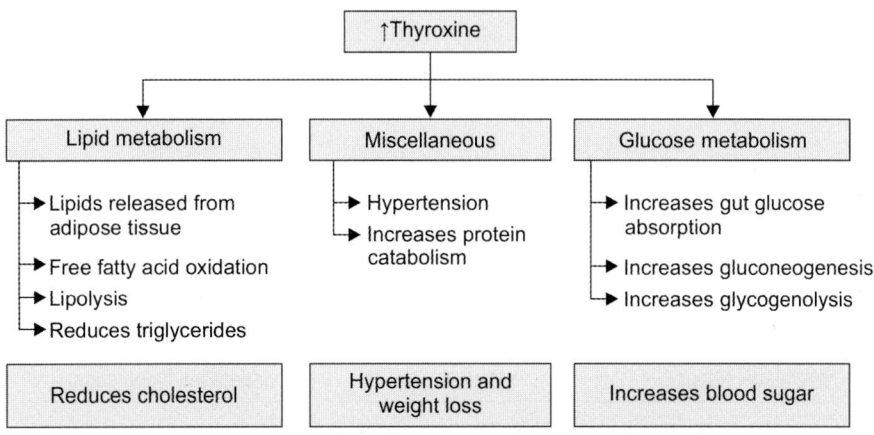

**FLOWCHART 1:** Effects of thyroid hormones on components of metabolic syndrome.

## Effect of Growth Hormone on Metabolic Health

Growth hormone (GH) causes a release of fatty acids from adipose tissue and increases fat utilization. GH has multiple effects that influence carbohydrate metabolism including: (1) decreased glucose uptake in tissues such as skeletal muscle and fat; (2) increased glucose production by the liver; and (3) increased insulin secretion.

Growth hormone antagonizes the action of insulin to stimulate the uptake and utilization of glucose in skeletal muscle and fat and to inhibit gluconeogenesis (glucose production) by the liver. Therefore, GH leads to impaired insulin sensitivity and this leads to increased blood glucose concentration and a compensatory increase in insulin secretion. Acromegaly or excess secretion of GH can be associated with significant insulin resistance and produce metabolic disturbances very similar to those found in patients with type 2 diabetes mellitus. At the same time, striking similarities exist between the clinical spectrum of adult GH deficiency and MetS. It is yet to be determined whether GH deficiency is a cause or a consequence of any of the components of MetS and the effects of GH replacement on metabolic health are highly debated. The effects of GH on individual components of MetS have been summarized in Flowchart 2.

## Effects of Glucocorticoids on Metabolic Health

The effect of glucocorticoids on metabolism is to stimulate gluconeogenesis, decreases glucose utilization, and promotes mobilization of fatty acids from adipose tissue. This increases the concentration of free fatty acids in the plasma, which also increases their utilization for energy. Despite the fact that glucocorticoids can cause fatty acid mobilization from adipose tissue, glucocorticoids have variable effects on different adipose tissue depots, with a net gain in fat in upper body and visceral adipose tissue. Therefore, cortisol excess is associated with central obesity with thinning of extremities and a Cushingoid habitus. The effects of glucocorticoids on individual components of MetS have been summarized in Flowchart 3.

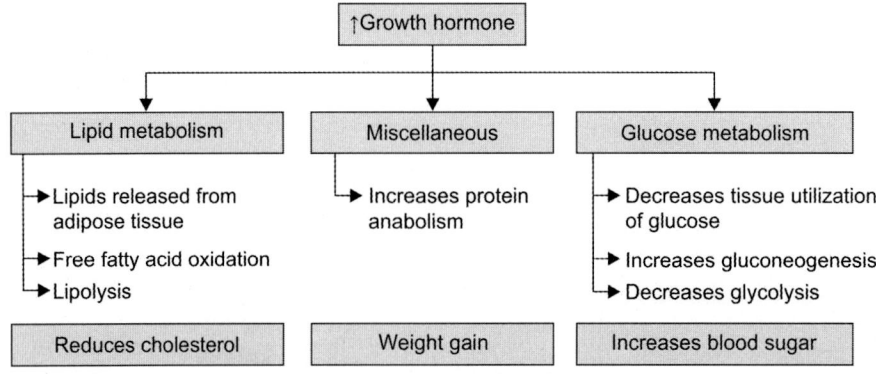

**FLOWCHART 2:** Effect of growth hormone on components of metabolic syndrome.

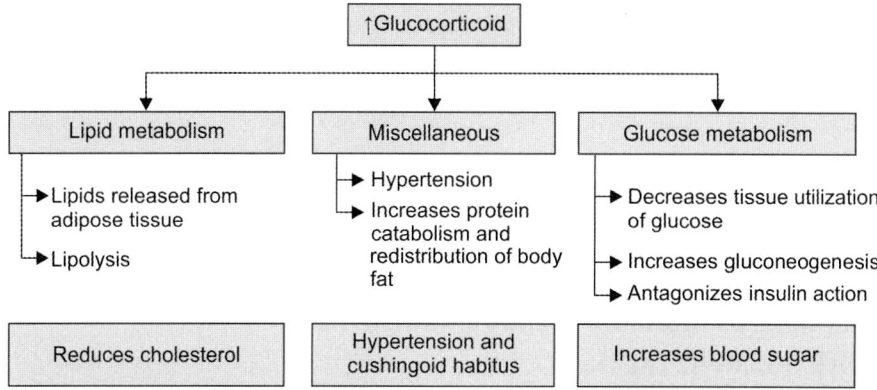

**FLOWCHART 3:** Effect of glucocorticoids on components of metabolic syndrome.

## Effects of Gonadal Hormones on Metabolic Health

Testosterone plays a compelling role in the maintenance of bone and muscle development, glucose homeostasis, and lipid metabolism in addition to the maintenance of sexual and reproductive health. Estrogen also contributes to lipid health and glucose homeostasis. Hypogonadism in both men and women is associated with increased visceral fat, inflammation and insulin resistance. While testosterone has a positive effect on metabolism in men, hyperandrogenism in women is associated with significant insulin resistance, as in polycystic ovary syndrome (PCOS).

## METABOLIC SYNDROME IN ENDOCRINOPATHY

The prevalence of MetS and endocrine disorders is rapidly increasing. While the rising prevalence of MetS is largely due to rapidly increasing prevalence of overweight and obesity, endocrine dysfunction is a significant contributor to metabolic disorders. Endocrine deficiency and excess disorders are associated with changes in glucose, lipid, and protein metabolism, endothelial dysfunction, chronic inflammation, hypertension and CVD. Both MetS and endocrinopathies affect general well-being and quality of life and have significant morbidity and contribute to increased cardiovascular and all-cause mortality. The relationship of endocrinopathies and MetS with CVD requires further scientific evidence to understand how best to reduce the burden of cardiometabolic disease.

For the purpose of augmenting comprehension and grasp, MetS and its association to various endocrinopathies will be depicted under the following sections, as depicted in Figure 1:
- Metabolic syndrome in endocrinopathies with hormone excess
- Metabolic syndrome in endocrinopathies with hormone deficiencies.

In addition, the authors discuss the similarities and the relationship between MetS and PCOS, which has often been regarded as the "ovarian component" of MetS.

```
┌─────────────────────────┐
│ Metabolic syndrome in   │
│ endocrinopathies with   │
│ hormone excess          │
└─────────────────────────┘
      ┌─────────────────────────┐
      │ Metabolic syndrome      │
      │ endocrinopathies with   │
      │ hormone deficiencies    │
      └─────────────────────────┘
```

**FIG. 1:** Classification of endocrinopathies in patients with metabolic syndrome.

## METABOLIC SYNDROME IN ENDOCRINOPATHIES WITH HORMONE EXCESS

Hormone excess states are less common than deficiency disorders. Several disorders of hormone excess present with a clinical phenotype resembling MetS and are associated with increased cardiovascular risk.

### Hyperthyroidism

The impact of thyroid hormones on fat metabolism, blood pressure, and glucose tolerance individually are well known, but its liaison with the elements of MetS is obscure. In a study by Gyawali et al. hyperthyroidism in any form in MetS (overt or subclinical) was seen in only 0.83% of the study population.[7] There was a similar shallow prevalence in other studies from North India, South India, Nepal and Nigeria.[8-11] Elevated free T4 levels in subjects with MetS may be a coincidence rather than an association.

### Acromegaly

There is inconsistent data with regard to the relationship between serum insulin-like growth factor-1 (IGF-1) levels and MetS. A number of studies in nonacromegalic patients have implied that increased levels of IGF-1 occur in patients with obesity or type 2 diabetes mellitus, while others have observed similarities between untreated GH deficiency (low IGF-1 levels) and some components of MetS. The pivotal findings common to both are obesity, insulin resistance, premature atherosclerosis, and increased mortality from CVD.

Conversely, it is well established that during treatment of patients with acromegaly, IGF-1 reduction not only reduces the clinical signs and symptoms of acromegaly, but also reduces morbidities such as insulin resistance, glucose intolerance and CVD.[12]

In acromegaly, prolonged exposure to GH and IGF-1 causes insulin resistance and secondary diabetes. In the general population, insulin resistance and diabetes are most often associated with increased body fat, a hallmark of MetS. However, in acromegaly, despite a favorable body habitus, patients often develop insulin resistance and diabetes. The mechanisms involved in the appearance of insulin resistance and diabetes in acromegaly are poorly understood. GH has a positive effect on insulin sensitivity by stimulating the secretion of IGF-1 from the liver, but it also has direct antagonistic effects to insulin. Hence GH and IGF-1 expend opposite effects on glucose homeostasis.[13]

## Cushing's Syndrome

An assemblage of clinical studies summarizing the prevalence of various clinical signs and symptoms of Cushing's syndrome showed that obesity was found in 95% of the patients, hypertension in 75% and glucose intolerance in 60%.[14] Many also had elevated triglyceride levels (around 20% of the cases) and reduced high-density lipoprotein (HDL) cholesterol levels (36% of the cases).[15,16] It has been estimated that almost two-thirds of Cushing's syndrome patients fulfill three of the five criteria for MetS. Whatever the cut-off points used to define MetS, Cushing's syndrome represents an archetype of MetS.[17] Another possible contributing factor for the development of MetS in patients with Cushing's syndrome is the finding of associated GH deficiency in these patients.[18]

Metabolic syndrome is extremely common in Cushing's syndrome. Glucocorticoids induce hyperglycemia by increasing hepatic gluconeogenesis and disrupting the insulin signaling in the liver, skeletal muscle, and adipose tissue with a consequent decrease of peripheral uptake and disposal of glucose. Central fat accumulation is coupled with dysregulation of adipokine secretion and facilitated by glucocorticoid-related increased appetite, enhanced adipogenesis and altered lipid storage. Hyperlipidemia, a major cardiovascular risk factor, is associated to the increased mobilization of free fatty acids from the adipose tissue and increased hepatic lipogenesis. The patient of Cushing's syndrome with obesity, DM, dyslipidemia, hypertension, procoagulant phenotype and severe structural and functional alterations of the heart and vessels is the prototype of a patient with increased cardiovascular risk.[19]

## METABOLIC SYNDROME IN ENDOCRINOPATHIES WITH HORMONE DEFICIENCIES

Several hormone deficiency disorders are associated with obesity, insulin resistance, dysmetabolism and cardiovascular risk.

## Hypothyroidism

Thyroid dysfunction is one of the commonest endocrine disorders in patients with MetS. There is an existence of considerable overlap in the basic pathophysiological mechanisms contributing to atherosclerotic cardiovascular disease (ASCVD) in MetS and hypothyroidism. The duo are harbingers for CVD and the presence of both conditions may compound the risk for CVD.

Various studies have shown an association between patients with MetS and hypothyroidism. The prevalence of hypothyroidism in MetS ranges from 26% to 30%.[10,20] Conversely, the prevalence of MetS was 51.8% in hypothyroid subjects in one study.[21] The thyroid-stimulating hormone (TSH) levels in patients with MetS were found to be higher than the normal population. A linear association was observed between TSH levels and lipid profile across the MetS group.[22] While thyroxine replacement has clear beneficial role in individuals with overt hypothyroidism, it is still ambiguous whether all patients with high normal TSH or subclinical hypothyroidism with deranged cholesterol levels should be treated with thyroid hormone replacement to avert the development of MetS.[23] There is an intimate interaction of thyroid hormone with all the components of MetS, but there is no good evidence to prove that its supplementation is beneficial.

## Adrenal Insufficiency

Scientific studies are scarce in this subject. According to a study in Sweden, 33% of patients with Addison's disease on treatment with glucocorticoids had MetS, a high rate explained by the relatively high glucocorticoid dose used for replacement.[24] Patients with Addison's disease receiving standard replacement therapy have higher frequency of MetS in a younger age compared to well-matched controls. This may be explained by the relatively supraphysiological doses of glucocorticoids used for replacement.[25]

## Hypogonadism

Hypogonadism is likely a fundamental component of MetS. In particular, it is difficult to opine whether it is a cause or a consequence of MetS. Theoretically, testosterone replacement in men with hypogonadism carries a considerable therapeutic advantage. Testosterone may not only treat hypogonadism, but may also have potential to slow or halt the progression from MetS to overt CVD.[26]

Further evidence of the link is provided by a study that found that men with prostate cancer on long-term androgen suppression therapy had significantly higher rates of MetS than those who did not.[27] Hypogonadism associated with the MetS may be related to a low-grade inflammatory state, which leads to a reduced testosterone synthesis.[28,29]

In a meta-analysis of 20 studies, patients with MetS showed significantly lower testosterone compared with healthy individuals.[30] In another study, oral testosterone treatment in men with type 2 diabetes mellitus and androgen deficiency improved glucose homeostasis and body mass index.[31] In a study from Tunisia, MetS was found in 27.5% of hypogonadal men.[32] The impact of hypogonadism on MetS concerns the role of testosterone replacement therapy, not only on the reproductive aspect but also on the metabolic parameters.

## Hypopituitarism

There is a paucity of scientific evidence to demonstrate the association between hypopituitarism and MetS. A study from Italy demonstrated a 33.3% prevalence of MetS in patients with hypopituitarism following a traumatic brain injury.[33] Another study from Poland demonstrated a 41.7% prevalence rate in patients with hypopituitarism receiving supplemental hormonal therapy.[34] These studies had limitations to them and is safe to comment that more scientific evidence is required.

## METABOLIC SYNDROME AND POLYCYSTIC OVARY SYNDROME: THE METABOLIC MENACE

Metabolic syndrome and PCOS have been portrayed as the zenith of metabolic dysfunction disorders. Each of the syndromes are related by virtue of insulin resistance being a core component in them. Many patients exhibit characteristics that are common to both MetS and PCOS. There is a significant association between the two syndromes which has been recorded by various authors.[35-38] Within all its phenotypic heterogeneity compounded with an ever-increasing incidence of DM, the overlap between the two syndromes will continue to get stronger and wider. Authors have long postulated that MetS and PCOS are a part of a larger spectrum and not distinct disorders, with few even suggesting renaming PCOS as "metabolic reproductive syndrome" to provide a greater focus on the contribution of metabolic dysfunction toward the disease.[39] The reproductive and metabolic manifestations of PCOS are depicted in Flowchart 4. White adipose tissue dysfunction has been seen to contribute to the MetS-PCOS phenotype.[40-42]

The heterogeneity among patients having PCOS have long been acknowledged; some authors have noted the absence of insulin resistance in some women with PCOS.[43,44] Clearly, a greater understanding of these syndromes is needed before a more concrete integrated management strategy can be adopted.

Yet, while the defining criteria for MetS and PCOS remain distinct and do not overlap, the similarity in their core pathophysiology and clinical features cannot be ignored. Apart from insulin resistance, obesity and dyslipidemia have also been interlinked to each of the two syndromes—demonstrating the dysmetabolic aspect of PCOS which runs a similar course with MetS.

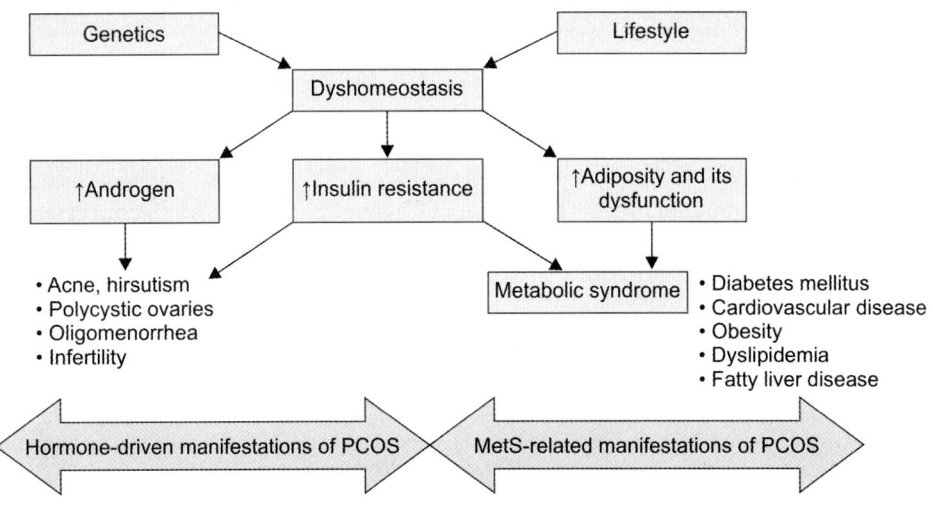

(MetS: metabolic syndrome; PCOS: polycystic ovary syndrome)

**FLOWCHART 4:** The MetS-PCOS overlap.

Patients with PCOS and MetS were different from those lacking MetS in terms of increased hyperandrogenemia, lower serum sex-hormone binding globulin, and higher prevalence of acanthosis nigricans, all features that may reflect more severe insulin resistance.[45] CVD morbidity and DM which are defining of MetS are prevalent in PCOS as well.[46,47] PCOS is seen in 27% of premenopausal women with type 2 diabetes mellitus.[48] Moreover, PCOS patients have an elevated risk of MetS, more so in subsets/phenotypes of PCOS with hyperandrogenism.[49] With this information in hand, there is lot of scope for a therapeutic strategy that addresses these similarities and can be central to reduction of cardiometabolic risk in PCOS.[50]

## CONCLUSION

There is no denying the fact that further scientific evidence is necessary to establish protocols for screening for endocrinopathies in patients with MetS. MetS exponentially increases the risk for developing CVD. Not only is it vital to identify and pick out the various critical parameters forging MetS, but it is as imperative to be aware of the various endocrinopathies linked to it. Specific treatment for endocrinopathies does influence and correct distinct metabolic risk factors. Cushing's syndrome, hypothyroidism, and hypogonadism are frequent offenders in patients with MetS and hence efforts should be made to screen them for these disorders and vice versa. The overlap between MetS and PCOS is too great to ignore; insulin resistance being pivotal to their pathophysiology. Common therapeutic methodology can be implemented in the future to tackle these threats.

## REFERENCES

1. Alberti KG, Zimmet P, Shaw J The metabolic syndrome—a new worldwide definition. Lancet. 2005;366:1059-62.
2. Guyton AC, Hall JE. Textbook of Medical Physiology, 11th edition. Philadelphia: Elsevier Saunders; 2006. p. 936.
3. Iwen KA, Schröder E, Brabant G. Thyroid hormones and the metabolic syndrome. Eur Thyr J. 2013;2(2):83-92.
4. Waring AC, Rodondi N, Harrison S, et al. Thyroid function and prevalent and incident metabolic syndrome in older adults: the Health, Ageing and Body Composition Study. Clin Endocrinol (Oxf). 2012;76(6):911-8.
5. Roos A, Bakker SJ, Links TP, et al. Thyroid function is associated with components of the metabolic syndrome in euthyroid subjects. J Clin Endocrinol Metab. 2007;92(2):491-6.
6. Maratou E, Hadjidakis DJ, Kollias A, et al. Studies of insulin resistance in patients with clinical and subclinical hypothyroidism. Eur J Endocrinol. 2009;160(5):785-90.
7. Gyawali P, Takanche JS, Shrestha RK, et al. Pattern of thyroid dysfunction in patients with metabolic syndrome and its relationship with components of metabolic syndrome. Diab Metabol J. 2015;39(1):66-73.
8. Jayakumar RV. Hypothyroidism and metabolic syndrome. Thyroid Res Pract. 2013;10 (Suppl S1):1-2.
9. Dhanju AS, Neki NS, Singh A, et al. A study on association between thyroid stimulating hormone levels and metabolic syndrome components. Ann Int Med Den Res. 2016;2(3):102-5.
10. Khatiwada S, Sah SK, Rajendra KC, et al. Thyroid dysfunction in metabolic syndrome patients and its relationship with components of metabolic syndrome. Clin Diab Endocrinol. 2016;2:3.
11. Ogbera AO, Kuku S, Dada O. The metabolic syndrome in thyroid disease: a report from Nigeria. Indian J Endocrinol Metab. 2012;16:417-22.

12. Matta M, Bongard V, Grunenwald S, et al. Clinical and metabolic characteristics of acromegalic patients with high IGF1/normal GH levels during somatostatin analog treatment. Eur J Endocrinol. 2011;164(6):885-9.
13. Olarescu NC, Bollerslev J. The impact of adipose tissue on insulin resistance in acromegaly. Trends Endocrinol Metab. 2016;27(4):226-37.
14. Newell-Price J, Bertagna X, Grossman AB, et al. Cushing's syndrome. Lancet. 2006;367(9522):1605-17.
15. Faggiano A, Pivonello R, Spiezia S, et al. Cardiovascular risk factors and common carotid artery caliber and stiffness in patients with Cushing's disease during active disease and 1 year after disease remission. J Clin Endocrinol Metab. 2003;88:2527-33.
16. Pivonello R, Faggiano A, Lombardi G, et al. The metabolic syndrome and cardiovascular risk in Cushing's syndrome. Endocrinol Metab Clin North Am. 2005;34:327-39, viii.
17. Chanson P, Salenave S. Metabolic syndrome in Cushing's syndrome. Neuroendocrinology. 2010;92(suppl 1):96-101.
18. Pecori Giraldi F, Andrioli M, De Marinis L, et al. Significant GH deficiency after long-term cure by surgery in adult patients with Cushing's disease. Eur J Endocrinol. 2007;156:233-9.
19. Ferraù F, Korbonits M. Metabolic comorbidities in Cushing's syndrome. Eur J Endocrinol. 2015;173;M133-M157.
20. Kota SK, Meher LK, Krishna S, et al. Hypothyroidism in metabolic syndrome. Indian J Endocrinol Metabol. 2012;16(Suppl 2):S332-S333.
21. Kannan L, Pomerantz S, Chernoff A. Hypothyroidism and the metabolic syndrome. Endocrinol Metab Int J. 2017;5(2):00115.
22. Meher LK, Raveendranathan SK, Kota SK, et al. Prevalence of hypothyroidism in patients with metabolic syndrome. Thyroid Res Pract. 2013;10:60-4.
23. Kc R, Khatiwada S, Deo Mehta K, et al. Cardiovascular risk factors in subclinical hypothyroidism: A case control study in Nepalese population. J Thyroid Res. 2015;2015:305241.
24. Bergthorsdottir R, Ragnarsson O, Skrtic S, et al. Mortality and morbidity in patients with Addison's disease. Doctor of Philosophy (Medicine). University of Gothenburg: Sahlgrenska Academy; 2015.
25. Bergthorsdottir R, Ragnarsson O, Johannsson G. Patients with Addison's disease have increased frequency of the metabolic syndrome: a case–control study. Presented at European Congress of Endocrinology, Copenhagen, Denmark. Endocrine Abstracts. 2013;32:P30.
26. Makhsida N, Shah J, Yan G, et al. Hypogonadism and metabolic syndrome: implications for testosterone therapy. J Urol. 2005,174(3).827-34.
27. Braga-Basaria M, Dobs AS, Muller DC, et al. Metabolic syndrome in men with prostate cancer undergoing long-term androgen-deprivation therapy. J Clin Oncol. 2006;24:3979-83.
28. Gorbachinsky I, Akpinar H, Assimos D. Metabolic syndrome and urologic diseases. Rev Urol. 2010;12:e157-80.
29. Kalyani RR, Dobs AS. Androgen deficiency, diabetes, and the metabolic syndrome in men. Curr Opin Endocrinol Diabetes Obes. 2007;14:226-34.
30. Corona G, Monami M, Rastrelli G, et al. Testosterone and metabolic syndrome: a meta-analysis study. J Sex Med. 2011;8:272-83.
31. Boyanov MA, Boneva Z, Christov VG. Testosterone supplementation in men with type 2 diabetes, visceral obesity and partial androgen deficiency. Aging Male. 2003;6:1-7.
32. Naifar M, Rekik N, Messedi M, et al. Male hypogonadism and metabolic syndrome. Andrologia. 2015;47(5):579-86.
33. Prodam F, Gasco V, Rovere S, et al. Hypopituitarism and features of the metabolic syndrome in patients with traumatic brain injury (TBI). Presented at European Congress of Endocrinology, Berlin, Germany. Endocrine Abstracts. 2008;16:P434.
34. Zwolak A, Swirska J, Dudzinska M, et al. The prevalence of metabolic syndrome in adult patients with long-standing hypopituitarism who receive adequate supplemental therapy. Endocrine Abstracts. 2016;41:EP944.
35. Glueck CJ, Papanna R, Wang P, et al. Incidence and treatment of metabolic syndrome in newly referred women with confirmed polycystic ovarian syndrome. Metabolism. 2003;52(7):908-15.
36. Teede HJ, Hutchison S, Zoungas S, et al. Insulin resistance, the metabolic syndrome, diabetes, and cardiovascular disease risk in women with PCOS. Endocrine. 2006;30(1):45-53.

37. Pasquali R. Metabolic syndrome in polycystic ovary syndrome. Front Horm Res. 2018;49:114-30.
38. Shah D, Rasool S. PCOS and metabolic syndrome: The worrisome twosome? Endocrinol Metab Synd. 2015;4:169.
39. Teede H, Gibson-Helm M, Norman RJ, et al. Polycystic ovary syndrome: perceptions and attitudes of women and primary health care physicians on features of PCOS and renaming the syndrome. J Clin Endocrinol Metab. 2014;99(1):E107-11.
40. Spinedi E, Cardinali DP. The polycystic ovary syndrome and the metabolic syndrome: A Possible chronobiotic-cytoprotective adjuvant therapy. Int J Endocrinol. 2018;2018:1349868.
41. Moran LJ, Misso ML, Wild RA, et al. Impaired glucose tolerance, type 2 diabetes and metabolic syndrome in polycystic ovary syndrome: a systematic review and meta-analysis. Hum Reprod Update. 2010;16(4):347-63.
42. Yildiz BO, Azziz R. Ovarian and adipose tissue dysfunction in polycystic ovary syndrome: report of the 4th special scientific meeting of the Androgen Excess and PCOS Society. Fertil Steril. 2009;94(2):690-3.
43. Rotterdam ESHRE/ASRM-Sponsored PCOS Consensus Workshop Group. Revised 2003 consensus on diagnostic criteria and long-term health risks related to polycystic ovary syndrome. Fertil Steril. 2004;81(1):19-25.
44. Azziz R, Carmina E, Dewailly D, et al. The Androgen Excess and PCOS Society criteria for the polycystic ovary syndrome: the complete task force report. Fertil Steril. 2009;91(2):456-88.
45. Apridonidze T, Essah PA, Iuorno MJ, et al. Prevalence and characteristics of the metabolic syndrome in women with polycystic ovary syndrome. J Clin Endocrinol Metab. 2005;90(4):1929-35.
46. Reaven GM. Insulin resistance, hyperinsulinemia, hypertriglyceridemia, and hypertension. Parallels between human disease and rodent models. Diabetes Care. 1991;14(3):195-202.
47. Ford ES, Giles WH, Dietz WH. Prevalence of the metabolic syndrome among US adults: findings from the third National Health and Nutrition Examination Survey. JAMA. 2002;287(3):356-9.
48. Peppard HR, Marfori J, Iuorno MJ, et al. Prevalence of polycystic ovary syndrome among premenopausal women with type 2 diabetes. Diabetes Care. 2001;24:1050-2.
49. Moran L, Teede H. Metabolic features of the reproductive phenotypes of polycystic ovary syndrome. Hum Reprod Update. 2009;15(4):477-88.
50. Sharpless JL. Polycystic ovary syndrome and the metabolic syndrome. Clin Diabetes. 2003;21(4):154-61.

# CHAPTER 11

# Endocrine Syndromes in Diabetes

*Alpesh Goyal, Saptarshi Bhattacharya, Shahjada Selim*

## INTRODUCTION

Diabetes mellitus (DM) is a heterogeneous group of disorders characterized by chronic hyperglycemia and other metabolic perturbations resulting from either a defect in insulin secretion, insulin action or both. The two most common forms of DM [type 1 and type 2 DM (T1DM and T2DM)] are polygenic in nature, with multiple and complex genetic determinants interacting with various environmental factors to result in a given phenotype. However, a certain subset of patients may present with "syndromic form of diabetes", which cannot be classified into either of these prevalent forms. These include monogenic DM syndromes with defective insulin secretion [maturity-onset diabetes of the young or MODY, neonatal diabetes mellitus (NDM), Wolfram syndrome and thiamine-responsive megaloblastic anemia], monogenic DM syndromes with defective insulin action (insulin receptoropathies and lipodystrophic diabetes), other genetic syndromes associated with DM (Turner syndrome, Klinefelter syndrome, Down syndrome, myotonic dystrophy, Huntington chorea, Friedreich ataxia, Bardet–Biedl syndrome, Alström syndrome and porphyria), immune-mediated DM syndrome (stiff-man syndrome), and autoimmune polyglandular syndromes (APS) (Box 1). The clinical phenotype associated with various forms of syndromic diabetes and a clinical approach to diagnosis and management in such patients has been outlined in this chapter.

## MONOGENIC DIABETES SYNDROMES

Diabetes resulting from mutation in a single gene is referred to as monogenic DM. Patients with monogenic DM are often misdiagnosed as either T1DM or T2DM. Although rare, it is being increasingly recognized nowadays as a result of improved awareness, and increased availability of molecular tools for the genetic diagnosis. A correct diagnosis of this rare form of DM is important since it may have important implications on treatment, genetic counseling and prognosis.

> **BOX 1** **Endocrine syndromes in diabetes.**
>
> - **Monogenic diabetes:**
>   - Defect in insulin secretion:
>     - Maturity-onset diabetes of the young
>     - Neonatal diabetes mellitus
>     - Mitochondrial diabetes
>     - Wolfram syndrome
>     - Thiamine-responsive megaloblastic anemia syndrome (Rogers syndrome)
>   - Defect in insulin action:
>     - Type A insulin resistance
>     - Leprechaunism (Donohue syndrome)
>     - Rabson–Mendenhall syndrome
>     - Lipodystrophic diabetes
> - **Other genetic syndromes associated with diabetes:**
>   - Turner syndrome
>   - Down syndrome
>   - Klinefelter syndrome
>   - Bardet–Biedl syndrome
>   - Alström syndrome
>   - Prader–Willi syndrome
>   - Myotonic dystrophy
>   - Huntington chorea
>   - Friedreich ataxia
>   - Porphyria
> - **Immune-mediated diabetes syndrome:**
>   - Stiff-man syndrome
> - **Autoimmune polyglandular syndromes (APS):**
>   - APS-1
>   - APS-2
>   - IPEX syndrome
>
> (IPEX: immunodysregulation, polyendocrinopathy, enteropathy, X-linked inheritance)

Monogenic DM syndromes may result from gene mutations affecting insulin secretion or insulin action.[1]

## Monogenic Diabetes due to Defective Insulin Secretion

### Maturity-onset Diabetes of the Young

Maturity-onset diabetes of the young is an autosomal dominant form of diabetes typically characterized by:[1-3]

- Youth-onset diabetes with age at onset less than 25–35 years
- Strong positive family history of diabetes in two or three consecutive generations
- Absence of insulin autoantibodies
- A good residual insulin secretion as evidenced by excellent glycemic control on low doses of insulin or preserved C-peptide response well beyond the typical honeymoon period.

Globally, MODY accounts for about 2–3% of all patients diagnosed with diabetes. It may occur due to gene mutations causing defect in transcription factors (hepatocyte nuclear factor or *HNF1α, HNF4α, HNF1β*, insulin promoter factor-1 or IPF-1 and neuronal differentiation 1 or NeuroD1), glucose sensing enzyme (glucokinase or GCK) or lipolytic enzyme (carboxyl ester lipase or CEL). The clinical features of various MODY subtypes have been summarized in Table 1. Recently, there has been a change in the nomenclature of MODY, whereby it is named by the genetic defect instead of the number sign (GCK-MODY or HNF1α-MODY instead of MODY2 or MODY3). Greater than 85% cases of MODY are caused by mutations in the gene encoding HNF1α (MODY3), GCK (MODY2), and HNF4α (MODY1).[1]

## TABLE 1  Monogenic forms of diabetes associated with defective insulin secretion.

| Syndrome | Gene involved | Clinical phenotype and treatment |
|---|---|---|
| **Maturity-onset diabetes of the young** | | |
| MODY1 | HNF4α | Progressive insulin secretory defect; on OGTT, 2-h glucose rise by >5 mmol/L (90 mg/dL); decreased renal threshold for glucosuria; history of LGA and transient neonatal hypoglycemia may be present; sulfonylurea responsive; most common type after MODY3 and MODY2 |
| MODY2 | GCK | Nonprogressive, stable fasting hyperglycemia; incidental detection; on OGTT, 2-h glucose rise by <3 mmol/L (54 mg/dL); microvascular complications rare; treatment not indicated except during pregnancy (with unaffected baby in utero) to prevent macrosomia and hypoglycemia after birth; most common type after MODY3; homozygous mutation associated with permanent NDM |
| MODY 3 | HNF1α | Progressive insulin secretory defect; on OGTT, 2-h glucose rise by >5 mmol/L (90 mg/dL); sulfonylurea responsive; most common type |
| MODY4 | IPF1/PDX1 | Heterozygous mutations cause MODY; compound heterozygous or homozygous mutations cause NDM with pancreatic agenesis and exocrine insufficiency; and insulin requiring; rare |
| MODY5 | HNF1β | Also known as RCAD (renal cysts and diabetes); renal cysts, genitourinary abnormalities, pancreatic atrophy, hyperuricemia, gout and renal failure unrelated to diabetes control; do not respond well to sulfonylurea and may require early insulin therapy; uncommon; homozygous mutation associated with permanent NDM |
| MODY6 | NEUROD1 | Phenotype characterized by obesity and insulin resistance; need insulin for glycemic control; rare |
| MODY7 | KLF11 | Insulin requiring; rare |
| MODY8 | CEL | Exocrine pancreatic insufficiency; increased pancreatic fat deposition; insulin requiring; rare |
| MODY9 | PAX4 | Impaired β-cell development; insulin requiring; rare |
| MODY10 | INS | Mild defect causes MODY; progressive severe defects cause type 1 DM, type 2 DM and NDM; insulin requiring; rare |
| MODY11 | BLK | Insulin requiring; rare |
| **Neonatal diabetes** | | |
| Transient | 6q24 imprinting defects KCNJ11, ABCC8, INS | Remission of DM with high risk of relapse later in life |
| Permanent | KCNJ11, ABCC8, INS HNF1β, GCK, IPF1/PDX1 | Persistent DM; sulfonylurea therapy effective in patients with KCNJ11 or ABCC8 mutation; insulin in others |
| Syndrome | EIF2AK3, FOXP3 | Spondyloepiphyseal dysplasia, renal dysfunction, recurrent acute liver failure, neutropenia (EIF2AK3, Wolcott–Rallison syndrome); immune dysregulation, polyendocrinopathy, enteropathy, X-linked inheritance (FOXP3 and IPEX syndrome); both insulin-requiring |

*Continued*

*Continued*

| Syndrome | Gene involved | Clinical phenotype and treatment |
|---|---|---|
| **Mitochondrial diabetes** | | |
| | 3243A > G mitochondrial DNA point mutation | MIDD (maternally inherited diabetes and deafness); cardiac conduction defect and cardiomyopathy; short stature; pigmentary retinopathy; lactic acidosis; glomerulopathy; myopathy; encephalopathy and stroke-like episodes; insulin requiring; avoid metformin |
| **Wolfram syndrome** | | |
| | WFS | DIDMOAD (diabetes insipidus, DM, optic atrophy and deafness); optic atrophy and DM are usually first manifestations followed by central DI and deafness in second decade; widespread neurodegeneration with incontinence, cerebellar ataxia and myoclonus by fourth decade; insulin requiring; desmopressin for DI |
| **Thiamine-responsive megaloblastic anemia syndrome (Rogers syndrome)** | | |
| | SLC19A2 | Triad of megaloblastic anemia, sensorineural hearing loss and DM; defective thiamine transporter protein; DM and anemia respond to thiamine supplements in early disease course; however, need insulin therapy and blood transfusions after puberty |

(DM: diabetes mellitus; DI: diabetes insipidus; LGA: large for gestational age; MODY: maturity-onset diabetes of the young; NDM: neonatal diabetes mellitus; OGTT: oral glucose tolerance test)

The presence of certain associated clinical features (such as renal cysts and genitourinary abnormalities in MODY5, history of macrosomia and neonatal hypoglycemia in MODY1, and fatty infiltration of pancreas in MODY8) may help in narrowing down the subtype in a given patient with suspected MODY. Definitive diagnosis is achieved using molecular testing for a given genetic mutation. Patients with MODY3 and MODY1 respond to sulfonylurea therapy; however, due to the progressive nature of β-cell defect, a proportion (about one-third) of them ultimately require insulin therapy. MODY2 is characterized by stable and nonprogressive fasting hyperglycemia, which does not require treatment except during pregnancy (in the setting of an unaffected fetus negative for GCK mutation, to prevent fetal macrosomia and hypoglycemia after birth).[4]

## Neonatal Diabetes Mellitus

Neonatal diabetes mellitus is defined as diabetes diagnosed within the first 6 months of life. A small proportion of cases may, however, present till the age of 12 months, and NDM should therefore be considered a possible diagnosis in infants with diabetes between 6 and 12 months of age (especially those with negative insulin autoantibodies).[5] Children with NDM have intrauterine growth retardation (IUGR) at birth (implying the role of insulin in fetal growth) and show poor or absent C-peptide response at the time of diagnosis. NDM may be transient (45%), permanent (45%), or syndromic (10%) (Table 1).

Transient NDM is characterized by a diagnosis of DM in the first few weeks of life, remission of DM at about 12 weeks and increased risk for relapse of DM later in life. About half of the patients with transient NDM have relapse of DM during adolescence or adulthood. Around 70% cases of transient NDM are caused by abnormalities in imprinted genes located on chromosome 6q24, while other 30% are caused by mutations in genes encoding Kir6.2 subunit of ATP-sensitive potassium channel or KATP channel (*KCNJ11* gene), sulfonylurea receptor 1 or SUR1 subunit of KATP channel (*ABCC8* gene) and insulin (*INS* gene*)*.

Permanent NDM is caused by mutations in the genes *KCNJ11*, *ABCC8*, *INS*, *HNF1β* and *GCK*. Genetic diagnosis is important because patients with proven *KCNJ11* and *ABCC8* mutations can be successfully transitioned to oral sulfonylurea therapy in 85–90% cases. The dose of sulfonylurea (per kilogram body weight) is higher in patients with NDM compared to MODY or T2DM. However, such patients achieve excellent glycemic control, which has been shown to be maintained over a period of 10 years in a large multinational cohort involving patients with Kir6.2 NDM.[6]

Syndromic NDM may be seen with mutations in *FOXP3* gene causing IPEX (immunodysregulation, polyendocrinopathy, enteropathy, X-linked inheritance) syndrome and *EIF2AK3* causing Wolcott-Rallison syndrome (Table 1).

## Mitochondrial Diabetes

Maternally inherited diabetes and deafness (MIDD) is a rare mitochondrial disorder characterized by the presence of maternally transmitted diabetes and sensorineural hearing loss. It is caused by point mutation in mitochondrial DNA (3243A > G). The gene mutation is nearly always inherited from the mother and many members on the maternal side may be affected. Diabetes is related to β-cell defect and is variable in severity, commonly being misdiagnosed as T1DM. Other systemic manifestations including seizures, encephalopathy, lactic acidosis, glomerulopathy, cardiomyopathy, myopathy, short stature and pigmentary retinopathy may be present.[7,8]

## Monogenic Diabetes due to Defective Insulin Action

### Insulin Receptoropathies

Insulin receptoropathies refer to the inherited syndromes of insulin resistance caused by mutations in the genes encoding the insulin receptor. These include—leprechaunism (Donohue syndrome), Rabson–Mendenhall syndrome and type A insulin resistance syndrome (Table 2).

Leprechaunism (Donohue syndrome) represents the most severe form of insulin receptoropathy. Children with this syndrome rarely survive beyond the age of 1–2 years.[1] Young females with type A insulin resistance come to medical attention primarily due to the presence of severe acanthosis nigricans and hyperandrogenism.[9] Rabson-Mendenhall syndrome has an intermediate phenotype between leprechaunism and type A insulin resistance with documented survival into childhood or early adulthood.

## TABLE 2: Monogenic forms of diabetes associated with defective insulin action.

| Syndrome | Gene involved | Clinical phenotype and treatment |
|---|---|---|
| **Primary insulin-signaling defects** | | |
| Leprechaunism (Donohue syndrome) | INSR | Most severe; complete absence of insulin receptor; severe intrauterine growth restriction; postprandial hyperglycemia and fasting hypoglycemia; facial dysmorphism; absence of subcutaneous fat; protuberant abdomen; enlarged genitals in males and cystic ovaries in females; exogenous insulin usually ineffective; and death 1–2 years after birth in most cases |
| Rabson–Mendenhall syndrome | INSR | Milder form; residual insulin action present; postprandial hyperglycemia and fasting hypoglycemia; dysplastic nails and teeth; pineal hyperplasia; and responds to insulin |
| Type A insulin resistance syndrome | INSR | Relatively mild and more common than other two forms; presents in young females with hyperandrogenism, severe acanthosis nigricans, insulin resistance and glucose intolerance |
| **Insulin resistance due to adipose tissue abnormalities (lipodystrophic syndromes)** | | |
| Congenital generalized lipodystrophy (CGL) | AGPAT2, BSCL2, CAV1 | Generalized absence of fat; muscular prominence; acromegaloid features; hypertrophic cardiomyopathy; liver steatosis and steatohepatitis; hepatosplenomegaly; increased appetite; accelerated growth; secondary PCOS; hypertriglyceridemia and resultant pancreatitis; difficulty in finding subcutaneous tissue for insulin therapy; and recombinant leptin (Metreleptin) therapy approved for use, but highly expensive |
| Familial partial lipodystrophy | PPARG, LMNA, PLIN1 | Loss of body fat from extremities; truncal fat loss in some; fat deposition at nonlipodystrophic sites as abdomen, perineal region, under the chin and back of the neck; may be misdiagnosed as Cushing syndrome |

(PCOS: polycystic ovary syndrome)

## Lipodystrophic Diabetes

Genetic lipodystrophies are characterized by variable degree of fat loss and may be classified into—(1) congenital generalized lipodystrophy (CGL) and (2) familial partial lipodystrophy (FPL).

Congenital generalized lipodystrophy, also called as Berardinelli–Seip syndrome, is characterized by complete absence of adipose tissue, extreme muscularity, severe hypoleptinemia, severe insulin resistance, excessive appetite, acromegaloid features, severe hypertriglyceridemia, recurrent acute pancreatitis, hepatosplenomegaly, steatohepatitis, and secondary polycystic ovary syndrome (PCOS). CGL is caused by mutations in *AGPAT2* (CGL type 1), *BSCL2* (CGL type 2), and *PTRF* (CGL type 3). While patients with CGL type 1 lack only metabolically active adipose tissue (located in subcutaneous tissue, abdomen, thorax, and bone marrow), CGL type 2 is characterized by loss of both metabolic and mechanical adipose tissue (located in palms and soles, under scalp, orbital and periarticular region). In addition, patients with type 2 CGL may have mild mental retardation and cardiomyopathy.[10,11]

Patients with FPL have fat loss from upper and lower extremities, with variable degree of truncal fat loss. The diagnosis is often revealed on careful clinical examination of extremities, especially gluteal region. Patients with FPL may gain fat at nonlipodystrophic sites (such as under the chin, over back of the neck, abdomen and perineal region) as a secondary phenomenon. Due to characteristic fat redistribution, such patients may be initially misdiagnosed as Cushing syndrome. FPL is caused by mutation in *LMNA* (FPL type 2, Dunnigan variety), *PPARG* (FPL type 3), and *PLIN1* (FPL type 4). The exact molecular basis of FPL type 1 (Koberling variety) is not known.[12,13]

## OTHER GENETIC SYNDROMES ASSOCIATED WITH DIABETES

Several genetic syndromes are associated with diabetes supporting the fact that DM represents a heterogeneous group of disorders. Although rare, these syndromes provide an insight into etiopathogenesis of the common forms of diabetes. The degree of glucose intolerance may range in severity from mild-to-severe.[14] These genetic syndromes may be classified on the basis of (1) predominant pathological mechanism—insulin secretion defect (Turner syndrome, Klinefelter syndrome, and Down syndrome) or insulin action defect (Alström syndrome and Prader–Willi syndrome) or (2) associated organ system involvement—cardiovascular system (Turner syndrome, Down syndrome and Alström syndrome), central nervous system (Down syndrome, Huntington chorea and Friedreich ataxia), peripheral nervous system (porphyria and myotonic dystrophy), gastrointestinal system (porphyria and Turner syndrome), ocular system (Bardet–Biedl syndrome and myotonic dystrophy) and auditory system (Turner syndrome and Alström syndrome) (Box 2).

## AUTOIMMUNE POLYGLANDULAR SYNDROMES

Autoimmune polyglandular syndromes comprise of a group of disorders characterized by functional insufficiency of multiple endocrine organs due to autoimmune destruction resulting from loss of self-tolerance. The term APS is a bit of misnomer since the autoimmune destructive process may also involve nonendocrine organs (resulting in manifestations such as pernicious anemia, celiac disease, alopecia and vitiligo). A progressive T cell-mediated organ destruction accompanied by production of organ-specific autoantibodies is the characteristic immune phenotype of APS.

Autoimmune polyglandular syndromes can be classified based on the genetic defect and clinical features into three subtypes—(1) APS-1, (2) APS-2 and (3) IPEX syndrome (Table 3). APS-1 or autoimmune polyendocrine-candidiasis-ectodermal dystrophy (APECED) is a rare monogenic disorder caused by mutation in autoimmune regulator (AIRE). The disorder is inherited in an autosomal recessive manner and usually manifests during childhood or adolescence. The major manifestations of this syndrome are chronic mucocutaneous candidiasis, hypoparathyroidism and Addison's disease; presence of two of these is required for the diagnosis. APS-2 is far more common than APS-1 and has onset later in life compared to APS-1 or IPEX. It is diagnosed in the presence of at least two of the following three major manifestations—(1) Addison's disease, (2) autoimmune thyroid disease and (3) T1DM. It is a polygenic

## BOX 2: Syndromic diabetes classification according to organ system involvement.

**Central nervous system**
- Mitochondrial diabetes (cerebellar ataxia, stroke-like episodes, seizures, dementia and psychosis)
- Wolfram syndrome (neurodegeneration, incontinence, cerebellar ataxia, myoclonus and dementia)
- Neonatal diabetes (KCNJ11 and ABCC8) (developmental delay and epilepsy)
- Rabson–Mendenhall syndrome (pineal hyperplasia)
- Friedreich ataxia (cerebellar ataxia)
- Huntington chorea (chorea, dystonia, parkinsonism and dementia)
- Prader–Willi syndrome (intellectual disability)
- Bardet–Biedl syndrome (intellectual disability)
- Down syndrome (gross developmental delay and intellectual disability)
- Klinefelter syndrome (learning disabilities and behavioral problems)

**Peripheral nervous system**
- Mitochondrial diabetes (myopathy)
- Porphyria (motor neuropathy)
- Friedreich ataxia (axonal sensory neuropathy)
- Myotonic dystrophy (myotonia, progressive muscle weakness)
- Prader–Willi syndrome (decreased fetal movements, hypotonia)
- Stiff-man syndrome (progressive muscular rigidity and painful muscular spasms)
- APS-2 (myasthenia gravis)

**Ocular system**
- Mitochondrial diabetes (pigmentary retinopathy)
- Wolfram syndrome (optic atrophy)
- Bardet–Biedl syndrome (pigmentary retinopathy)
- Myotonic dystrophy (cataract)
- Turner syndrome (epicanthal folds, ptosis, amblyopia, hypertelorism, and strabismus)
- Down syndrome (epicanthal folds, up-slanting palpebral fissure, and Brushfield iris spots)
- Alström syndrome (retinal dystrophy)

**Auditory system**
- Wolfram syndrome (sensorineural hearing loss)
- Mitochondrial diabetes (sensorineural hearing loss)
- Thiamine-responsive megaloblastic anemia syndrome (sensorineural hearing loss)
- Turner syndrome (recurrent otitis media, conductive and sensorineural hearing loss)
- Alström syndrome (sensorineural hearing loss)

**Cardiovascular system**
- Mitochondrial diabetes (conduction defects and cardiomyopathy)
- Lipodystrophic diabetes (hypertrophic cardiomyopathy)
- Turner syndrome (bicuspid aortic valve, aortic root abnormalities and hypertension)
- Down syndrome (endocardial cushion defects)
- Alström syndrome (dilated cardiomyopathy)
- Friedreich ataxia (hypertrophic cardiomyopathy)
- Myotonic dystrophy (conduction defects)

*Continued*

## CHAPTER 11: Endocrine Syndromes in Diabetes

*Continued*

**Renal and genitourinary system**
- MODY (type 5) (renal cysts, genitourinary abnormalities and renal failure unrelated to glycemic control)
- Mitochondrial diabetes (focal segmental glomerulosclerosis and lactic acidosis)
- Turner syndrome (horseshoe kidney, double collecting system and renal agenesis)
- Bardet–Biedl syndrome, Wolcott–Rallison syndrome (renal dysfunction)
- Alström syndrome (progressive renal dysfunction)

**Gastrointestinal system**
- MODY (type 5, 8) (exocrine pancreatic insufficiency)
- Lipodystrophic diabetes (hepatic steatosis and steatohepatitis, pancreatitis, hepatosplenomegaly)
- Turner syndrome (inflammatory bowel disease and celiac disease)
- APS-1 and APS-2 (celiac disease and pernicious anemia)
- IPEX syndrome (enteropathy)
- Porphyria (recurrent abdominal pain)
- Wolcott–Rallison syndrome (recurrent acute liver failure)
- Alström syndrome (progressive liver dysfunction)

**Hematological system**
- Thiamine-responsive megaloblastic anemia syndrome (megaloblastic anemia)
- Wolcott–Rallison syndrome (neutropenia)
- IPEX syndrome (autoimmune hemolytic anemia and thrombocytopenia)
- Down syndrome (leukemia)

**Skin and musculoskeletal system**
- IPEX syndrome (eczema)
- Wolcott–Rallison syndrome (spondyloepiphyseal dysplasia)
- Rabson–Mendenhall syndrome (dental dysplasia, hair and nail abnormalities)
- Bardet–Biedl syndrome (polydactyly)
- APS-1 (mucocutaneous candidiasis and ectodermal dystrophy)

**Endocrine system**
- Rabson–Mendenhall syndrome (short stature)
- Turner syndrome and Down syndrome (hypothyroidism, short stature and hypogonadism)
- Mitochondrial diabetes (short stature)
- IPEX syndrome (autoimmune thyroiditis)
- Klinefelter syndrome (tall stature and hypogonadism)
- Wolfram syndrome (central diabetes insipidus)
- Prader–Willi syndrome (obesity, hypogonadism and short stature)
- Bardet–Biedl syndrome (obesity and hypogonadism)
- Alström syndrome (obesity, short stature, hypertriglyceridemia and hypogonadism)
- Lipodystrophic diabetes (secondary PCOS and hypertriglyceridemia)
- Myotonic dystrophy (infertility)
- APS-1 (hypoparathyroidism and Addison's disease)
- APS-2 (autoimmune thyroid disease and Addison's disease)
- IPEX (autoimmune thyroid disease)

(APS: autoimmune polyglandular syndrome; IPEX: immunodysregulation, polyendocrinopathy, enteropathy, X-linked inheritance; MODY: maturity-onset diabetes of the young; PCOS: polycystic ovary syndrome)

**TABLE 3**: Comparison of autoimmune polyglandular syndromes.

| Parameter | APS-1 | APS-2 | IPEX |
|---|---|---|---|
| Age at onset | Childhood and adolescence | Adolescence and young adulthood | Infancy |
| Prevalence | Less common (1:100,000) | Most common (1:1,000) | Least common (1:1,000,000) |
| Genetics | • Monogenic<br>• AIRE gene<br>• Autosomal recessive | • Polygenic<br>• HLA-DR3, HLA-DR4 and non-HLA genes (CTLA4, PTPN22, and IL2Rα) | • Monogenic<br>• FOXP3 gene |
| Gender | Male = Female | Female > Male | Male |
| Main manifestations | Mucocutaneous candidiasis, hypoparathyroidism and Addison's disease (two-thirds) | Addison's disease, autoimmune thyroid disease and type 1 DM (two-thirds) | Autoimmune enteropathy, neonatal type 1 DM, eczema |
| Other manifestations | Primary ovarian insufficiency, autoimmune thyroid disease, type 1 DM, alopecia, enamel hypoplasia, nail dystrophy, vitiligo, gastritis, hepatitis, pneumonitis, malabsorption syndrome, pernicious anemia and keratopathy | Myasthenia gravis, pernicious anemia, celiac disease, alopecia, vitiligo, hypogonadism | Autoimmune thyroid disease, autoimmune hemolytic anemia and thrombocytopenia |
| Type 1 DM | <20% | ≈50% | >50–60% |
| Immune phenotype | Autoantibodies against interferon-ω, interferon-α, IL-17 family of cytokines and other organ-specific autoantibodies | Autoantibodies against 21-hydroxylase, TPO, Tg, TSHR, GAD65, Insulin, IA-2, tTG, gastric parietal cell, acetylcholine receptor | Autoantibodies against GAD65, elevated IgE lymphocytosis, eosinophilia |

(AIRE: autoimmune regulator; APS: autoimmune polyglandular syndrome; CTLA4: cytotoxic T-lymphocyte-associated protein 4; DM: diabetes mellitus; FOXP3: forkhead box P3; GAD65: glutamic acid decarboxylase 65; HLA: human leukocyte antigen; IPE: immunodysregulation, polyendocrinopathy, enteropathy, X-linked inheritance; IL-17: interleukin-17; IL2Rα: interleukin-2 receptor alpha; IgE: immunoglobulin E; PTPN22: protein tyrosine phosphatase, non-receptor type 22; TPO: thyroid peroxidase; Tg: thyroglobulin; TSHR: thyroid-stimulating hormone receptor; IA-2: islet antigen-2; tTG: tissue transglutaminase)

disorder caused by mutation in both major histocompatibility complex (MHC) and non-MHC genes. Other disease manifestations of APS-2 include celiac disease, pernicious anemia, myasthenia gravis, hypogonadism, alopecia and vitiligo. Some authors further subdivide APS-2 into—APS-3 (autoimmune thyroid disease plus another autoimmune illness, except Addison's disease) and APS-4 (any other combination of autoimmune diseases); and others prefer to avoid this categorization due to similarity in genetics and pathophysiology of APS-3 and APS-4 (with APS-2).[15,16] As already discussed, IPEX manifests in infancy with autoimmune enteropathy, NDM, eczematous dermatitis, autoimmune thyroid disease and cytopenias. It is inherited in X-linked recessive manner and is caused by mutation in FOXP3 gene, resulting in defective regulatory T-cell function.

## DIAGNOSIS AND MANAGEMENT

A high index of suspicion for diagnosing syndromic diabetes should be kept in patients presenting with diabetes at young age with associated dysmorphic features and other anomalies. A classification of syndromic diabetes according to involvement of various organ systems has been presented in Box 2. Diagnosis should be confirmed with the help of appropriate investigations such as karyotyping (chromosomal aneuploidies), hormonal profile (Turner and Klinefelter syndrome) and urine test for porphyrins (porphyria). For diagnosis of DM, the diagnostic criteria remain same as in other forms of diabetes (FPG ≥126 mg/dL and/or 2-hour plasma glucose following 75 g glucose ≥200 mg/dL and/or random plasma glucose ≥200 mg/dL in presence of symptoms of hyperglycemia and/or glycated hemoglobin ≥6.5%).[17]

Management of patients with syndromic forms of diabetes often requires a multidisciplinary team approach. The basic principles of management of diabetes remain similar to any other form of diabetes. Certain forms such as MODY (MODY 3 and 1) and NDM (*KCNJ11* and *ABCC8* mutation) may respond to sulfonylureas. Patients with mitochondrial diabetes may initially be treated with diet or sulfonylureas; however, metformin is contraindicated due to risk of lactic acidosis. Due to progressive insulinopenia, most patients with mitochondrial diabetes require insulin after about 2 years of DM diagnosis.[18]

The importance of healthy diet and regular physical activity should be emphasized in patients with FPL in order to prevent fat accumulation at nonlipodystrophic sites. Metformin can be used safely; it helps to reduce insulin resistance and appetite in these patients. The use of thiazolidinediones may be associated with excessive fat accumulation at nonlipodystrophic sites in patients with FPL, and hence is best avoided.[1] Due to the presence of severe insulin resistance, high-dose insulin therapy may be needed, necessitating the use of concentrated insulin (U-500 insulin). The lack of subcutaneous adipose tissue for insulin administration may be another important issue in patients with generalized lipodystrophy. Subcutaneous metreleptin (recombinant human leptin) therapy has been shown to reduce appetite and improve glycemic control, steatosis and dyslipidemia in severely hypoleptinemic patients with CGL; however, the efficacy is only modest in patients with FPL. Metreleptin has been approved by the US Food and Drug Administration (FDA) for use in patients with generalized lipodystrophy to improve metabolic outcomes; however, cost is a limiting factor in most cases.[19,20]

Patients with T1DM (in the setting of APS) are at high risk of developing autoimmune disease affecting other endocrine (autoimmune thyroid disease, Addison's disease, and premature ovarian insufficiency) and nonendocrine tissues (celiac disease, pernicious anemia and vitiligo). The presence of an associated autoimmune disease should be suspected in the setting of (1) unexplained glycemic variability, recurrent hypoglycemia (celiac disease, hypothyroidism and adrenal insufficiency), (2) malabsorption, refractory anemia (autoimmune gastritis, pernicious anemia and celiac disease), (3) unexplained growth failure (hypothyroidism and celiac disease), and (4) amenorrhea, oligomenorrhea, infertility or hypoestrogenic symptoms (primary ovarian insufficiency). Hashimoto's thyroiditis and celiac disease are the two most common autoimmune diseases accompanying T1DM. It is therefore recommended that a routine screening for these autoimmune disorders (thyroid function test and tissue transglutaminase antibody test) be performed at the time of diagnosis and at periodic intervals (1–2 yearly) in such individuals.[21,22]

The target for blood glucose control should be individualized considering following factors—age, duration of diabetes, risk of hypoglycemia, associated comorbidities, self-management skills, life expectancy and overall quality of life.

## SYNDROMES ASSOCIATED WITH POOR GLYCEMIC CONTROL

### Mauriac Syndrome

Mauriac syndrome is typically described in adolescents and young adults with poorly controlled T1DM. Typically, such patients present with growth retardation, delayed pubertal maturation, protuberant abdomen, moon facies, hepatomegaly related to glycogen deposition in liver, transaminitis, dyslipidemia and proximal muscle wasting.[23,24] A history of recurrent hospital admissions for diabetic ketoacidosis (DKA) is frequently present. Due to its association with poor glycemic control, microvascular complications such as nephropathy and retinopathy are seen with increased frequency in such patients.

The pathologic basis for hepatic glycogen deposition is related to two factors— (1) hyperglycemia and (2) administration of large amounts of insulin. While hyperglycemia promotes entry of glucose into liver (through insulin-independent GLUT2 transporter), and its phosphorylation via the enzyme GCK, increased insulin leads to polymerization of glucose-6-phosphate into glycogen through the enzyme glycogen synthase. Since DKA is treated with high doses of intravenous followed by subcutaneous insulin (and is associated with hyperglycemia), hepatic glycogen deposition is facilitated in patients with history of recurrent DKA episodes.[25]

The growth retardation in patients with Mauriac syndrome is multifactorial, with possible etiologies being inadequate glucose delivery to the tissues, decreased insulin-like growth factor-1 (IGF-1) levels, resistant or defective hormone receptor action, and hypercortisolism. Liver biopsy shows presence of large, swollen, glycogen-laden hepatocytes and glycogenated nuclei without significant fatty change, inflammation, and lobular spotty necrosis or fibrosis. Good glycemic control can help arrest the growth and pubertal failure, and reverse the metabolic manifestations associated with this rare syndrome.[25]

## CONCLUSION

A substantial proportion of patients with diabetes, who cannot be classified as either T1DM or T2DM, belong to the category of syndromic diabetes. Such atypical forms of diabetes should be suspected in an individual having onset of diabetes at young age with associated dysmorphic features, other organ system involvement or other endocrinopathies. Accurate diagnosis is important because it can have implications on treatment, prognosis, and genetic counseling (in selected cases). Besides, a number of endocrine syndromes accompany poorly controlled diabetes, the manifestations of which may be effectively reversed with good metabolic control.

# REFERENCES

1. Sperling MA, Garg A. Monogenic forms of diabetes. In: Cowie CC, Casagrande SS, Menke A, et al. (Eds). Diabetes in America, 3rd edition. Bethesda, MD: National Institutes of Health; 2017. pp. 7.1-7.27.
2. Anık A, Çatlı G, Abacı A, Böber E. Maturity-onset diabetes of the young (MODY): an update. J Pediatr Endocrinol Metab. 2015;28(3-4):251-63.
3. Thanabalasingham G. Diagnosis and management of maturity onset diabetes of the young (MODY). BMJ. 2011;343:d6044.
4. Murphy R. Monogenic diabetes and pregnancy. Obstet Med. 2015;8(3):114-20.
5. Bryan AL, Bryan J. Neonatal diabetes mellitus. Endocr Rev. 2008;29:265-91.
6. Bowman P, Sulen Å, Barbetti F, et al. Effectiveness and safety of long-term treatment with sulfonylureas in patients with neonatal diabetes due to *KCNJ11* mutations: An international cohort study. Lancet Diabetes Endocrinol. 2018;6:637-46.
7. Murphy R, Turnbull DM, Walker M, et al. Clinical features, diagnosis and management of maternally inherited diabetes and deafness (MIDD) associated with the 3243A>G mitochondrial point mutation. Diabet Med. 2008;25:383-99.
8. Meas T, Laloi-Michelin M, Virally M, et al. Mitochondrial diabetes: clinical features, diagnosis and management. Rev Med Interne. 2010;31:216-21.
9. Semple RK, Savage DB, Cochran EK, et al. Genetic syndromes of severe insulin resistance. Endocr Rev. 2011;32:498-514.
10. Garg A. Acquired and inherited lipodystrophies. N Engl J Med. 2004;350:1220-34.
11. Friguls B, Coroleu W, del Alcazar R, et al. Severe cardiac phenotype of Berardinelli-Seip congenital lipodystrophy in an infant with homozygous E189X BSCL2 mutation. Eur J Med Genet. 2009;52:14-6.
12. Hegele RA. Familial partial lipodystrophy: A monogenic form of the insulin resistance syndrome. Mol Genet Metabol. 2000;71:539-44.
13. Shackleton S, Lloyd DJ, Jackson SN, et al. LMNA, encoding lamin A/C, is mutated in partial lipodystrophy. Nat Genet. 2000;24:153-6.
14. Robinson S, Kessling A. Diabetes secondary to genetic disorders. Baillieres Clin Endocrinol Metab. 1992;6:867-98.
15. Betterle C, Dal Pra C, Mantero F, et al. Autoimmune adrenal insufficiency and autoimmune polyendocrine syndromes: autoantibodies, autoantigens, and their applicability in diagnosis and disease prediction. Endocr Rev. 2002;23:327-64
16. Husebye ES, Anderson MS, Kämpe O. Autoimmune polyendocrine syndromes. N Engl J Med. 2018;378:1132-41.
17. American Diabetes Association. Standards of medical care in diabetes—2014. Diabet Care. 2014;37: S14-80.
18. Maassen JA, 'T Hart LM, Van Essen E, et al. Mitochondrial diabetes: molecular mechanisms and clinical presentation. Diabetes. 2004;53(suppl 1):S103-9.
19. Brown RJ, Araujo-Vilar D, Cheung PT, et al. The diagnosis and management of lipodystrophy syndromes: a multi-society practice guideline. J Clin Endocrinol Metab. 2016;101(12):4500-11.
20. Ajluni N, Dar M, Xu J, et al. Efficacy and Safety of Metreleptin in Patients with Partial Lipodystrophy: Lessons from an Expanded Access Program. J Diabetes Metab. 2016;7:659
21. Kota SK, Meher LK, Jammula S, et al. Clinical profile of coexisting conditions in type 1 diabetes mellitus patients. Diabetes Metab Syndr. 2012;6:70-6.
22. Kordonouri O, Klingensmith G, Knip M, et al. ISPAD Clinical Practice Consensus Guidelines 2014. Other complications and diabetes-associated conditions in children and adolescents. Pediatr Diabetes. 2014;15(Suppl 20):270-8.
23. Madhu SV, Jain R, Kant S, et al. Mauriac syndrome: A rare complication of type 1 diabetes mellitus. Indian J Endocrinol Metab. 2013;17(4):764-5.
24. Kim MS, Quintos JB. Mauriac syndrome: Growth failure and type 1 diabetes mellitus. Pediatr Endocrinol Rev. 2008;5:989-93.
25. Giordano S, Martocchia A, Toussan L, et al. Diagnosis of hepatic glycogenosis in poorly controlled type 1 diabetes mellitus. World J Diabetes. 2014;5:882-8.

# CHAPTER 12

# Hypoglycemia in Endocrinopathies

*Belinda George, Ankia Coetzee*

## INTRODUCTION

In normal physiological conditions, plasma glucose is kept within a relatively narrow range. Given the fact that the central nervous system (CNS) relies almost exclusively on glucose as fuel, the task of maintaining euglycemia is assigned to highly sophisticated structures. Normal glucose homeostasis is dependent on a delicate interplay between cellular receptors and chemical messengers, and the conductor of this metabolic orchestra is the neuroendocrine system.[1] If each constituent that contributes to glucose control functions optimally, the melody performed is one of harmonious normoglycemia.

However, if disturbances occur in one of the critical components or concurrent disturbances exist, life-threatening glucose abnormalities follow. It remains a challenge to mimic the normal well-balanced physiological processes that regulate the glucose-insulin counterregulatory loop with pharmacologic agents. Drugs used to treat diabetes mellitus are in fact the most common reason for hypoglycemia encountered in clinical practice.[2] Overall, the human body's inability to appropriately downregulate insulin levels or action and/or the incapability to counteract insulin effects leads to hypoglycemia, in people with and without diabetes.

On the other hand, hypoglycemia is often erroneously accused as being responsible for a multitude of unrelated sensory perceptions or symptoms. It remains of cardinal importance that the clinician confirms if hypoglycemia is present and verify that low blood glucose is in fact accountable for the symptoms. The context in which low blood glucose occurs should also be carefully contemplated. If hypoglycemia in an otherwise well person is confirmed, further investigation aimed at the identification of the cause should follow.

## WHIPPLE'S TRIAD

When evaluating a patient with a history suggestive of hypoglycemia, the devil is unfortunately in the detail. The clinician must remain vigilant to initiate and guide

investigations appropriately. Whipple's criteria date back to the 1930s when it became apparent that a few patients could be cured from the symptoms of shakiness, sweating and syncope by pancreatic surgery. It had also become known that a large proportion of patients with analogous symptom complexes could not be cured with surgery. Allen O Whipple, a pancreatic surgeon, proposed in 1938 that no pancreatic surgery was to be performed if certain conditions were not met.[3] Whipple's triad was born and remains relevant in endocrine practice today. It requires that three criteria should be met to differentiate between "true" hypoglycemia and its imitators.[3] The triad consists of:
1. The symptoms attributed to hypoglycemia should be compatible with the physiological responses associated with low blood glucose
2. Low plasma glucose should be confirmed and if low
3. Symptoms should resolve by normalizing the glucose concentration.

## ARTIFACTUAL HYPOGLYCEMIA

In practice, point-of-care glucose measurement is often a convenient alternative to laboratory glucose determination. Whenever point-of-care testing (POCT) devices are used and finger-prick glucose results are interpreted, it should be borne in mind that readings depend on the acquisition of capillary blood, which in turn depends on normal capillary blood flow.[4,5] Discrepancies between venous and capillary glucose values occur with increased glucose extraction in conditions such as Raynaud's phenomenon, acrocyanosis, Eisenmenger's syndrome, shock and peripheral vascular disease.[5-7] In addition, POCT glucose devices are designed for self-monitoring in patients with diabetes, and even though the performance of these meters may be acceptable in the context of self-monitoring in diabetes, a low plasma glucose is to be confirmed with plasma glucose estimation to satisfy the Whipple's triad criteria.[3]

## MAINTAINING EUGLYCEMIA

In otherwise well individuals, glucose supply is carefully regulated and a graded sequence of responses occurs with a reduction in plasma glucose concentration. Each of these responses opposes a further drop in glucose and ultimately attempts to ensure adequate glucose supply to the CNS. Counterregulation is a stepwise process, and the release of hormones that counteract hypoglycemia in fact occurs before the development of symptoms at an estimated glucose level of ~ 3.7 mmol/L (68 mg/dL ± 1 mg/dL).[8] The autonomic nervous system response in healthy individuals ensues at glucose levels of ~ 3.3 mmol/L (58 mg/dL ± 2 mg/dL) and is characterized by sympathetic and parasympathetic responses.[8] Tremors, anxiety, palpitations and sweating are due to sympathetic stimulation and hunger is the response to parasympathetic stimulation.[8,9] Cerebral impairment in normal individuals first appears at glucose levels below ~ 2.8 mmol/L (49–51 mg/dL).[8] If counterregulatory responses are unable to promptly reverse hypoglycemia and prevent a further decrease in glucose, neuroglycopenic symptoms such as convulsions, coma, brain damage and death may follow. Not all individuals follow the classic sequence however, and symptoms of hypoglycemia can differ. Other factors such as age, cerebral blood flow, the rate of glucose decrease and glucose transport across the blood–brain barrier can influence the symptoms and reactions to hypoglycemia, also in otherwise well individuals.[9]

Increase in plasma glucose concentration in the fed state is primarily regulated by insulin. If the amount of insulin released does not match the amount required, or if a mismatch occurs between the timing of the insulin and glucose peak, a state of disequilibrium with either hyper- or hypoglycemia transpires. In the fasting state, when intestinal glucose absorption is interrupted between meal times, glucose must be produced endogenously. The first protective response against hypoglycemia is to decrease insulin release while glucose concentrations are still in the normal range.[10] Insulin reciprocally regulates glucagon secretion and the second defense is to increase glucagon release in order to facilitate glucose production by the liver.[10] First, the liver produces and releases glucose by hepatic glycogen breakdown and when glycogen stores (~100 g) are depleted, it does this by means of gluconeogenesis.[11] Amino acids (alanine) from muscle, lactate from blood and glycerol from lipolysis are all substrates for hepatic gluconeogenesis.[12] In addition to providing glycerol, adipose tissue releases free fatty acids during lipolysis, and provides ketone bodies which serves as an alternate source of fuel to the CNS.[13]

The magnitude of the kidney's contribution to endogenous glucose production has been debated and is confounded by the glucose use of the renal medulla.[14] With no glycogen stores, the kidney is dependent on gluconeogenesis with glutamine being the substrate for gluconeogenesis as opposed to alanine in the liver. Insulin inhibits gluconeogenesis and an appropriate fall in insulin levels and corresponding increase in glucagon sets glucose production in motion. Hypoglycemia sufficient to result in the secretion of catecholamines, engages the kidney in this process of hypoglycemic counterregulation, and further stimulates renal gluconeogenesis.[15]

The insulin and glucagon systems are functionally and anatomically interrelated and collectively form the main buffer against hypoglycemia in normal individuals. In the setting of absent or suboptimal insulin and glucagon release and effect, the sympathoadrenal system becomes significantly important and is the third line of defense.[8,16] Autonomic nervous system activation occurs at glucose concentrations of ~ 3.7 mmol/L (68 mg/dL ± 1 mg/dL) whereas autonomic symptoms first ensue at somewhat lower concentrations, indicating that hormonal counterregulation in fact precedes symptoms of hypoglycemia.[15,16] Neuroglycopenia, assessed by means of cognitive testing in normal individuals, turns out to be detectable at glucose levels of ~2.8 mmol/L (49–51 mg/dL).[8,16]

The extent of the contribution of growth hormone (GH) and adrenocorticotropic hormone (ACTH) from the anterior pituitary to hypoglycemia prevention is less clear. ACTH increase, with a resultant cortisol release, occurs at glucose levels accompanying the first signs of neuroglycopenia.[17,18] The mechanism whereby cortisol opposes insulin action is by facilitating lipolysis and promoting protein catabolism with resultant gluconeogenesis in the liver and kidney.[14,17] GH also antagonizes insulin effect by increasing lipolysis and GH release occurs at similar glucose levels as that of glucagon. If all other factors and protective mechanisms prevail, isolated GH and ACTH deficiencies are infrequently the cause of life-threatening hypoglycemia.[18,19] However, if metabolic glucose demands are high, and counterregulatory mechanisms are blunted or flawed, pathological states of endocrine organs such as the pituitary and/or adrenal glands may be associated with hypoglycemia.

## PATHOLOGICAL CAUSES OF HYPOGLYCEMIA

The various pathologies causing hypoglycemia could be attributed broadly to be either mediated by insulin or insulin-like effects or secondary to absence of endocrine defenses. The most common cause of hypoglycemia encountered in clinical practice is often related to unwanted therapeutic effects of agents used to treat diabetes mellitus, mediated by either exogenous or endogenous hyperinsulinemia. Endogenous unregulated secretion of insulin from a pancreatic tumor (insulinoma) is the most common cause for hypoglycemia in a seemingly well patient without diabetes mellitus. Although these two conditions are the most common, hypoglycemia may be encountered as part of various other endocrinopathies in clinical practice (Table 1).

### Endogenous Hyperinsulinemia

The conditions leading to endogenous hyperinsulinemic hypoglycemia (EHH) are broadly classified into congenital and acquired. Among the causes of congenital hypoglycemia, potassium channel mutations leading to unregulated insulin secretion and causing hypoglycemia in the newborn is the most common cause of EHH. However, in adults, insulin secreting tumors of the pancreas or insulinomas comprise the largest etiological group. Other etiologies such as autoimmune hypoglycemia, nesidioblastosis and reactive hypoglycemia may also be encountered occasionally in clinical practice.

### Insulinoma

The estimated incidence of insulinoma is approximately four per one million patient years. They are usually solitary, well-encapsulated benign lesions, with more than 90% of them being small (<2 cm in size). Once hyperinsulinemic hypoglycemia is confirmed, imaging is essential to localize the tumor and assess its extent. Frequently

**TABLE 1** Common causes of hypoglycemia in people without diabetes mellitus.

| Seemingly well individual | Unwell individual |
|---|---|
| Insulinoma | Organ failure and/or sepsis |
| Nesidioblastosis | Nonislet cell tumor hypoglycemia |
| Hormone deficiency—cortisol, growth hormone, glucagon and catecholamines* | |
| Insulin autoimmune syndrome* | |
| Insulin and/or drugs such as insulin secretagogues | |
| Accidental or surreptitious hypoglycemia | |

*Clinical picture depends on underlying pathological condition.

used imaging modalities are contrast-enhanced CT or MRI of the abdomen. Endoscopic ultrasound is an emerging imaging modality with good sensitivity and specificity. Positron emission tomography (PET)-CT with 68Gallium (Ga)-DOTA-exendin-4 has been reported in recent studies as a good imaging modality to localize insulinomas.

### Noninsulin Pancreatogenous Hypoglycemia Syndrome (NIPHS)

The NIPHS should be considered in patients presenting with EHH without a history of bypass surgery and negative imaging studies. Diazoxide, octreotide, or distal pancreatectomy in refractory cases may be necessary. Surgical specimens have revealed nesidioblastosis; however, no gene mutations seen in congenital hyper-insulinemia have been reported in these patients.

### Insulin Autoimmune Syndrome (IAS)

The IAS is an uncommon cause of hyperinsulinemic hypoglycemia caused by auto-antibodies directed against endogenous insulin in insulin naïve patients. It was originally described by Hirata et al. from Japan, and is still considered to be the third most common cause of spontaneous hypoglycemia among them. There have been several case reports from India as well.[20] Autoimmune conditions like Graves' disease and rheumatoid arthritis may coexist. Recent exposure to drugs containing sulfhydryl group is thought to be a risk factor, with methimazole and carbimazole being frequently encountered culprits. These medications have been proposed to induce antibodies against the insulin molecule by interacting with the disulfide bonds of insulin. When endogenous insulin is bound to insulin antibodies, there is sequestration of insulin, leading to reduction in the amount of bioavailable insulin. In the early postprandial phase, this sequestration of insulin may lead to hyperglycemia, stimulating further insulin secretion from the pancreas. Subsequently, if the insulin is released from the antibody complex during the late postprandial or fasting state, hypoglycemia ensues.

This phenomenon leads to the insulin C-peptide dissociation seen in IAS. After β-cell stimulation by glucose or other insulin secretagogues, both insulin and C-peptide are released from the pancreas into the portal circulation in a 1:1 molar ratio. However, endogenous insulin undergoes extensive hepatic extraction, significantly reducing its concentration in peripheral circulation. C-peptide, on the other hand, undergoes predominantly renal clearance and passes the liver with zero or negligible hepatic extraction. Hence, the insulin C-peptide molar ratio (ICMR) should always be less than 1. The two conditions where ICMR exceeds 1 are IAS and surreptitious or inadvertent exogenous insulin administration leading to an insulin C-peptide mismatch.[20] Typically, patients with IAS tend to have very high insulin values detected at the time of hypoglycemia and have high titers of anti-insulin antibodies. Assay interference from circulating antibodies may also contribute to the falsely elevated serum insulin levels seen as most assays used in clinical practice are immunoassays that are susceptible to such interferences.

Autoimmune hypoglycemia may occur even in patients who develop antibodies against the insulin receptor (IR) leading to prolonged binding of these antibodies to the IR. They may act as blocking antibodies presenting with hyperglycemia and features of severe insulin resistance. Less commonly, they may act like insulin agonists and produce hypoglycemia by binding to the IR.

## Nonislet Cell Tumor Hypoglycemia (NICTH)

The NICTH syndrome is a rare cause of hypoglycemia mediated by insulin-like growth factor-II (IGF-II) secreted by large mesenchymal tumors. These pro-IGF-II molecules bind poorly of its binding proteins; the free form penetrates into tissues and binds to IR causing hypoglycemia.

## Postprandial Reactive Hypoglycemia

Impaired glucose tolerance or initial years of type 2 diabetes mellitus (T2DM) is often associated with loss of the first-phase insulin secretion in response to nutrients. This may result in higher glucose excursions in the early postprandial period, and then by lower glucose nadirs in the late postprandial phase. Occasionally, patients may present with features of reactive hypoglycemia in this situation.

Postprandial reactive hypoglycemia (PRH) may develop due to an exaggerated insulin secretory response in individuals with insulin resistance and manifest with troublesome adrenergic symptoms in the postprandial phase.[21] Hypoglycemia is relatively mild and neurocognitive symptoms rarely develop. In fact, in most cases, plasma glucose values rarely fall below the threshold to label hypoglycemia. High carbohydrate diet and alcohol intake may trigger the symptoms. Increased sensitivity to insulin, defective glucose response and renal glucosuria are other factors considered in causation of these episodes, especially in lean individuals or those who have had significant weight loss. Extended oral glucose tolerance test has been used to diagnose reactive hypoglycemia, but other causes of endogenous or exogenous hyperinsulinemia need to be excluded. These individuals can be managed with dietary modification with intake of small, more frequent meals and restriction of refined carbohydrates. Alpha-glucosidase inhibitors may be used for troublesome symptoms.

## Counter-regulatory Hormone Deficiency

As mentioned earlier, the extent to which the other hormones like ACTH and GH contribute to prevention of hypoglycemia is not clearly understood.

### Hypopituitarism

Isolated deficiency of these hormones does not usually present with hypoglycemia, except in infancy. However, combined deficiencies of these hormones as seen in pituitary diseases, particularly in the presence of acute onset of adrenal insufficiency (apoplexy or acute Sheehan's syndrome), could manifest with hypoglycemia.[22]

### Adrenal Insufficiency

Primary adrenal insufficiency is also less likely to present with hypoglycemia as dyselectrolytemia and hypotension due to mineralocorticoid deficiency will usually precede glucocorticoid deficiency-mediated hypoglycemia. However, recurrent hypoglycemia in a patient with type 1 diabetes mellitus (T1DM) may be a pointer toward autoimmune adrenalitis. Hypoglycemia may be encountered rarely in patients who are on replacement steroids for adrenal insufficiency. Malabsorption from the gut, drug interactions (particularly enzyme inducers that enhance steroid metabolism), and inadequate replacement doses predisposing to nocturnal hypoglycemia should be considered in these situations.

## Thyroid Disorders Associated with Hypoglycemia

As thyroid hormone is involved in energy homeostasis and affects almost all cellular activities in the body, functional disorders of thyroid gland can cause alterations in the glycemic milieu. Hypothyroidism causes several neural, hormonal and metabolic derangements that may predispose to hypoglycemia.[23] Delay in gastric emptying, impaired absorption of glucose from the gut and reduced portal blood flow all contribute to lower plasma glucose values. Insulin secretion from the islets is usually proportionate to the circulating plasma glucose values; however, degradation and clearance of insulin from the circulation may be delayed contributing to relative hyperinsulinemia. The counterregulatory mechanisms are also blunted in hypothyroidism. Norepinephrine levels are slightly increased due to increased production; however, epinephrine levels remain unchanged. The increase in central sympathetic outflow is thought to be a compensatory mechanism for reduced sensitivity to circulating catecholamines. This attenuated response in target tissues like the liver to catecholamines occur because of downregulation of β-adrenergic receptors and some postreceptor defects leading to impaired glycogenolysis, gluconeogenesis and lipolysis.

Cortisol deficiency may occur in hypothyroid patients either as associated autoimmune adrenalitis or there may be a relative cortisol deficiency which manifests itself in the presence of stress or infections contributing to hypoglycemia. Though the production of cortisol is reduced in hypothyroidism, metabolic clearance of the hormone is also reduced leading to adequate basal levels of circulating cortisol. Cortisol deficiency may also be seen in patients with central hypothyroidism as part of panhypopituitarism where both cortisol and GH deficiency may contribute to hypoglycemia. Primary hypothyroidism may also lead to suppression of GH secretion as a result of the increased hypothalamic somatostatinergic tone, which exerts a negative effect on somatotrophs. Although these mechanisms shift the glycemic range to the lower side, in the absence of stressors or precipitating factors, plasma glucose levels are usually maintained within normal limits. The occurrence of frank and recurrent hypoglycemia should prompt the physician to screen the patient for coexisting diseases like Addison's disease or hypopituitarism. In those patients receiving insulin for diabetes control, reduction in dosage may be necessary in view of the reduced degradation and clearance of insulin from the system.

Hyperthyroidism and thyrotoxicosis, on the other hand, are rarely associated with hypoglycemia. The direct effect of thyroid hormones on metabolic parameters and gastric absorption are more likely to cause transient impaired glucose tolerance. Severe hepatic failure with lactic acidosis, congestive cardiac failure and anorexia associated with thyroid storm have been rarely reported to present with hypoglycemia. The most common etiology for hypoglycemia in these patients, however, is the insulin autoimmune syndrome or Hirata disease associated with methimazole or carbimazole therapy.

## Glucagon Deficiency

As glucagon is the most important and first counterregulatory hormone increasing in defense of falling plasma glucose levels, one would expect glucagon deficiency to manifest as hypoglycemia.[24] However, in reality, this is a very rare condition with only about two cases of neonatal and adult hypoglycemia being attributed to glucagon deficiency syndrome in reported literature.[25] In diabetic patients with pancreatic diseases like cystic fibrosis, calcific pancreatitis and atrophic pancreas, the risk of therapeutic hypoglycemia is substantially increased due to lack of endogenous glucagon secretion. Similarly, in patients with long-standing T1DM, one may encounter refractory hypoglycemia compounded by glucagon deficiency as β-cell failure causes loss of the decrement in insulin levels which normally signals an increase in alpha-cell-mediated glucagon secretion during hypoglycemia.[26,27]

## Catecholamine Deficiency

Being the next line of defense against hypoglycemia, catecholamine deficiency also may lead to hypoglycemia, particularly in patients in whom the first line of defense is impaired, e.g. T1DM. In such patients, the risk of therapeutic hypoglycemia markedly increases to as high as 25-fold. Isolated catecholamine deficiency in the absence of diabetes mellitus usually does not present with hypoglycemia, though there are few reports of ketotic hypoglycemia in neonates and children attributed to catecholamine deficiency on the basis of low levels of urinary epinephrine.

Catecholamine excess, on the other hand, is usually associated with mild glucose intolerance or hyperglycemia. However, there are few case reports of hypoglycemia occurring in patients with pheochromocytoma. Catecholamines control glucose homeostasis by increasing glycogenolysis and gluconeogenesis via action on β-adrenoceptors; they also act on pancreatic islets via the alpha-adrenoceptors which suppresses release of insulin. As this is the predominant action in the pancreas, the net effect is usually transient increase in plasma glucose levels.[28] However, the direct action of adrenaline on β-receptors of the pancreatic islets is to stimulate release of insulin; this may become important in disease states associated with depleted glycogen stores or severe hepatic impairment leading to failure of gluconeogenesis. In such a situation, excess adrenaline may paradoxically lead to hypoglycemia. IGF-II-secreting pheochromocytoma could be another rare condition causing the NICTH syndrome. More frequently, hypoglycemia has been reported following surgical excision of pheochromocytoma, which has been postulated to be caused by sudden withdrawal of catecholamine excess resulting in rebound hyperinsulinemia and improved insulin sensitivity.

## Liver and Kidney Diseases

The liver being the most important site for glycogenolysis and gluconeogenesis, the two main mechanisms in place to increase endogenous glucose production, one would expect hypoglycemia in the presence of liver disease. However, in reality, hypoglycemia is rare even in the presence of significant hepatic infiltration or dysfunction. It is often multifactorial with poor nutritional intake, anorexia and infection contributing significantly to the development of hypoglycemia. This is partly due to hepatorenal reciprocity, which ensures that when gluconeogenesis from the liver is reduced, the kidneys are able to step up endogenous glucose production significantly above their usual 15–20% contribution. Another reason for developing hypoglycemia, particularly secondary to cardiac failure, is reduced hepatic perfusion leading to hypoxic injury of hepatocytes. This phenomenon is called Pasteur effect, where decreased oxygenation would drive anaerobic glycolysis and lactate accumulation leading to an increased NADH/NAD ratio. As nicotinamide adenine dinucleotide (NAD) is an essential cofactor required for several gluconeogenic enzymes, this altered ratio would suppress gluconeogenesis.[25]

Similar to the liver, the kidney is the other organ involved in maintaining plasma glucose levels in the normal range, and patients with diabetes are likely to develop renal compromise over time as diabetic nephropathy develops. Many factors like altered drug metabolism, delayed gastric emptying, malnutrition, infection, dialysis, etc. contribute to hypoglycemia in these individuals. Loss of alanine during dialysis, and use of high glucose dialysate (especially in peritoneal dialysis) leading to exaggerated secretion of insulin which is degraded or excreted slowly by kidneys are additional factors that may worsen the risk of hypoglycemia in patients undergoing dialysis.

## Metabolic and Storage Diseases Causing Nonhyperinsulinemic Hypoglycemia

The predominant storage fuel for immediate use is glycogen which is stored in liver, kidney and muscle. In times of need, if stored glycogen is not easily broken down to release glucose, one would expect fasting hypoglycemia, which is seen in association with glycogen storage diseases (GSDs). The steps involved in the synthesis or breaking down of glycogen that may be dysregulated and lead to fasting hypoglycemia in humans include glycogen phosphorylase-liver isoenzyme deficiency, debranching enzyme deficiency, glucose-6-phosphatase deficiency and glucose-6-phosphate translocase deficiency and are enlisted in Table 2.

Following utilization of glycogen in the immediate phase, if dietary glucose is not available, the body next initiates gluconeogenesis; the most important substrate for this are fatty acids stored in the adipose tissue. Inability to mobilize and oxidize fatty acids would lead to hypoglycemia with prolonged fasting especially among those vulnerable, like children and malnourished adults with diminished glycogen reserve. The most common fatty acid oxidation defect among humans is medium-chain acyl-CoA dehydrogenase (MCAD) deficiency. Deficiency of other enzymes necessary for gluconeogenesis like pyruvate carboxylase, phosphoenolpyruvate carboxykinase (PEPCK) and fructose-1,6-bisphosphatase may also present with hypoglycemia. Other rare metabolic diseases causing hypoglycemia include organic

| TABLE 2 | Metabolic storage diseases associated with hypoglycemia. |
|---|---|
| Glycogen storage diseases (GSDs) | • Glycogen phosphorylase—liver isoenzyme deficiency (Hers disease, type VI GSD)<br>• Debranching enzyme deficiency (Cori disease; type III GSD)<br>• Glucose-6-phosphatase deficiency (Von Gierke disease, type Ia GSD)<br>• Glucose-6-phosphate translocase deficiency (Von Gierke disease, type Ib GSD)<br>• Glycogen synthase deficiency (GSD type 0) |
| Defects of fatty acid and glucose metabolism | • Medium-chain acyl-CoA dehydrogenase (MCAD) deficiency<br>• Deficiency of pyruvate carboxylase<br>• Deficiency of phosphoenolpyruvate carboxykinase<br>• Deficiency of fructose-1,6-bisphosphatase |
| Others | • Organic aciduria<br>• Galactosemia<br>• Hereditary fructose intolerance<br>• Glucose transporter type 2 receptor mutations |

aciduria, galactosemia, hereditary fructose intolerance and glucose transporter type 2 (GLUT2) receptor mutations.[29]

## Miscellaneous Causes

### Postbariatric Surgery

Disruption of the entero-insular axis following bariatric surgery leads to amplification of the glucagon-like peptide-1 (GLP-1) effect with resultant postprandial hyperinsulinemia. Obese nondiabetic patients are particularly at risk of developing reactive hypoglycemia in this setting. Low or complex carbohydrate diet with or without alpha-glucosidase inhibitors can ameliorate symptoms; refractory cases may need octreotide, continuous feeding, or partial pancreatectomy.

### Alcohol

Ethanol is a well-known cause for fasting hypoglycemia in malnourished alcoholics and healthy adolescents following alcohol intoxication. The liver uses up NAD during oxidation of ethanol, skewing the NADH to NAD ratio; NAD being an essential factor for gluconeogenesis, fasting hypoglycemia ensues.

### Litchi-associated Seasonal Toxic Encephalopathy

Consumption of only litchi fruit without an evening meal in malnourished glycogen-deprived children has been linked to fatal hypoglycemia in India. The causative factor has been postulated to be the presence of hypoglycin and methylene cyclopropyl glycine (MCPG) in litchi fruit akin to its cousin, the ackee fruit, which has been associated with Jamaican vomiting sickness (toxic hypoglycemic encephalopathy). These toxins are known to cause hypoglycemia by disrupting various gluconeogenic enzymes and inhibiting β-oxidation of fatty acids.[30]

## APPROACH TO HYPOGLYCEMIA

If a seemingly well patient presents with episodic hypoglycemic symptoms, the most probable cause is endogenous hyperinsulinemia. If these episodes are frequent with high suspicion of hypoglycemia, an attempt to draw the critical sample during any such spontaneous event should be made. If not, the patient may be subjected to a 72-hour supervised fast for the development of hypoglycemia. The critical sample collected at the time of hypoglycemia should be assayed for plasma glucose, insulin, C-peptide and β-hydroxybutyrate. If facilities are available, sampling should also be done for proinsulin, serum cortisol and oral hypoglycemic agent (sulfonylurea and glinides) screening.[29] A low serum cortisol in the setting of hypoglycemia is not always suggestive of adrenal insufficiency, as recurrent hypoglycemia may lower the glycemic threshold for cortisol secretion. If serum ketone assays are not available, urine ketone estimation may be used as an alternative. In children, additional evaluation of serum lactate and blood gas analysis for acidosis are beneficial in narrowing down the etiology.[30] Following collection of a critical sample, the hypoglycemia should be initially corrected with 1 mg glucagon given intravenously with assessment of glucose response. Critical diagnostic findings are plasma insulin concentrations of at least 3 µU/mL (18 pmol/L), plasma C-peptide concentrations of at least 0.6 ng/mL (0.2 nmol/L), and plasma proinsulin concentrations of at least 5.0 pmol/L when the fasting plasma glucose concentrations are below 55 mg/dL. Plasma β-hydroxybutyrate levels of 2.7 mmol/L or less and an increase in the plasma glucose concentration of at least 25 mg/dL (1.4 mmol/L) after glucagon (indicating preserved hepatic glycogen stores) suggests hyperinsulinemia (Flowchart 1).

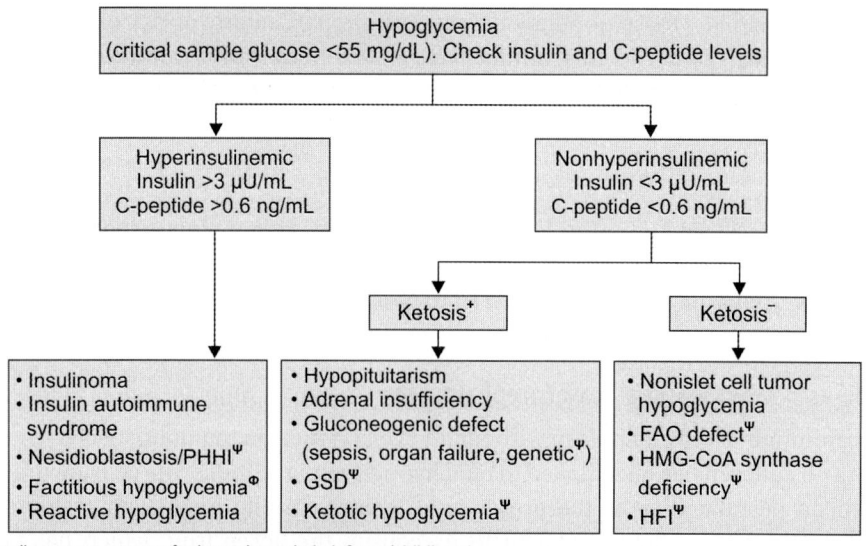

$^\Psi$usually seen as causes for hypoglycemia in infancy/childhood.
$^\Phi$except in exogenous insulin-mediated hypoglycemia, where C-peptide is suppressed.
(FAO: fatty acid oxidation; GSD: glycogen storage disease; HFI: hereditary fructose intolerance; HMG-CoA: 3-hydroxy-3-methylglutaryl-coenzyme A; PHHI: persistent hyperinsulinemic hypoglycemia of infancy)

**FLOWCHART 1:** Approach to hypoglycemia.

## CONCLUSION

Hypoglycemia is a commonly encountered clinical problem and occurs most often in the setting of antidiabetes medications or due to unregulated insulin secretion. However, there are other uncommon causes encountered infrequently which need to be identified and treated appropriately. As multiple endocrine systems are part of the orchestra continuously playing to maintain harmonious normoglycemia, it is not surprising to encounter hypoglycemia in various endocrinopathies. Correcting the primary disease will usually ameliorate hypoglycemia; dual deficiencies or coexisting diseases need to be considered in case of persistent or recurrent hypoglycemia.

## REFERENCES

1. Tesfaye N, Seaquist ER. Neuroendocrine responses to hypoglycemia. Ann N Y Acad Sci. 2010; 1212(1):12-28.
2. Marks V, Teale JD. Drug-induced hypoglycemia. Endocrinol Metab Clin North Am. 1999;28(3):555-77.
3. Whipple AO. The surgical therapy of hyperinsulinism. J Int Chir. 1938;3(1):237-76.
4. MacDuff A, Grant IS. Facticious hypoglycaemia in hypotension. Emerg Med J. 2002;19(4):376.
5. Wickham NW, Achar KN, Cove DH. Unreliability of capillary blood glucose in peripheral vascular disease. Pract Diabetes Int. 1986;3(2):100.
6. Khoury M, Yousuf F, Martin V, et al. Pseudohypoglycemia: a cause for unreliable finger-stick glucose measurements. Endocr Pract. 2008;14(3):337-9.
7. Theofilogiannakos EK, Giannakoulas G, Ziakas A, et al. Pseudohypoglycemia in a patient with the Eisenmenger syndrome. Ann Int Med. 2010;152(6):407-8.
8. Mitrakou A, Ryan C, Veneman T, et al. Hierarchy of glycemic thresholds for counterregulatory hormone secretion, symptoms, and cerebral dysfunction. Am J Physiol. 1991;260(1 Pt 1):E67-74.
9. Cryer PE. Symptoms of hypoglycemia, thresholds for their occurrence, and hypoglycemia unawareness. Endocrinol Metab Clin North Am. 1999;28(3):495-500.
10. Rizza R, Cryer P, Gerich J. Role of glucagon, catecholamines, and growth hormone in human glucose counterregulation. Effects of somatostatin and combined - and -adrenergic blockade on plasma glucose recover and glucose flux rates after insulin-induced hypoglycemia. J Clin Invest. 1979;64(3):62-71.
11. Wasserman DH. Four grams of glucose. Am J Physiol Endocrinol Metab. 2009;296(1):E11-21.
12. Garber AJ, Menzel PH, Boden G, et al. Hepatic ketogenesis and gluconeogenesis in humans. J Clin Invest. 1974;54(4):981-9.
13. Amiel SA, Archibald HR, Chusney G, et al. Ketone infusion lowers hormonal responses to hypoglycaemia: evidence for acute cerebral utilization of a non-glucose fuel. Clin Sci (Lond). 1991;81(2):189-94.
14. Mitrakou A. Kidney: its impact on glucose homeostasis and hormonal regulation. Diabetes Res Clin Pract. 2011;93 Suppl 1:S66-72.
15. Hoffman RP. Sympathetic mechanisms of hypoglycemic counterregulation. Curr Diabetes Rev. 2007;3(3):185-93.
16. Bolli GB, Fanelli CG. Physiology of glucose counterregulation to hypoglycemia. Endocrinol Metab Clin North Am. 1999;28(3):467-93.
17. Davis SN, Shavers C, Costa F, et al. Role of cortisol in the pathogenesis of deficient counterregulation after antecedent hypoglycemia in normal humans. J Clin Investig. 1996;98(3):680-91.
18. De Feo P, Perriello G, Torlone E, et al. Contribution of cortisol to glucose counterregulation in humans. Am J Physiol. 1989;257(1 Pt 1):E35-42.
19. De Feo P, Perriello G, Torlone E, et al. Demonstration of a role for growth hormone in glucose counterregulation. Am J Physiol. 1989;256(6 Pt 1):E835-43.
20. Manjunath PR, George B, Mathew V, et al. "Riding High on Low Fuel" - Our Experience with Endogenous Hyperinsulinemic Hypoglycemia. Indian J Endocrinol Metab. 2017;21(5):655-9.

21. Galati SJ, Rayfield EJ. Approach to the patient with postprandial hypoglycemia. Endocr Pract. 2014;20(4):331-40.
22. Pahadiya HR, Lakhotia M, Gandhi R, et al. Fasting intolerance and recurrent hypoglycemia: Ponder for Sheehan's. Indian J Endocrinol Metab. 2016;20(5):739-40.
23. Kalra S, Unnikrishnan AG, Sahay R. The hypoglycemic side of hypothyroidism. Indian J Endocrinol Metab. 2014;18(1):1-3.
24. Dick AP, Harik SI. Distribution of the glucose transporter in the mammalian brain. J Neurochem. 1986;46(5):1406-11.
25. Spanakis EK, Cryer PE, Davis SN. Hypoglycemia during therapy of diabetes. In: Feingold KR, Anawalt B, Boyce A (Eds). Endotext [Internet]. South Dartmouth: MDText.com, Inc.; 2000.
26. Yale JF, Paty B, Senior PA. Hypoglycemia. Can J Diabetes. 2018;42 (Suppl 1):S104-8.
27. Kahkoska AR, Buse JB. Primum Non Nocere: Refocusing Our Attention on Severe Hypoglycemia Prevention. Diabetes Care. 2018;41(8):1557-9.
28. Thonangi RP, Bhardwaj M, Kulshreshtha B. A case report of reactive hypoglycemia in a patient with pheochromocytoma and it's review of literature. Indian J Endocrinol Metab. 2014;18(2):234-7.
29. Gandhi K. Approach to hypoglycemia in infants and children. Transl Pediatr. 2017;6(4):408-20.
30. Shrivastava A, Kumar A, Thomas JD, et al. Association of acute toxic encephalopathy with litchi consumption in an outbreak in Muzaffarpur, India, 2014: a case-control study. Lancet Glob Health. 2017;5(4):e458-66.

# CHAPTER 13

# Glucovigilance in Endocrine Therapy

Altamash Sheikh, Sandeep Chaudhary

## INTRODUCTION

The concept of glucocrinology is an interesting one as it opens a Pandora's box for the endocrinologist and the treating physician.[1] There exists a close bidirectional harmony between the endocrine system and metabolism, with endocrinopathies creating a significant burden of metabolic disorders and vice versa. Likewise, medications used to treat diabetes have endocrine effects beyond glucose metabolism and endocrine drugs have effects on metabolic health. It is, therefore, prudent to understand the effects of drugs or medications used in the treatment of endocrine/hormonal disorders on glucose physiology, insulin secretion and action and overall metabolic health. This is particularly so because endocrine drugs are usually required over long periods of time and can have an important bearing on cardiometabolic risk of an individual. As diabetes is one of the most important and prevalent problems of current era, it will be of vital importance to maintain pharmacovigilance (PV) of glucose metabolism in endocrine therapy.

Pharmacovigilance or drug safety refers to the science relating to the detection, assessment, understanding and prevention of adverse effects or any other drug-related problems and the implication of this knowledge in clinical practice.[2] Thus, glucovigilance in endocrine therapy would refer to the pharmacological science of the impact of various endocrine drugs on glucose metabolism.

This is of vital importance as endocrine disorders may themselves be associated with abnormal glucose metabolism, and their treatment may have a positive or negative impact on metabolic health, further compounded by unique effects of various drugs on glucose metabolism. We shall discuss glucovigilance in relation to therapy of disorders of the various endocrine axes including the pituitary and hypothalamus, parathyroid and bone mineral metabolism, thyroid, adrenals, gonads and adipose tissue.

## EFFECTS OF ENDOCRINE THERAPY ON GLYCEMIC HEALTH

Endocrine drugs or hormones may affect glucose metabolism in many ways. For ease of understanding, we discuss the effects of various endocrine drugs on glucose homeostasis under the following sections:
- Drugs that may increase glucose levels (detrimental: worsen or exacerbate hyperglycemia)
- Drugs that may reduce glucose levels (beneficial: improve hyperglycemia)
- These will be elaborated in the subsequent sections and are summarized in Tables 1 and 2.

**TABLE 1** Beneficial effects of endocrine drugs on glucose homeostasis.

| Endocrine therapy | Effects on glucose homeostasis |
| --- | --- |
| Levothyroxine | • Improved insulin sensitivity and reduced risk of hypoglycemia<br>• Improved red cell turnover with improved accuracy of HbA1c in identification of hyperglycemia |
| Antithyroid drugs—carbimazole, methimazole | • Improved glucose homeostasis with amelioration of thyrotoxicosis<br>• Can trigger insulin autoimmune hypoglycemia |
| Bromocriptine-QR | • Reduces FPG and HbA1c<br>• Approved for use in diabetes |
| Cabergoline | Reduces both FPG, PPG and HbA1c. May improve glucose homeostasis in diabetic individuals |
| Mifepristone | • Nonselective glucocorticoid receptor (GR) antagonist<br>• Improved glycemic control in Cushing's syndrome |
| 11β-HSD1 inhibitors | Significant reductions in HbA1c and FPG, under development |
| Bisphosphonates | Significant 50% reduction in risk of incident T2DM in retrospective cohorts. But no effect on glycemic control in randomized trials |
| Denosumab | Modest FPG lowering in patients not on OHA |

(11β-HSD1: 11β-hydroxysteroid dehydrogenase type 1; FPG: fasting plasma glucose; HbA1c: hemoglobin A1c; OHA: oral hypoglycemic agent; PPG: postprandial glucose; T2DM: type 2 diabetes mellitus)

**TABLE 2** Detrimental effects of endocrine drugs on glucose homeostasis.

| Endocrine therapy | Effects on glucose homeostasis |
| --- | --- |
| Glucocorticoids | • Impair insulin sensitivity and secretion<br>• Can cause new-onset diabetes, unmask underlying latent diabetes, or worsen glycemic control in diabetic individuals<br>• Greater rise in postprandial blood glucose |
| $\beta_2$-adrenergic agonists | • Impair insulin sensitivity<br>• Can contribute to stress hyperglycemia |
| Growth hormone | • Increase insulin resistance<br>• Can cause new-onset diabetes, especially in individuals at high risk of diabetes |
| *Somatostatin analogs*: Octreotide, lanreotide and pasireotide | • Impair insulin secretion<br>• Can lead to worsening of glycemic control<br>• Pasireotide particularly associated with a high risk of new-onset diabetes or worsening of glycemic control |
| Combined oral contraceptives | High-dose estrogen can increase insulin resistance and cause rise in blood glucose. Effect is negligible with low-doses of contraceptives |

# ENDOCRINE DRUGS WITH A DETRIMENTAL IMPACT ON GLYCEMIC CONTROL

Many endocrine drugs have a significant negative impact on insulin sensitivity and/or insulin secretion, increase hepatic glucose production, or have a direct cytotoxic effect on β-cells. Therefore, they can lead to new-onset diabetes or worsen glycemic control in a diabetic individual. Drug-induced diabetes refers to a new-onset hyperglycemic state concurring with the definition of diabetes and caused by the use of a drug.[3] Drugs that cause or worsen hyperglycemia can increase the risk of symptomatic acute hyperglycemic emergencies and the long-term risk of micro- and macrovascular complications, if one is not vigilant to the possibility.

- *Glucocorticoids*: These are used in a variety of endocrine disorders such as primary or secondary adrenal insufficiency, congenital adrenal hyperplasia, thyrotoxicosis, thyroid eye disease and thyroid storm. Glucocorticoids are also used for their immunosuppressive and anti-inflammatory effects, often in supraphysiological doses.

  Glucocorticoids have a diabetogenic effect primarily by the development of insulin resistance. They increase hepatic gluconeogenesis and decrease peripheral glucose disposal in muscle and adipose tissue and result in the development of insulin resistance in muscle, liver and adipose tissue. Another possible mechanism for insulin resistance is impaired postreceptor insulin-signaling in insulin-sensitive tissues. Decreased insulin-induced vasodilation in muscle leads to reduced glucose delivery to muscle beds and reduced clearance.[4] Action of insulin is blunted by corticosteroids and further promotion of gluconeogenesis is probably due to the activation of liver X receptor-β (LXR-β) involved in phosphoenolpyruvate carboxykinase (PEPCK) gene transcription. In addition, glucocorticoids also reduce pancreatic insulin secretion by a direct effect on β-cells. There is also a net increase in lipid mobilization with increased circulating free fatty acids and lipotoxicity.

  Several factors increase the risk of steroid-induced hyperglycemia. The risk is higher with the use of more potent longer-acting glucocorticoids, especially when used in supraphysiological doses.[5] Therefore, when glucocorticoids are used as replacement therapy in adrenal insufficiency or congenital adrenal hyperplasia, an attempt must be made to minimize the dose of glucocorticoid used. More physiological replacement regimens with hydrocortisone (15–20 mg/day) given in divided doses to mimic normal circadian rhythm is associated with less risk of hyperglycemia.[6] Prednisolone and dexamethasone are associated with a greater risk of adverse metabolic effects. Addition of fludrocortisone can also help to minimize the dose of glucocorticoids. Newer preparations of hydrocortisone (dual release hydrocortisone with an immediate release outer coating and extended release inner core) are associated with less glycemic effects and are underdevelopment.[5]

  However, despite attempts to optimize glucocorticoid doses, most patients on long-term glucocorticoids are often exposed to supraphysiological replacement and are at risk of adverse metabolic and cardiovascular effects.[5] Steroid-induced hyperglycemia is even more common with higher doses of glucocorticoids used in inflammatory and immunosuppressive doses such as in chronic obstructive lung disease, chronic inflammatory disorders, malignancies and posttransplantation. High-dose glucocorticoids, even in the short-term, may lead to increased risk of acute severe hyperglycemic emergencies, including diabetic ketoacidosis and hyperosmolar hyperglycemic state, recurrent infections, poor wound healing, longer hospital stay and complication rates and an overall increased risk of mortality.[6]

This calls for a need for regular blood glucose monitoring and greater metabolic vigilance. Regular blood glucose monitoring should be commenced with initiation of glucocorticoids. Furthermore, it is important to remember that monitoring of fasting plasma glucose (FPG) may not be able to detect hyperglycemia, as glucocorticoids cause predominantly postprandial hyperglycemia, which is more marked in the postlunch period when the glucocorticoid dose is scheduled in the morning. Therefore, self-monitoring of blood glucose (SMBG) throughout the day is advised.

Hyperglycemia is managed with appropriate nutrition counseling, higher protein intake and increased physical activity. Insulin sensitizers such as metformin can improve glycemic control. However, many patients with glucocorticoid-induced hyperglycemia will require insulin for glycemic control. Insulin regimens are guided by SMBG profiles. It is important to remember that when using insulin, most patients will require higher doses of prandial insulin and lower doses of basal insulin. Prandial dose requirements are usually higher in the afternoon and evening meals, as compared to morning meal.[7] Intermediate-acting insulin given once or twice daily may be a useful regimen in some patients. Dipeptidyl peptidase-4 (DPP-4) inhibitors and glucagon-like peptide-1 (GLP-1) agonists have also been found to be useful.[7] However, the pharmacological treatment of hyperglycemia is tailored to meet individual glycemic pattern and the clinical picture

- *Growth hormone (GH)*: Growth hormone acts as via insulin-like growth factor-1 (IGF-1) which has insulin-mimetic effects, and GH deficiency is associated with visceral obesity and insulin resistance. However, GH is an important counterregulatory hormone that increases glycogenolysis and gluconeogenesis in the liver and kidney. In addition, GH causes insulin resistance by disrupting the insulin-signaling in target tissues and reducing peripheral glucose uptake.[8] GH also increases lipolysis with resultant increase in circulating free fatty acids, which further exacerbates insulin resistance. There may be a compensatory increase in insulin secretion from the β-cells, but GH also increases glucose-stimulated insulin secretion directly. However, the persistent rise in free fatty acids may result in increased β-cell apoptosis due to lipotoxicity.

    Growth hormone deficiency is associated with central obesity and insulin resistance with an increased risk of hyperglycemia and dyslipidemia. GH deficiency in adults is associated with increased cardiovascular risk. These metabolic perturbations improve with adequate GH replacement therapy, with improvement in fat distribution, muscle mass, blood pressure and lipids.[8] However, many studies report that GH replacement is associated with insulin resistance, reversible mild glucose intolerance, or even diabetes. Risk factors for

GH-induced hyperglycemia include age, obesity, family history of diabetes, higher doses of GH, and longer treatment duration. Higher doses (≥0.01 mg/kg/day) and longer duration were more significantly associated with hyperglycemia, despite a reduction in visceral fat.[8]

On the other hand, low-dose GH treatment (<0.01 mg/kg/day) is associated with positive changes in body composition and insulin sensitivity and minimal effects on glycemic parameters, even with long-term use. A mild but nonsignificant increase in FPG and hemoglobin A1c (HbA1c) levels has been reported in individuals with preexisting diabetes.[8] Overall, GH replacement therapy was not found to be associated with an increased risk of diabetes as compared to untreated GH deficient adults, but it may contribute to hyperglycemia in individuals at risk of diabetes.

Large prospective studies in children on GH treatment, on the other hand, have demonstrated that the incidence of type 2 diabetes mellitus (T2DM) is six times higher compared to general population.[9] This risk is more marked in individuals with other risk factors for diabetes, such as obesity, Turner syndrome, Prader-Willi syndrome, positive family history, or concomitant glucocorticoid treatment. Another French study that included only children with isolated GH deficiency did not demonstrate such a risk.[9] New-onset diabetes has been described in patients treated with supraphysiological doses of human GH, such as for human immunodeficiency virus (HIV) wasting syndrome [acquired immunodeficiency syndrome (AIDS) cachexia].

Therefore, one needs to be vigilant about the effects of GH treatment on glucose homeostasis when using GH over long periods of time. This is especially so because the risk of insulin resistance and diabetes is per se higher in individuals who are being prescribed GH therapy (e.g. GH deficiency, Turner syndrome, Prader-Willi syndrome). Lower doses of GH therapy are preferred than high-dose GH regimens

- *β-adrenergic agonists/catecholamines*: Acute administration of β-adrenergic agonists including epinephrine and norepinephrine, and synthetic β-agonists is associated with increase in both gluconeogenesis and glycogenolysis. In fact, catecholamines are one of the most important defenses against hypoglycemia. β-adrenergic agonists stimulate protein kinase A, with phosphorylation of the insulin receptor. The resultant reduction in insulin receptor tyrosine kinase activity causes a decrease in insulin signaling.[3,10] β-adrenergic agonists are often used in intensive care for their inotropic and vasoactive effects and they may contribute to stress hyperglycemia, among other factors. It has been demonstrated that epinephrine is more strongly associated with hyperglycemic effect than norepinephrine. Norepinephrine also increases peripheral glucose uptake and utilization[10]
- *Combined oral contraceptives (COCs) and hormone replacement therapy (HRT)*: COCs are associated with weight gain and an increase in insulin resistance. However, the hyperglycemic risk was more with higher-dose estrogen preparations. The effect of low-dose estrogen (20–35 μg) COCs on glucose metabolism seems to be minimal. No significant adverse effect of COCs on glucose homeostasis was documented in a meta-analysis.[11] Progestogens also seem to have minimal

effect on glucose levels. However, depot medroxyprogesterone acetate may worsen insulin resistance due to its effect on the glucocorticoid receptor (GR). Levonorgestrel and antiandrogenic progestins are associated with less metabolic risk.

Hormone replacement therapy in women with Turner syndrome, premature ovarian insufficiency and postmenopausal women also does not affect glycemic control. In fact, the risk of diabetes is increased in hypogonadal women and HRT was associated with a reduced risk of diabetes in menopausal women in Women's Health Initiative and the Heart and Estrogen/progestin Replacement Study (HERS) trials.[12]

However, glucovigilance is justified when using estrogen in women at high risk of diabetes, such as those with positive family history, obesity, polycystic ovary syndrome, previous gestational diabetes mellitus, or glucose intolerance

- *Anabolic androgens*: Synthetic steroid derivatives with androgenic properties, like oxymetholone and danazol, can impair glucose tolerance, probably by inducing insulin resistance at the postreceptor site and increasing glucagon secretion.[13] On the other hand, dehydroepiandrosterone (DHEA) improves insulin secretion and sensitivity and DHEA replacement in postmenopausal women and those with adrenal insufficiency was associated with insignificant improvements in metabolic profile[14]
- *Somatostatin receptor ligands*: Long-acting somatostatin analogs such as octreotide long-acting release (LAR) and lanreotide, which have a predominant effect on somatostatin receptors 2 and 5 (SSTR2 > SSTR5), have been used in acromegaly and other neuroendocrine tumors. They are known to have varied effects on glucose homeostasis. While somatostatin analogs may reduce insulin resistance in acromegaly by inhibiting the secretion of GH, they also impair insulin secretion.[15] Therefore, they can worsen glycemic control and even lead to overt diabetes. Use of insulin secretagogues rather than insulin sensitizers may be more effective in individuals who develop frank hyperglycemia on somatostatin analogs.[15] However, the effects on glucose metabolism are reversible on discontinuation of treatment.

    Pasireotide, which has a high affinity for SSTR1, SSTR2, SSTR3 and SSTR5, is being increasingly used in the management of acromegaly and Cushing's disease. It is associated with a significantly high risk of diabetes, due to reduced secretion of GLP-1, gastric inhibitory polypeptide (GIP) and insulin. It may have a direct inhibitory effect on pancreatic β-cells. New-onset hyperglycemia or worsening hyperglycemia occurs in 50–75% of Cushing's disease patients treated with pasireotide, usually within 3 months of initiation of treatment.[16] Hyperglycemia may be reversible upon discontinuation of the drug. Therefore, close monitoring of glycemic parameters is required in patients on pasireotide treatment. Insulin sensitizers such as metformin and incretin-based drugs including DPP-4 inhibitors and GLP-1 agonists may be useful in the management of hyperglycemia due to pasireotide.[16] Some patients may require insulin initiation
- *Antihypertensive agents*: Certain antihypertensive drugs may worsen glycemic control. Thiazide diuretics can impair insulin secretion when given at high dosages, possibly due to potassium depletion. However, more importantly,

they impair hepatic insulin sensitivity and increase hepatic glucose output.[17] Nonselective β-blockers can reduce peripheral blood flow and reduce peripheral glucose uptake, but this risk is less with cardioselective β-blockers. β-blockers may also impair insulin secretion.[17] Both thiazide diuretics and β-blockers have been associated with an increased risk of diabetes in observational studies. Lower doses of thiazides and cardioselective β-blockers are associated with lower risk.[18,19] On the other hand, calcium-channel blockers, angiotensin-converting enzyme (ACE) inhibitors and angiotensin II receptor blockers (ARBs) are metabolically neutral. ACE inhibitors and ARBs may improve insulin sensitivity.[18]

However, the effect of thiazides and β-blockers on glycemic control is only mild and not associated with an increased cardiovascular risk. While one must remain vigilant of the possible effect of these drugs on glycemic control, optimization of blood pressure control in endocrine disorders is important as part of multifactorial risk reduction and will often require the use of multiple drugs

- *Lipid-lowering drugs*: These can have a significant impact on glucose homeostasis. Statins are associated with an increased risk of hyperglycemia and new-onset diabetes. This effect seems to be related to their low-density lipoprotein (LDL) lowering effect, with resultant increase in insulin resistance and decreased insulin secretion. This effect seems to be dose-dependent and is more with higher-intensity statins.[20]

    Proprotein convertase subtilisin/kexin type 9 (PCSK9) inhibitors are also associated with a mild increase in FPG, though this has not been associated with increased risk of diabetes.[20] Niacin is also associated with hyperglycemia, though the exact mechanism is not clearly understood. Niacin may act via niacin receptors in the β-cells to reduce glucose-stimulated insulin secretion.[20]

    On the other hand, colesevelam, a bile acid sequestrant, has a positive effect on glycemic control and may improve insulin sensitivity. Fibrates seem to have a neutral effect on glucose metabolism, but have been found to reduce the risk of retinopathy in diabetes.

## ENDOCRINE DRUGS WITH BENEFICIAL EFFECTS ON GLUCOSE METABOLISM

Many endocrine therapies have a positive impact on glycemic control. Optimal treatment of endocrine disorders associated with impaired glucose metabolism results in improvement in glycemic control. This is true for both surgical and pharmacological management of endogenous glucocorticoid excess (Cushing's syndrome), acromegaly, pheochromocytoma, primary hyperaldosteronism, primary hyperparathyroidism, thyrotoxicosis, prolactinoma, polycystic ovary syndrome and syndromic obesity. Many endocrine therapies have a positive effect on glucose homeostasis, and in fact have been used as antidiabetic medications. These include bromocriptine, cabergoline, mifepristone, 11β-hydroxysteroid dehydrogenase type 1 (11β-HSD1) inhibitors and metreleptin.

- *Bromocriptine*: It is an oral agonist of dopamine receptor type 2. It has been used in the management of prolactinoma, acromegaly, infertility and galactorrhea as a slow-release formulation. It has been demonstrated that the hypothalamic effects of quick-release (QR) preparation of bromocriptine were associated with lowering of blood glucose levels. It seems to act by enhancing early morning central nervous system dopaminergic activity, with a resultant increase in insulin sensitivity and reduction in liver glucose output.[21]

Bromocriptine-QR add-on therapy lowers HbA1c compared with placebo, with significant reduction in FPG and minimal effect on postprandial glucose.[22] It may lead to nausea and vomiting, but the risk of hypoglycemia is minimal. Though it can lead to postural hypotension, it does not seem to have adverse cardiovascular effects. Bromocriptine-QR is an alternative option to currently available antidiabetic agents for adults with T2DM.

- *Cabergoline*: It is a long-acting dopamine agonist with high affinity for dopamine receptors type 2. The mechanism of benefit seems to be similar to that seen with bromocriptine. Cabergoline has been associated with reduction in fasting as well as postprandial blood glucose (PPBG) and HbA1c.[23] Compared to bromocriptine, cabergoline has fewer gastrointestinal side effects, especially when used in lower doses and has better patient tolerability. It is also associated with improvement in insulin sensitivity, lipid abnormalities and markers of cardiovascular risk. In one study, treatment with cabergoline was compared to gliclazide and was associated with significant ($p < 0.05$) and comparable reductions in fasting blood glucose (FBG), PPBG and HbA1c.[24] Cabergoline may be useful as a long-acting antidiabetic agent in T2DM. However, more studies are needed to elucidate the mechanisms of the dopamine agonist effect on glucose metabolism
- *Mifepristone*: It is a high-affinity, nonselective GR antagonist with 10 times greater affinity for the GR than cortisol and four times greater affinity than dexamethasone. It was associated with significant reduction in the area under curve on an oral glucose tolerance test (OGTT) in patients with Cushing's syndrome.[25] It is also associated with reduction in diastolic blood pressure. It is United States Food and Drug Administration (USFDA)-approved for the reduction of hyperglycemia (both T2DM and glucose intolerance) in patients with Cushing's syndrome[26]
- *11β-hydroxysteroid dehydrogenase type 1 inhibitors*: 11β-HSD regulates to inter-conversion between active cortisol and inactive cortisone in several tissues. The two isoforms of 11β-HSD (1 and 2) are expressed in a tissue-specific manner. 11β-HSD2 inactivates cortisol by converting it to cortisone and is expressed in kidneys and colon. On the other hand, 11β-HSD1 increases the conversion of cortisone to active cortisol. 11β-HSD1 seems to be involved in the pathogenesis of obesity and insulin resistance. Inhibition of 11β--HSD1 leads to reduced glucocorticoid effect on liver, adipose tissue and vascular tissue. 11β-HSD1 inhibitors are a novel therapeutic target in the management of obesity and T2DM and are currently in phase II trials.[27]

They reduce hepatic gluconeogenesis, improve peripheral glucose uptake and have a positive effect on lipid metabolism. In early studies, they are associated with small reduction in FPG, HbA1c, weight, hypercholesterolemia and hypertriglyceridemia.[28] Also, positive effects are observed primarily in obese/overweight, explaining the significance of 11β-HSD1 activity in adipose tissue.[28] However, the magnitude of effect seems to be small. Current research is focused

on the development of tissue-specific 11β-HSD1 inhibitors for the management of T2DM
- *Metreleptin*: Metreleptin, an analog of leptin, has been used in the management of congenital and acquired lipodystrophies. Subcutaneous metreleptin is associated with significant improvements in body composition, insulin sensitivity, hyperglycemia and dyslipidemia and liver histology. 12 months of metreleptin treatment was associated with significant reduction in HbA1c, triglycerides and hepatic transaminases.[29] Therefore, it may be a very useful agent in patients with secondary diabetes due to lipodystrophy
- *Antiosteoporosis drugs*: Recent research indicates that bone secretes several osteokines that have a role in glucose metabolism and undercarboxylated osteocalcin improves insulin sensitivity and secretion. However, bisphosphonates or denosumab did not have any effect on glycemic parameters in FIT, FREEDOM and HORIZON-PFT trials.[30] Teriparatide also does not seem to impact glucose metabolism.

On the other hand, long-term retrospective data suggests that bisphosphonate use was associated with a small initial increase followed by a progressive sustained 50% decrease in the risk of incident diabetes.[31] The beneficial effects were seen irrespective of age and body mass index (BMI) or glucocorticoid exposure and was consistent for all bisphosphonates evaluated. In addition, denosumab was associated with modest reduction in FPG in patients not on antidiabetic medications.[30] Thus, future larger and specified clinical trials will tell us whether blocking receptor activator nuclear factor κ-B ligand (RANKL) has any clinically important effect on glucose metabolism.

## DRUGS THAT MAY CAUSE HYPOGLYCEMIA OR HYPOGLYCEMIA UNAWARENESS

- *Antithyroidal drugs*: Untreated or uncontrolled hyperthyroidism may lead to poor glycemic control, and even recurrent diabetic ketoacidosis. Antithyroid drug treatment with methimazole or carbimazole can help resolve hyperglycemia due to improvement in thyrotoxic state. However, these drugs have also been associated with the occurrence of spontaneous insulin autoimmune hypoglycemia, also called Hirata syndrome, in rare cases. Insulin autoimmune syndrome develops due to the production of antibodies that bind to insulin in circulation. The individual may have hyperglycemia with postprandial hypoglycemia. Drugs with sulfur or sulfhydryl groups have been implicated in the pathogenesis and antithyroid drugs such as methimazole and carbimazole have been reported to be causative[32]
- *β-blockers*: Nonselective β-blockers such as propranolol are used to manage hyperadrenergic symptoms in patients with thyrotoxicosis. Metoprolol and bisoprolol are alternative drugs. While β-blockers may have a mild diabetogenic effect in general, it does not seem to be clinically significant. However, they may increase the risk of hypoglycemia by reducing counterregulatory effects of catecholamines. Hypoglycemia has been reported with even topical ocular use of β-blockers in type 1 diabetic individuals. However, more importantly, β-blockers

may mask the adrenergic symptoms in response to hypoglycemia and increase the risk of hypoglycemia unawareness.[33] Cardioselective β-blockers cause less hypoglycemia unawareness and may be preferred in diabetic individuals. It is important to recognize hypoglycemia for prompt treatment.

## DRUGS USEFUL IN THE MANAGEMENT OF HYPOGLYCEMIA

- *Somatostatin analogs*: Somatostatin analogs such as octreotide and lanreotide suppress insulin secretion. The hyperglycemic effects of octreotide have been exploited in the management of hypoglycemia, especially for stabilization of glucose levels prior to surgery in patients with insulinoma or cases of malignant insulinoma, in the management of persistent hyperinsulinemic hypoglycemia of infancy, postbariatric surgery nesidioblastosis, autoimmune hypoglycemia and even refractory sulfonylurea-induced hypoglycemia[34]
- *Diazoxide*: It is a nondiuretic benzothiadiazine derivative with a potent vasodilator effect and was initially developed as an antihypertensive. It acts on the cell membrane to open the ATP-dependent potassium (K-ATP) channel, leading to membrane hyperpolarization and inhibition of insulin secretion. It can cause hyperglycemia with two or three doses only. It is approved for the management of hyperinsulinemic hypoglycemia including preoperative glucose stabilization prior to insulinoma surgery, malignant insulinoma and persistent hyperinsulinemic hypoglycemia of infancy.[35] Side effects include hypertrichosis, fluid retention, pulmonary hypertension, leukopenia and hyperuricemia
- *Glucocorticoids*: Adrenal insufficiency, both primary or secondary, is associated with increased risk of hypoglycemia. Adequate glucocorticoid replacement leads to amelioration of hypoglycemia. In addition, glucocorticoids have been used in the medical management of endogenous hyperinsulinism, particularly in patients with insulin autoantibody syndrome. Short-term use of glucocorticoids was associated with reduction of insulin antibody titers and reduced episodes of hypoglycemia[36]
- *β₂-agonists*: β₂-agonists such as terbutaline can increase glucose levels and have been considered for the prevention of nocturnal hypoglycemia, along with alanine. The effect is more pronounced in the nocturnal period when terbutaline was administered at night. Though they are seldom used for hypoglycemia prevention, they may be useful in individuals with hypoglycemia unawareness.[37] However, adrenergic sensitivity may be reduced in long-standing diabetes, limiting their clinical utility. No long-term trials have evaluated the role of β₂-agonists in the prevention of nocturnal hypoglycemia or hypoglycemia unawareness.

## TREATMENT OF ENDOCRINE DYSFUNCTION MAY UNMASK LATENT DIABETES

Endocrine disorders like Addison's disease, hypothyroidism and hypopituitarism may be associated with lower blood glucose levels and even increased risk of hypoglycemia. Once adequate hormone replacement treatment with glucocorticoids and/or thyroxine is commenced, it may unmask underlying latent hyperglycemia.

Therefore, glucovigilance may become important.[38] This is also important since these disorders may be autoimmune in origin and associated with type 1 diabetes mellitus. Insulin dose modification may be required once glucocorticoid or thyroid hormone replacement is initiated.

In addition, hypothyroidism may be associated with reduced red blood cell turnover, with a falsely increased HbA1c.[39] Therefore, in such cases, measurement of fasting and postprandial glucose should guide therapy decisions for coexistent diabetes until thyroxine replacement has been optimized and HbA1c can be reliably estimated.

## CONCLUSION

Endocrine disorders are associated with significant alterations in glucose and energy metabolism. Therefore, the importance of glucovigilance in the endocrine practice cannot be overemphasized. At the same time, many hormone-based and other therapies used in the medical management of endocrine disorders can have significant impact on glycemia. This calls for a need for continued glucovigilance, during long-term care. A high index of suspicion for dysglycemia in endocrine therapy is required. Monitoring and treatment of hyperglycemia related to endocrine therapy needs to be individualized. A regular follow-up and a personalized therapeutic approach are needed to improve clinical care with vigilance toward early detection and management of drug-induced hyperglycemia.

Monitoring of FPG and HbA1c may miss many cases as some of these drugs, such as glucocorticoids, lead to predominant postprandial hyperglycemia. OGTT and SMBG may be more useful. More physiological replacement such as for glucocorticoids and female HRT may be associated with less risk of hyperglycemia. Similarly, lower doses of thiazides and cardioselective β-blockers are associated with less effect on glycemic control. Management of hyperglycemia will require specific strategies that address the underlying pathophysiology. Glucocorticoid-induced hyperglycemia often requires insulin initiation, with higher doses of prandial insulin. Hyperglycemia caused by pasireotide is more responsive to incretin-based therapies.

An understanding of the glucocrinology of endocrine therapies has also paved the way for development of novel therapeutic strategies in the management of diabetes. Bromocriptine and 11β-HSD1 inhibitors are under exploration for their potential role in metabolic disorders. Research is also focused on understanding the effects of osteokines on glucose health. Similarly, the hyperglycemic effects of somatostatin receptor agonists and diazoxide have been exploited in the management of hyperinsulinemic hypoglycemia.

## REFERENCES

1. Kalra S, Priya G, Gupta Y. Glucocrinology. J Pak Med Assoc. 2018;68(6):963-5.
2. Pitts PJ, Louet HL, Moride Y, et al. 21st century pharmacovigilance: efforts, roles, and responsibilities. Lancet Oncol. 2016;17(11):e486-92.
3. Repaske DR. Medication-induced diabetes mellitus. Pediatr Diabetes. 2016;17(6):392-7.
4. Alduaiji NM, Alduayji MM. Steroid Induced Diabetes. Diabetes Obes Int J. 2017;2(4):000165.

5. Mazziotti G, Formenti AM, Frara S, et al. Management of Endocrine Disease: Risk of overtreatment in patients with adrenal insufficiency: current and emerging aspects. Eur J Endocrinol. 2017;177(5):R231-48.
6. Suh S, Park MK. Glucocorticoid-Induced Diabetes Mellitus: An Important but Overlooked Problem. Endocrinol Metab (Seoul). 2017;32(2):180-9.
7. Tamez-Pérez HE, Quintanilla-Flores DL, Rodríguez-Gutiérrez R, et al. Steroid hyperglycemia: Prevalence, early detection and therapeutic recommendations: A narrative review. World J Diabetes. 2015;6(8):1073-81.
8. Kim SH, Park MJ. Effects of growth hormone on glucose metabolism and insulin resistance in human. Ann Pediatr Endocrinol Metab. 2017;22(3):145-52.
9. Child CJ, Zimmermann AG, Scott RS, et al. Prevalence and incidence of diabetes mellitus in GH-treated children and adolescents: analysis from the GeNeSIS observational research program. J Clin Endocrinol Metab. 2011;96(6):E1025-34.
10. Phadke D, Beller JP, Tribble C. The Disparate Effects of Epinephrine and Norepinephrine on Hyperglycemia in Cardiovascular Surgery. Heart Surg Forum. 2018;21(6):E522-6.
11. Goodman NF, Cobin RH, Futterweit W, et al. American Association of Clinical Endocrinologists, American College of Endocrinology and Androgen Excess and PCOS Society Disease State Clinical Review: Guide to the Best Practices in the Evaluation and Treatment of Polycystic Ovary Syndrome - Part 2. Endocr Pract. 2015;21(12):1415-26.
12. Stuenkel CA. Menopause, hormone therapy and diabetes. Climacteric. 2017;20(1):11-21.
13. Bruce R, Godsland I, Stevenson J, et al. Danazol induces resistance to both insulin and glucagon in young women. Clin Sci (Lond). 1992;82(2):211-7.
14. Aoki K, Terauchi Y. Effect of Dehydroepiandrosterone (DHEA) on Diabetes Mellitus and Obesity. Vitam Horm. 2018;108:355-65.
15. Paragliola RM, Salvatori R. Novel Somatostatin Receptor Ligands Therapies for Acromegaly. Front Endocrinol (Lausanne). 2018;9:78.
16. Colao A, De Block C, Gaztambide MS, et al. Managing hyperglycemia in patients with Cushing's disease treated with pasireotide: medical expert recommendations. Pituitary. 2014;17(2):180-6.
17. Blackburn DF, Wilson TW. Antihypertensive medications and blood sugar: theories and implications. Can J Cardiol. 2006;22(3):229-33.
18. Barzilay JI, Davis BR, Whelton PK. The glycemic effects of antihypertensive medications. Curr Hypertens Rep. 2014;16(1):410.
19. Mills GA, Horn JR. Beta-blockers and glucose control. Drug Intell Clin Pharm. 1985;19(4):246-51.
20. Zafrir B, Jain M. Lipid-lowering therapies, glucose control and incident diabetes: evidence, mechanisms and clinical implications. Cardiovasc Drugs Ther. 2014;28(4):361-77.
21. Liang W, Gao L, Li N, et al. Efficacy and Safety of Bromocriptine-QR in Type 2 Diabetes: A Systematic Review and Meta-Analysis. Horm Metab Res. 2015;47(11):805-12.
22. Garber AJ, Blonde L, Bloomgarden ZT, et al. The role of bromocriptine-QR in the management of type 2 diabetes expert panel recommendations. Endocr Pract. 2013;19(1):100-6.
23. Bahar A, Kashi Z, Daneshpour E, et al. Effects of cabergoline on blood glucose levels in type 2 diabetic patients: A double-blind controlled clinical trial. Medicine. 2016;95(40):e4818.
24. Morcos JA, Ebeid AM, Khodeir SA, et al. Co-Administration of Cabergoline and Gliclazide Improve Glycemic Parameters and Lipid Profile in T2DM. J Diabetes Metab. 2017;8(9):759.
25. Fleseriu M, Biller BM, Findling JW, et al. Mifepristone, a glucocorticoid receptor antagonist, produces clinical and metabolic benefits in patients with Cushing's syndrome. J Clin Endocrinol Metab. 2012;97(6):2039-49.
26. Morgan FH, Laufgraben MJ. Mifepristone for management of Cushing's syndrome. Pharmacotherapy. 2013;33(3):319-29.
27. Dube S, Norby BJ, Pattan V, et al. 11beta-hydroxysteroid dehydrogenase types 1 and 2 activity in subcutaneous adipose tissue in humans: implications in obesity and diabetes. J Clin Endocrinol Metab. 2015;100(1):E70-6.
28. Li X, Wang J, Yang Q, et al. 11β-Hydroxysteroid Dehydrogenase Type 1 in Obese Subjects With Type 2 Diabetes Mellitus. Am J Med Sci. 2017;354(4):408-14.
29. Brown RJ, Meehan CA, Cochran E, et al. Effects of Metreleptin in Pediatric Patients With Lipodystrophy. J Clin Endocrinol Metab. 2017;102(5):1511-9.

30. Schwartz AV, Schafer AL, Grey A, et al. Effects of antiresorptive therapies on glucose metabolism: results from the FIT, HORIZON-PFT, and FREEDOM trials. J Bone Miner Res. 2013;28(6):1348-54.
31. Toulis KA, Nirantharakumar K, Ryan R, et al. Bisphosphonates and glucose homeostasis: a population-based, retrospective cohort study. J Clin Endocrinol Metab. 2015;100(5):1933-40.
32. Censi S, Mian C, Betterle C. Insulin autoimmune syndrome: from diagnosis to clinical management. Ann Transl Med. 2018;6(17):335.
33. Martín-Timón I, Del Cañizo-Gómez FJ. Mechanisms of hypoglycemia unawareness and implications in diabetic patients. World J Diabetes. 2015;6(7):912-26.
34. Bodnar TW, Acevedo MJ, Pietropaolo M. Management of non-islet-cell tumor hypoglycemia: a clinical review. J Clin Endocrinol Metab. 2014;99(3):713-22.
35. Fukutomi M, Shimodera M, Maeda Y, et al. Safety and effectiveness, including intelligence prognosis, of diazoxide in pediatric patients with hyperinsulinemic hypoglycemia: special survey in Japan (long-term, all-case survey). Clin Pediatr Endocrinol. 2018;27(3):131-43.
36. Hunter A, Graham U, Lindsay JR. Insulin Autoimmune Syndrome: a rare case of hypoglycaemia resolving with immunosuppression. Ulster Med J. 2018;87(1):34-6.
37. Cooperberg BA, Breckenridge SM, Arbelaez AM, et al. Terbutaline and the prevention of nocturnal hypoglycemia in type 1 diabetes. Diabetes Care. 2008;31(12):2271-2.
38. Anantarapu S, Vaikkakara S, Sachan A, et al. Effects of thyroid hormone replacement on glycated hemoglobin levels in non diabetic subjects with overt hypothyroidism. Arch Endocrinol Metab. 2015;59(6):495-500.
39. Kalra S. Thyroid disorders and diabetes. J Pak Med Assoc. 2014;64(8):966-8.

# CHAPTER 14

# Glucovigilance Across Stages of Life

Beatrice Anne, Roberta Lamptey, Gagan Priya

## INTRODUCTION

A close bidirectional relationship exists between glucose and energy homeostasis and endocrine functions throughout life. The various endocrine axis regulate the dynamic alterations in metabolism and organ function that occur in individuals across the lifespan, from intrauterine life to neonatal period, infancy and childhood, adolescence, reproductive period and during aging.

Endocrine factors governing glucose homeostasis vary according to age and maturation. The steady state of glucose levels in the body is maintained by the interplay between these endocrine factors, and the hormones and processes involved in glucose metabolism. In this chapter, we review these physiological interactions between glucose metabolism and the hormones involved through various stages of life. This chapter also looks at disease processes associated with disorders of glucose regulation at different stages of life.

## GLUCOVIGILANCE IN NEONATES

### Glucose Physiology in Neonatal Period

The endocrine-metabolic milieu changes dramatically from in utero to birth and the neonatal period is a very vulnerable time for the neonate who is at risk of both hypoglycemia and hyperglycemia. In utero, glucose is the primary fuel for the developing fetus, and it is obtained through the maternal circulation via glucose transporter 1 (GLUT1)-mediated facilitated transport through the placenta. The circulating glucose concentrations in fetus are estimated to be slightly less than maternal plasma glucose, approximating 70–90 mg/dL (3.9–5 mmol/L).[1] Despite fetal glucose concentrations being slightly lower than maternal glucose concentrations, there is a lower threshold of insulin secretion in fetal life to allow for sufficient insulin secretion to maintain fetal growth. In fact, fetal insulin secretion plays little role in glucose homeostasis during intrauterine period, and glucose is primarily derived from maternal circulation.

During labor, a rise in stress hormones causes a slight increase in this glucose supply and cord blood glucose concentrations have been reported to be slightly high. After delivery, there is an abrupt cessation of this supply of nutrients from the placenta with a rapid decline in plasma glucose levels within 2-3 hours of birth, by almost 25-30 mg/dL (1.4-1.7 mmol/L), to as low as 55-60 mg/dL (3-3.3 mmol/L).[1]

Several physiological adaptations occur in this transition phase following birth, to ensure a constant supply of glucose for physiological needs of the newborn until the newborn is fed colostrum which is rich in fat and low in carbohydrates. Birth is accompanied by a decrease in plasma insulin levels and an increase in glucagon and cortisol levels in the newborn.[2] Insulin secretion is, however, not completely suppressed despite low glucose concentrations. Likewise, the low glucose concentrations are accompanied by low plasma ketone levels due to insulin-induced suppression of lipolysis and ketone production.[1] Ketogenesis is partially activated after 1-2 days of birth. Therefore, ketones are not an alternative fuel for brain in the event of significant neonatal hypoglycemia.

There is also a dramatic surge in the catecholamine levels induced by the stressors associated with delivery, including transient hypoxia, cold exposure, and cutting of the cord. This particular hormonal milieu promotes glycogenolysis, lipolysis and gluconeogenesis with the glucocorticoids also increasing the availability of gluconeogenic substrates. As a result, the blood glucose levels gradually increase over the next several hours to few days after birth to reach levels of 70-100 mg/dL (3.9-5.6 mmol/L) seen in infancy and childhood.[1]

The newborn period is reflected by a plasma glucose requirement of approximately 6 mg/kg/min as assessed by isotope tracer studies, compared to 2-3 mg/kg/min in adults.[2] The glucose requirement varies in newborns relative to prematurity and increasing age. In the physiological state, blood glucose levels of term newborn babies vary greatly ranging from 40 to 100 mg/dL, relative to the narrow glycemic range found in adults (70-100 mg/dL).[2] Significant controversy exists over the definitions of both hypoglycemia and hyperglycemia in the period immediately following birth.

## Neonatal Hypoglycemia

The American Association of Pediatrics defines neonatal hypoglycemia as blood glucose less than 47 mg/dL (2.61 mmol/L) whereas the Pediatric Endocrine Society (PES) recommends a blood glucose cutoff value of less than 50 mg/dL (2.77 mmol/L) in the first 48 hours after birth as the threshold for neonatal hypoglycemia.[1,3] In addition, the PES endorses a threshold of 60 mg/dL (3.33 mmol/L) in the first 48 hours if there is concern for a congenital hypoglycemia disorder.[3]

Lower blood glucose values can be seen in the healthy neonatal population in the first 24-48 postnatal hours. These lower values are usually transitional and non-pathologic as the newborn adapts to the new environment, and this has been called as "transitional neonatal hypoglycemia in normal newborn". This occurs due to incomplete suppression of insulin secretion at relatively lower plasma glucose concentrations. Transitional neonatal hypoglycemia usually resolves spontaneously by 2-3 days of life.[1] Preterm, intrauterine growth restriction, birth asphyxia,[2] erythroblastosis and maternal toxemia can result in more prolonged transient neonatal hypoglycemia, requiring further evaluation and management, due to immature β-cell regulation of insulin secretion.

The causes of persistent hypoglycemia include defects in the regulation of insulin secretion, inborn errors of metabolism (glucose, glycogen and fatty acid metabolism) and growth hormone (GH) or glucocorticoid deficiency states.[4] These are enlisted in Table 1. Congenital hyperinsulinism may occur due to activating mutations in glucokinase or hexokinase, which result in lower glucose thresholds for insulin secretion. These infants have glucose values remaining constant between 50 and 65 mg/dL (2.8–3.6 mmol/L).[3] While they have frequent symptoms of hypoglycemia, brain injury rarely occurs.

Guidelines do not recommend regular blood glucose monitoring in all newborns; however, screening of at-risk newborns is highly recommended. The PES recommends that for the first 24–48 hours, the focus should be on stabilizing glucose levels, and if low blood glucose values persist after 48 hours, further evaluation for persistent hypoglycemia is warranted.[3] While transitional neonatal hypoglycemia is considered physiological and self-limiting, it is important to detect disorders that result in

**TABLE 1** Causes of neonatal hypoglycemia.

| | Specific etiology |
|---|---|
| Transient neonatal hypoglycemia of newborn | • More prolonged hypoglycemia with preterm delivery, intrauterine growth retardation, asphyxia, maternal diabetes or hypertension, erythroblastosis, polycythemia |
| Congenital hyperinsulinism | • ABCC8 (encodes SUR1 subunit of KATP channel) gene mutation<br>• KCNJ11 (encodes Kir6.2 subunit of KATP channel) gene mutation<br>• GLUD1 gene (encodes glutamate dehydrogenase) mutation<br>• Glucokinase, HNF-1α and HNF-4α mutations<br>• Inactivating mutations of UCP2<br>• Short chain 3-hydroxyacyl-CoA dehydrogenase mutation<br>• SLC16A1 (encodes monocarboxylate transporter 1) gene mutation<br>• Insulin receptor gene mutation<br>• Beckwith–Wiedemann syndrome |
| Inborn errors of metabolism | • Glycogen storage disorders<br>• Glucose-6-phosphatase deficiency<br>• Congenital disorders of glycosylation<br>• Galactosemia<br>• Fatty acid oxidation defect<br>• Hereditary fructose intolerance<br>• Carnitine deficiency<br>• Amino acidemia |
| Hormone deficiencies | • Growth hormone deficiency<br>• Combined anterior pituitary hormone deficiency<br>• Adrenal insufficiency |

(*ABCC8*: ATP-binding cassette subfamily C member 8; *GLUD1*: glutamate dehydrogenase 1; HNF: hepatocyte nuclear factor; KATP channel: ATP-sensitive potassium channel; *KCNJ11*: potassium voltage-gated channel subfamily J member 11; *SLC16A1*: solute carrier family 16 member 1; SUR1: sulfonylurea receptor 1; UCP2: uncoupling protein 2) severe and persistent hypoglycemia in order to avoid permanent brain damage and developmental disability. Table 2 enumerates the clinical indicators that warrant screening and evaluation of newborns for hypoglycemia.

The evaluation and management of hypoglycemia differs from adults and specific guidelines are available from various pediatric societies. An algorithm to evaluate an infant with hypoglycemia is given in Flowchart 1.[4] A low blood glucose value by glucometer must be confirmed by laboratory measurement of plasma glucose. Clinical evaluation should assess for features of hypopituitarism (micropenis, cleft lip or cleft palate, midline facial defects, short stature, blue sclera), adrenal insufficiency (anorexia, hyperpigmentation, abdominal pain), glycogen storage diseases (hepatomegaly) or Beckwith–Wiedemann syndrome (macroglossia, hemihypertrophy, omphalocele). In addition to measurement of plasma glucose, the "critical sample" should include measurement of serum insulin and C-peptide levels, β-hydroxybutyrate, bicarbonate, lactate, free fatty acids, plasma carnitine and acyl-carnitine profile and GH and cortisol levels to aid in differential diagnosis.[3]

**TABLE 2**: Newborns at-risk for prolonged hypoglycemia, requiring screening and evaluation.

| Risk factors | Clinical indicators |
| --- | --- |
| Severe and symptomatic hypoglycemia | • Symptomatic hypoglycemia<br>• Severe hypoglycemia<br>• Inability to maintain plasma glucose >60 mg/dL after 48 hours of birth |
| Abnormal fetal growth | • Preterm delivery<br>• Small for gestational age<br>• Intrauterine growth retardation<br>• Large for gestational age |
| Perinatal stress | • Cesarean section for fetal distress<br>• Meconium aspiration<br>• Birth asphyxia<br>• Intrauterine growth retardation<br>• Maternal preeclampsia or eclampsia or diabetes<br>• Erythroblastosis fetalis<br>• Polycythemia<br>• Hypothermia |
| Family history | • Family history of congenital hyperinsulinism<br>• Family history of inborn errors of metabolism |
| Features of anterior pituitary deficiency | • Cleft palate or cleft lip<br>• Other midline facial defects<br>• Micropenis<br>• Short stature<br>• Blue sclera |
| Hepatosplenomegaly | • Glycogen storage diseases |

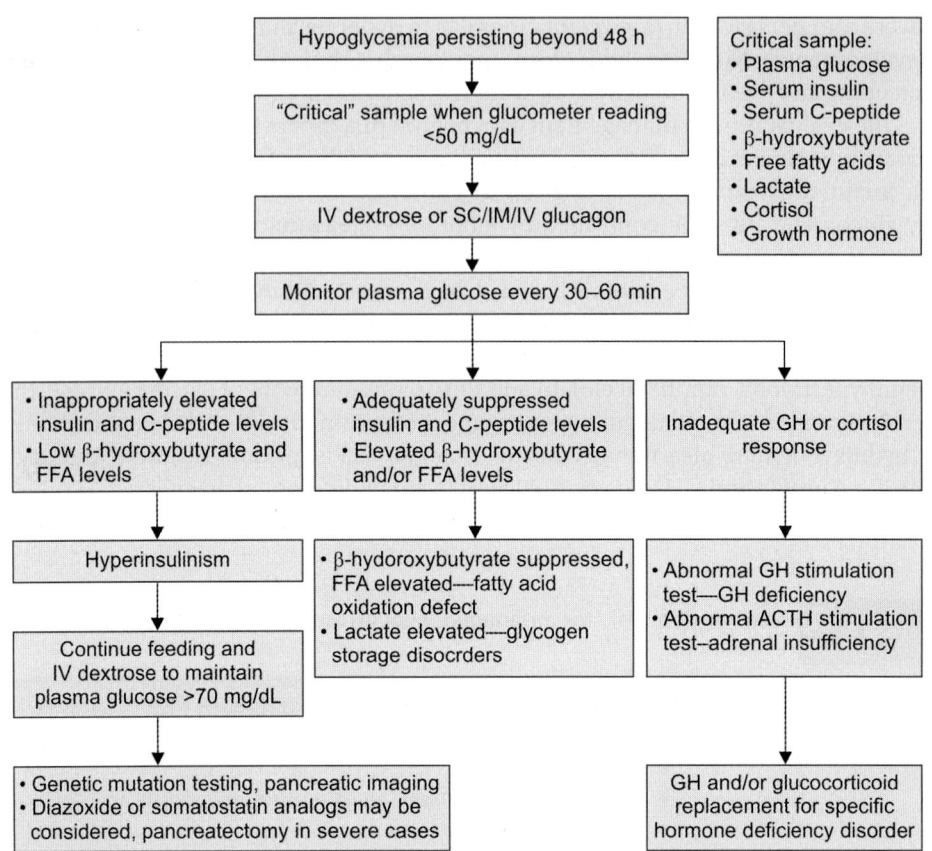

(ACTH: adrenocorticotropic hormone; FFA: free fatty acids; GH: growth hormone; IM: intramuscular; IV: intravenous; SC: subcutaneous)

**FLOWCHART 1:** Approach to neonatal hypoglycemia.

Management of persistent hypoglycemia includes maintenance of plasma glucose concentrations more than 70 mg/dL with frequent feeds. Severe symptomatic hypoglycemia requires intervention with intravenous dextrose infusion—initial dose of 200 mg/kg bolus, followed by 10% dextrose infusion.[3] In hyperinsulinism, intravenous, intramuscular or subcutaneous glucagon can be administered (0.5–1.0 mg).[3] Long-term management depends on underlying etiology. GH deficiency is treated with GH replacement, while adrenal insufficiency is managed with glucocorticoid replacement therapy. Newborns and infants with congenital hyperinsulinism are managed with diazoxide and octreotide and may require surgery in the form of subtotal or near-total pancreatectomy. Inborn errors of metabolism are treated with appropriate nutritional modification.[3]

## Neonatal Diabetes

Hyperglycemia in neonates is often the result of neonatal diabetes resulting from monogenic defects. However, transient neonatal hyperglycemia may also occur in premature and low or very-low birth weight (VLBW) infants. Hyperglycemia has been reported in 25–75% of preterm and low birth weight infants during first 3–5 days after birth, and this usually resolves in 2–3 days.[5] The possible causative factors of hyperglycemia in this subgroup of infants include immature β-cell function, relative lack of adipose tissue and skeletal muscle, inadequate counter-regulatory hormone response and inflammation, and these are listed in Table 3. The adverse effects of hyperglycemia include increased risk of sepsis (bacterial as well as fungal), intraventricular hemorrhage[6] and in premature infants, an increased risk of retinopathy of prematurity.[7] Significant hyperglycemia should be managed with insulin. However, there is lack of consensus about the level of blood glucose above

**TABLE 3**: Causes of hyperglycemia in newborn.

| Etiology | Pathogenesis/contributing factors | Treatment |
| --- | --- | --- |
| Neonatal hyperglycemia in preterm and low birth weight infants | • Immaturity of β-cells<br>• Less adipose tissue and skeletal muscle—decreased peripheral glucose utilization<br>• Hyperalimentation and drugs (parenteral glucose, glucocorticoids)<br>• Delay in establishment of enteral feeds—less incretin stimulation<br>• Respiratory failure and sepsis—increased counter-regulatory hormones<br>• Increased inflammatory markers and proinflammatory cytokines | • Symptomatic—management of severe hyperglycemia with insulin<br>• Resolves over 2–3 days |
| Mutations in KATP channel | Impaired insulin secretion:<br>• Activating mutations in *KCNJ11* (encodes Kir6.2 subunit)<br>• Activating mutations in *ABCC8* (encodes SUR1 subunit) | • Sulfonylureas (usually high doses required) |
| Mutations in *INS* gene | • Misfolding of insulin protein, with endoplasmic reticulum stress | • Require insulin therapy |
| Transient neonatal diabetes | • Overexpression of genes at chromosome 6q24 | • Transient, requires insulin<br>• Develop diabetes in adolescence |
| Rare forms | • Pancreatic hypoplasia (mutation in GATA6 and PDX1 transcription factors)<br>• EIF2AK3 mutations (β-cell death)<br>• FOXP3: Autoimmune (IPEX syndrome—immune dysregulation, polyendocrinopathy, enteropathy, X-linked syndrome) | • Insulin and pancreatic enzyme supplements<br>• Insulin therapy<br>• Insulin, stem cell transplantation |

(*ABCC8*: ATP-binding cassette subfamily C member 8; EIF2AK3: eukaryotic translation initiation factor 2 alpha kinase 3; FOXP3: forkhead box P3; GATA6: GATA-binding protein 6; KATP channel: ATP-sensitive potassium channel; *KCNJ11*: potassium voltage-gated channel subfamily J member 11; INS: insulin; PDX1: pancreatic and duodenal homeobox 1; SUR1: sulfonylurea receptor 1) which insulin should be initiated. Intravenous insulin may be considered if blood glucose remains above 250 mg/dL, at rates of 0.02–0.05 units/kg/h with hourly capillary glucose monitoring.[8] In general, hyperglycemia usually resolves over the next 2–3 days; if it persists beyond 7–10 days, evaluation for neonatal diabetes is warranted.[8]

Hyperglycemia occurring in the neonatal period and within 6 months of life could be due to neonatal diabetes. Neonatal diabetes is rare and often occurs due to monogenic defects—transient, permanent and syndromic. It may present in neonatal period or up to 12 months after birth.[9] Presenting symptoms may include polyuria, polydipsia, failure to thrive, altered mental status or diabetic ketoacidosis.

Most cases of permanent neonatal diabetes mellitus (PNDM) are caused by activating mutations in genes *KCNJ11* and *ABCC8* which encode the Kir6.2 and SUR1 subunits of the β-cell adenosine triphosphate (ATP)-sensitive potassium channel (KATP), respectively. These infants may also have attention deficit disorders, seizures and developmental delays.[8] Another important subtype of PNDM is the one caused by heterozygous mutations in the insulin gene (INS).[8] The majority of cases of transient neonatal diabetes are caused by mutations in the q24 region of chromosome 6 (6q24) affecting imprinted genes. These neonates usually present in the first week of life with severe hyperglycemia, in contrast to those with PNDM who tend to present at a median of around 4 weeks.[9] They require insulin treatment for about 3 months before going into remission, only to be followed by a recurrence of diabetes later in life. Most infants presenting with diabetes after 6 months age have autoimmune type 1 diabetes mellitus (T1DM).

Evaluation should include measurement of plasma glucose, serum insulin, C-peptide and ketones and an abdominal ultrasound to assess pancreatic morphology. Genetic evaluation should be considered in all cases of neonatal diabetes.[9] Assessment of antibodies against glutamic acid decarboxylase (GAD 65), insulin, islet antigen-2 (IA-2) and zinc transporter 8 (ZnT8) is suggested in infants presenting with diabetes after 6 months age.

Initial management of hyperglycemia is with intravenous insulin infusion at low rates, followed by later transition to subcutaneous insulin. Initial subcutaneous insulin administration includes small preprandial doses prior to alternate feeds, often requiring dilution of insulin to U-10 strength. Insulin requirements are usually low in infancy and glycemic targets are more relaxed (<200 mg/dL) to avoid hypoglycemia.[8] Continuous subcutaneous insulin infusion allows for delivery of small doses. Long-term treatment of PNDM is guided by evaluation, especially genetic testing. Sulfonylureas, often in high doses (1 mg/kg/day of glyburide), are used in the treatment of neonatal diabetes due to mutations in *KCNJ11* and *ABCC8* genes as they promote closure of the KATP channels. Sulfonylureas may also reduce the risk of neurodevelopmental disability resulting from KATP channel mutations in brain.[9] Therefore, genetic testing should be done in all cases of neonatal diabetes.[8] Neonatal diabetes due to mutations in INS requires insulin therapy.

Hence, glucovigilance in the neonatal period is of particular importance because this can have consequences on growth and metabolism beyond the neonatal period.

# GLUCOVIGILANCE IN CHILDHOOD AND ADOLESCENCE

## Glucose Homeostasis in Children and Adolescents

Childhood and adolescence are a period of active growth and maturation. Puberty especially is a period of dynamic metabolic and hormonal changes. Body composition changes occur in both girls and boys as puberty progresses. The gain in fat seen in girls is typically peripheral and not abdominal in distribution.[10] Changes in adiponectin and leptin have been documented as well. Leptin is a permissive hormone for initiation of puberty and its levels are elevated in youth at the onset of puberty. However, some sex differences have been noted in leptin dynamics. In girls, leptin continues to increase throughout puberty to adult concentrations, whereas in boys, leptin increases transiently and is then reduced.[11] In girls, the levels of adiponectin appear to change very little, whereas they decrease at pubertal onset and continue to decline as puberty progresses in boys.[11]

Insulin sensitivity reduces drastically around mid-puberty and recovers around puberty completion. One of the important mediators of insulin resistance at puberty is GH, which rises to maximal concentrations during puberty, enhancing the growth spurt. It has been postulated that GH modulates the signaling of phosphoinositide 3 kinase (PI3K), the rate-limiting enzyme in insulin signaling pathway that mediates its metabolic effects, thereby resulting in changes in insulin sensitivity.[12] Multiple studies have found a correlation between serum insulin like growth factor-1 (IGF-1) and insulin sensitivity during puberty but whether this increase in IGF-1 is a cause or effect of insulin resistance is still a matter of debate.[13] In addition, low plasma adiponectin levels in children and adolescents have been linked to obesity, insulin resistance, type 2 diabetes mellitus (T2DM), higher systolic blood pressure and other markers of cardiovascular disease.[14]

## Diabetes in Children and Adolescents

Diabetes can present during this period as T1DM, T2DM, maturity-onset diabetes of the young (MODY), cystic fibrosis-related diabetes and diabetes associated with syndromes like Down syndrome, Prader–Willi syndrome or Wolfram syndrome. Table 4 gives a brief overview of the common types of diabetes in this age group and their usual clinical features.[15]

While younger children with T1DM do not demonstrate insulin resistance in the absence of obesity, significant impairment in insulin sensitivity may occur in the peripubertal period, requiring increase in insulin dose. In T1DM, increased insulin resistance of puberty has been studied in the background of the dawn phenomenon, in which it has been shown that insulin requirements increase overnight and are maximal between 8 AM and 9 AM. This change in overnight insulin sensitivity has been directly correlated with the mean GH concentrations. The dawn phenomenon has been found to be maximal at puberty Tanner stages 3 and 4 in both sexes, although there might be individual variations. This is an important issue to be kept in mind by the clinicians treating pubertal children with T1DM, when adjusting insulin doses. Insulin requirements may reach 1.5–2 units/kg/day during puberty and then return to prepubertal doses at the end of teenage years. Failure to reduce insulin doses in

**TABLE 4** Clinical and diagnostic features of diabetes in youth.

| | Type 1 diabetes mellitus | Type 2 diabetes mellitus | Monogenic diabetes | FCPD |
|---|---|---|---|---|
| Age at onset | Any age after 6 months; most common in childhood and early adolescence | Adolescence and young adulthood; onset in children becoming more common, although unusual before puberty | • Any age; usually presents before 25 years of age<br>• Hyperglycemia in GCK defects can be present from birth | Usually in the second decade |
| Family history of diabetes | Usually sporadic (>85%) | Strongly positive; usually on both sides of the family | Positive for at least three generations, on one side of the family | Unusual |
| Overweight/obesity | Occurs at frequency similar to general population | Common | Occurs at frequency similar to general population | Usually lean |
| Features of insulin resistance | Unusual | Common | Unusual | Unusual |
| C-peptide levels | Low or undetectable, particularly after 2–3 years of diagnosis | May be supranormal, normal or low | Usually lower than normal | Low |
| Islet autoantibodies | Present in majority of patients | Usually absent | Usually absent | Usually absent |

(FCPD: fibrocalculous pancreatic diabetes; GCK: glucokinase)
*Source*: Unnikrishnan R, Shah VN, Mohan V Challenges in diagnosis and management of diabetes in the young. Clin Diabetes Endocrinol. 2016;10;2:18.

late adolescent girls may aggravate weight gain. The physiological insulin resistance in puberty is exaggerated in obese youth and they do not recover from this insulin resistance at completion of puberty.

Puberty also releases the brakes, on the onset of youth-onset T2DM, in this vulnerable population. The incidence of youth-onset T2DM is associated with rapid β-cell decline[16] and its timing is tightly linked with puberty. Puberty also negatively impacts metabolic health in obese youth.[17] In a 1-year longitudinal follow-up study of over 1,000 obese youth, puberty onset and further weight gain were the two strongest predictors of transition to metabolically unhealthy obesity.[18]

Other physiological changes also contribute to youth-onset T2DM. Longitudinal studies have shown that girls show a significantly greater decline in physical activity than boys during puberty, especially girls of certain ethnicities who are at greater risk for cardiometabolic disease.[19] The relationship between insulin sensitivity and cardiorespiratory fitness is bidirectional in that impaired insulin sensitivity can by itself cause a decline in cardiorespiratory fitness.[20] Hence, puberty-induced impairment in insulin sensitivity may prove detrimental to youth who are already obese and have poor physical activity. Management of youth-onset T2DM should be holistic. It must focus not only on lifestyle modification, and glycemic control but also managing mental health and dyslipidemia. Medical nutrition therapy is an effective conduit for the optimization of body weight and increasing physical activity. Metformin is the first-line drug of choice; however, diabetes in this age is associated with a rapid decline in insulin secretion and need for early insulin initiation.

Although the most common cause of hyperglycemia in middle and old age is T2DM, diabetes in children and adolescents may result from a wide spectrum of hyperglycemic disorders and a clear differential diagnosis is required for appropriate management. Glucovigilance assumes importance in childhood and adolescence, especially around the time of puberty because metabolic alterations at this time can influence metabolic and cardiovascular health in adulthood.

## GLUCOVIGILANCE IN THE REPRODUCTIVE PERIOD

### Glucose Homeostasis in Reproductive Age

The reproductive period is again a very important phase in both men and women, with respect to glycemic control and metabolic health. With the rising prevalence of overweight and obesity, there is a rising trend in lifestyle-related disorders including polycystic ovary syndrome (PCOS), metabolic syndrome and T2DM in the reproductive age group.

In menstruating women, it has been shown that the glycemic status varies with the phase of the menstrual cycle. In women with T1DM, use of continuous glucose monitoring to evaluate blood glucose levels through phases of the menstrual cycle has shown an increase in the frequency of hyperglycemia during the luteal phase.[21] This has been postulated to be due to hormonal effects or the premenstrual syndrome. These findings are clinically important as insulin dose requirements may increase in late luteal phase with wide fluctuations in blood glucose profile.

Insulin resistance is the key factor in the pathophysiology of PCOS. Compensatory hyperinsulinemia results in pleiotropic effects including cogonadotrophic stimulation of ovarian and adrenal steroidogenesis. Women with PCOS are at a fourfold increased risk of developing T2DM, that occurs at an earlier age. Moreover, the risk of gestational diabetes mellitus (GDM) increases more than six times in patients with PCOS.[22] This assumes great clinical importance because both pregestational diabetes and gestational diabetes have negative consequences on maternal and fetal health.

Oral contraceptive use is common in women in reproductive age group and high-dose contraceptives have been associated with impaired insulin sensitivity and increased glucose levels. Progestins may directly affect pancreatic insulin secretion, reduce insulin receptor expression and impair postreceptor insulin signaling.[23] In addition, progestins with androgenic activity may have a greater impact on glucose and lipid metabolism than neutral and antiandrogenic progestins. Currently used oral contraceptive formulations contain low doses of estrogen (20–35 μg) and third-generation progestins which have less impact on metabolic health. Clinicians must discuss the risks associated with OCP use as well as the need for glucovigilance.

The importance of glucovigilance in men in the reproductive age group deserves mention. Diabetes can impact reproductive health, and sexual dysfunction is an important complication of diabetes. In addition, obesity and diabetes are associated with reduced testosterone concentration and functional hypogonadism. These issues are discussed in the chapters "Reproductive Health in Diabetes" and "Sexual Dysfunction in Diabetes". Glucose metabolism is an important event in spermatogenesis. Any derangement during the critical period of spermatogenesis can have detrimental effects on the developing sperm.[24] Suboptimal glycemic control can affect sperm quality by several mechanisms:

- Impairment of spermatogenesis, reduced sperm count and motility
- Altering steroidogenesis and sperm motility
- Testicular and erectile dysfunction
- Impairment of sperm deoxyribonucleic acid (DNA) integrity
- Effect on ingredients of seminal plasma
- Epigenetic dysregulation during spermatogenesis.

## GLUCOVIGILANCE DURING PREGNANCY

Significant changes in insulin sensitivity and insulin secretion occur during pregnancy, with an increase in insulin secretion and a progressive increase in insulin resistance in later half of pregnancy. These are discussed in the chapter "Glucocrinology of Female Reproductive System". Hyperglycemia during pregnancy can be due to pre-existing diagnosed or undiagnosed diabetes (T1DM, T2DM and secondary diabetes) or GDM.

### Gestational Diabetes Mellitus

The American Diabetes Association (ADA) describes GDM as diabetes that is first diagnosed in the second or third trimester of pregnancy that is not clearly either pre-existing T1DM or T2DM.[25] The Hyperglycemia and Adverse Pregnancy Outcome (HAPO) study showed that the relationship between maternal hyperglycemia and macrosomia is continuous, without any distinct threshold.[25] Fetal complications like macrosomia, shoulder dystocia, birth injury, neonatal hypoglycemia, neonatal hyperbilirubinemia and polycythemia are associated with uncontrolled GDM. Mothers with GDM also have an excess risk of hypertensive disorders during pregnancy and a high risk of progression to overt diabetes later in life.

The International Association of Diabetes and Pregnancy Study Group (IADPSG) criteria is used to diagnose GDM and overt diabetes in pregnancy.[26] A fasting 75 g oral glucose tolerance test (OGTT) is carried out and one or more values should be above the recommended cutoffs to diagnose GDM. Table 5 describes the diagnostic criteria and treatment targets for diabetes during pregnancy. Depending on the blood glucose levels, the mainstay of therapy in GDM includes medical nutrition therapy, exercise, self-monitoring of blood glucose, insulin and metformin. In the postpartum period, women with GDM should be tested for persistent diabetes or prediabetes at 6 weeks with a 75-g OGTT using nonpregnancy criteria.

### Epigenetic Programming

The metabolic map is drawn in utero through fetal programming for the developing progeny. Various factors affect the metabolic milieu in this crucial period,

**TABLE 5** Diagnostic criteria and treatment targets in gestational diabetes mellitus.

| Diagnostic criteria | |
|---|---|
| **Gestational diabetes (75 g oral glucose tolerance test)** | |
| Fasting plasma glucose | ≥92 mg/dL |
| 1-hour plasma glucose | ≥180 mg/dL |
| 2-hour plasma glucose | ≥153 mg/dL |
| **Overt diabetes** | |
| Fasting plasma glucose | ≥126 mg/dL |
| Random plasma glucose | ≥200 mg/dL |
| HbA1c | ≥6.5% |
| **Treatment targets** | |
| Fasting glucose | <95 mg/dL |
| 1-hour postprandial glucose | <140 mg/dL |
| 2-hour postprandial glucose | <120 mg/dL |

(HbA1c: glycated hemoglobin)

including hormonal changes, lifestyle and environmental factors. The intrauterine environment influences the expression and functioning of genes in the fetus. A small change in this environment has the potential to permanently alter gene expression and therefore the structure and function of developing organ systems. These processes, which govern evolution of an individual phenotype from the genome, are called "epigenetic" changes and involve chemical modifications in the structure of chromatin, through either methylation of DNA or acetylation of histones, that influence gene expression.[27] The role of maternal diabetes in fetal programming gave rise to the concept of fuel-mediated teratogenesis ranging from disfiguring birth defects to a wide range of changes in the body habitus of the developing fetus. Maternal hyperglycemia and the consequent fetal programming of relevant genes in utero may also contribute to increased risk of diabetes in the offspring in the future. This was demonstrated by a study on Arizona Pima Indians, which showed that infants of mothers living with diabetes, had an increased risk of obesity and glucose intolerance. This is usually demonstrable by late childhood. Over half of the cases of diabetes in young Pima Indians were estimated to be attributable to maternal diabetes.[28]

In summary, glucovigilance in both men and women in the reproductive age group cannot be overemphasized because of the adverse effects of deranged blood glucose on fertility and conception. It is also crucial around this period because of the effects on the progeny through epigenetic modifications on the sperm as well as in the intrauterine environment.

# GLUCOVIGILANCE IN THE ELDERLY

The geriatric population is another group which requires glucovigilance due to the effects of aging on glucose metabolism and body composition.

## Glucose Physiology in the Elderly

Aging is associated with reduced insulin sensitivity as well as impaired insulin secretion due to several factors, enumerated in Table 6. Hyperinsulinemic-euglycemic clamp studies have shown a reduction in whole body insulin sensitivity in older adults. Aging is associated with an increase in abdominal fat mass and a reduction in the lean body mass or sarcopenia. In addition, declining physical activity and aging-associated changes in hormonal milieu [reduced IGF-1, sex steroids and dehydroepiandrosterone (DHEA) secretion] also contribute to impaired insulin sensitivity. There is increased oxidative stress and inflammation and an increased burden of concomitant diseases and use of "diabetogenic" medications.[29]

In normal physiology, insulin is secreted from β-cells as low-amplitude pulses approximately every 8–14 minutes and as larger amplitude ultradian pulses occurring every 60–140 minutes. Older adults, in both the fasting and the fed state show reduced amplitude of rapid as well as ultradian pulses. Aging impairs β-cell function and β-cell adaptation to insulin resistance. The mechanism of this β-cell dysfunction is not clearly understood, but both lifestyle and genetic factors seem to play a contributory role.[29] The expression of p16INK4a was shown to increase in aging mice and was associated with reduced replicative capacity of islet cells. Further, accumulation of DNA mutations with aging may also reduce β-cell regeneration.[30] With regard to incretins, there is no evidence that the secretion of gastric inhibitory polypeptide (GIP) and glucagon like peptide-1 (GLP-1) is reduced in the elderly, although β-cell may be less responsive to their stimulatory effects.[29]

It has been estimated that there is a rise of 1–2 mg/dL in fasting plasma glucose and 15 mg/dL in postprandial plasma glucose every decade, after 30 years of age.[30]

**TABLE 6** Factors causing impaired insulin sensitivity and insulin secretion with aging.

| Impaired β-cell function | Increased insulin resistance |
| --- | --- |
| • Reduced glucose-stimulated insulin response<br>• Loss of insulin secretion pulsatility<br>• Decreased sensitivity to incretins<br>• Reduced β-cell mass | • Increase in total body fat mass<br>• Loss of lean muscle mass/sarcopenia<br>• Reduced physical activity<br>• Chronic inflammation<br>• Mitochondrial dysfunction<br>• Increased circulating free fatty acids<br>• Reduced levels of IGF-1, DHEA and sex steroids (estrogen in women, testosterone in men)<br>• Intercurrent illness<br>• Medications: Glucocorticoids, thiazides, β-blockers, statins |

(DHEA: dehydroepiandrosterone; IGF-1: insulin-like growth factor-1)

These age-related changes lead to a significantly higher prevalence of impaired glucose tolerance and diabetes seen in the elderly.

## Geriatric Diabetes

The prevalence of diabetes in individuals 65 years and above is estimated to be 25.2% or 123 million. Typical hyperglycemic symptoms may not appear, and the individual may present with fatigue, anorexia, weight loss, blurred vision, gait instability, urinary incontinence, impaired cognition or confusion. The symptoms may be confused as usual signs of aging and require a high index of suspicion. Elderly people are more susceptible to the development of hyperglycemic hyperosmolar state with severe dehydration and electrolyte imbalance.[30] The spectrum of diabetes in this age group includes cases of new-onset diabetes, previously diagnosed diabetes or previously undiagnosed diabetes. Those with long-standing diabetes are more likely to have micro- or macrovascular complications and comorbidities that influence therapeutic choices. In addition, there are various geriatric syndromes associated with diabetes in the elderly. These include loss of muscle function, frailty and sarcopenia, functional limitations and disability, cognitive dysfunction, depression, visual and hearing impairment, chronic pain, injurious falls, stress incontinence and polypharmacy. Higher HbA1c levels show a significant positive correlation with the degree of disability.[31] A J-shaped association of HbA1c with mortality has been shown in studies, with increased mortality seen in both higher and lower HbA1c groups.[32] There is increased risk of hypoglycemia resulting from several factors: renal and hepatic impairment, malnutrition, dementia, frailty, impaired counter-regulatory response to hypoglycemia, failure to perceive autonomic symptoms and polypharmacy.

Several factors need to be considered in the management of geriatric diabetes including assessment of biomedical, functional, psychological and social factors, as enlisted in Table 7. The ADA recommends stratifying the elderly with diabetes

**TABLE 7** Clinical assessment of elderly with diabetes.

| Domain of assessment | Factors |
|---|---|
| Medical | • Glycemic burden<br>• Comorbidities<br>• Complications<br>• Nutritional status |
| Functional | • Cognitive abilities<br>• Functional abilities |
| Psychological | • Depression<br>• Mood<br>• Motivation |
| Social | • Self-care ability<br>• Support system<br>• Finances |

based on a functional classification into three categories (healthy, intermediate, poor health) as detailed in Table 8.[30] The importance of glucovigilance in the elderly is not only to target hyperglycemia but also to prevent hypoglycemia. Due to the reasons discussed above, less stringent targets for HbA1c and glycemic control are followed for frail elderly persons with diabetes. In this aspect, the deterioration in cardiac and renal parameters with aging also needs to be considered. In managing elderly patients with diabetes, it is of paramount importance not to be glucocentric.

Medical nutrition therapy along with strength training is particularly efficacious in the elderly. Medical nutrition therapy should focus on ensuring an adequate and balanced intake of calories. Cruciferous vegetables, lean proteins, and high-quality fats should be emphasized as well as optimal hydration. Supervised muscle strengthening exercises and maintenance of healthy body weight is recommended. Metformin remains the preferred initial antihyperglycemic agent, unless contraindicated or not tolerated. Drugs with a low risk of hypoglycemia are preferred. DPP-4 inhibitors have a low risk of hypoglycemia and can be used in those with renal or hepatic impairment and cardiovascular disease. Thiazolidinediones increase the risk of osteoporosis and upper-arm fractures particularly in postmenopausal women and are best avoided. SGLT-2 inhibitors may be associated with increased risk of genitourinary infections, volume depletion, acute kidney injury, bone loss and increased risk of falls and require caution. Sulfonylureas and insulin are associated with an increased risk of hypoglycemia and should be initiated in lower doses and cautiously titrated.[30] Cognitive decline, physical disability, visual and hearing impairment may significantly impact a person's self-care abilities, requiring the identification of support system from family and friends. Elderly are also at increased risk of adverse drug reactions and drug interactions due to impaired glomerular filtration rate and polypharmacy. All of these factors need to be assessed and incorporated into the treatment plan.

**TABLE 8** Functional classification of elderly individuals with diabetes.

| ADA category | IDF category | Prognosis | HbA1c goal |
|---|---|---|---|
| Healthy (few coexisting chronic illnesses, intact cognitive and functional status) | Functionally independent | Longer life-expectancy | <7.5% |
| Complex/intermediate (multiple coexisting chronic illnesses* or impairment in ≥2 ADL or mild-to-moderate cognitive impairment) | Functionally dependent, frailty or dementia | Intermediate remaining life-expectancy, high burden of treatment, risk of hypoglycemia and falls | <8% |
| Very complex/poor health (long-term care or end-stage chronic illnesses* or moderate to severe cognitive impairment or 2 + activities of daily living dependencies) | End-of-life care | Limited life-expectancy, benefits of intensive control uncertain | <8.5% |

*Chronic illness: Disease serious enough to require medications (arthritis, cancer, congestive heart failure, depression, emphysema, falls, hypertension, incontinence, stage 3 or worse chronic kidney disease, myocardial infarction, stroke).
(ADL: activities of daily living ; ADA: American Diabetes Association; HbA1c: glycated hemoglobin; IDF: International Diabetes Federation)

## CONCLUSION

In this chapter, we have reviewed the importance of glucovigilance across the lifespan of an individual. Although screening for diabetes was classically advised after a particular age and in certain ethnic groups, with the rising prevalence of obesity and metabolic syndrome, no age can be considered free of risk. The importance of glucovigilance in the different age groups is to identify the different types of diabetes and its accompanying adverse effects, be it on growth or maturation, fertility, fecundity, biopsychosocial health and overall quality of life. Clinicians treating various metabolic disorders across different age groups should focus on glucovigilance as well.

## REFERENCES

1. Stanley CA, Rozance PJ, Thornton PS, et al. Re-evaluating "transitional neonatal hypoglycemia": mechanism and implications for management. J Pediatr. 2015;166(6):1520-5.
2. Harding JE, Harris DL, Hegarty JE, et al. An emerging evidence base for the management of neonatal hypoglycaemia. Early Hum Dev. 2017;104:51-6.
3. Thornton PS, Stanley CA, De Leon DD, et al. Recommendations from the Pediatric Endocrine Society for Evaluation and Management of Persistent Hypoglycemia in Neonates, Infants, and Children. J Pediatr. 2015;167(2):238-45.
4. Gandhi K. Approach to hypoglycemia in infants and children. Transl Pediatr. 2017;6(4):408-20.
5. Shield JP, Scharfmann R. Development of the Pancreas and Neonatal Diabetes. Endocr Dev Basel, Karger; 2007. pp. 124-37.
6. Finberg L. Dangers to infants caused by changes in osmolal concentration. Pediatrics. 1967;40(6):1031-4.
7. Ertl T, Gyarmati J, Gaal V, et al. Relationship between hyperglycemia and retinopathy of prematurity in very low birth weight infants. Biol Neonate. 2006;89(1):56-9.
8. Lemelman MB, Letourneau L, Greeley SA. Neonatal Diabetes Mellitus: An Update on Diagnosis and Management. Clin Perinatol. 2018;45(1):41-59.
9. Ashcroft FM, Puljung MC, Vedovato N. Neonatal Diabetes and the K(ATP) Channel: From Mutation to Therapy. Trends Endocrinol Metab. 2017;28(5):377-87.
10. Dai S, Labarthe DR, Grunbaum JA, et al. Longitudinal analysis of changes in indices of obesity from age 8 years to age 18 years. Project HeartBeat! Am J Epidemiol. 2002;156(8):720-9.
11. Ahmed ML, Ong KK, Morrell DJ, et al. Longitudinal study of leptin concentrations during puberty: sex differences and relationship to changes in body composition. J Clin Endocrinol Metab. 1999;84(3):899-905.
12. Del Rincon JP, Iida K, Gaylinn BD, et al. Growth hormone regulation of p85alpha expression and phosphoinositide 3-kinase activity in adipose tissue: mechanism for growth hormone-mediated insulin resistance. Diabetes. 2007;56(6):1638-46.
13. Guercio G, Rivarola MA, Chaler E, et al. Relationship between the GH/IGF-I axis, insulin sensitivity, and adrenal androgens in normal prepubertal and pubertal boys. J Clin Endocrinol Metab. 2002;87(3):1162-9.
14. Kotnik P, Fischer PP, Wabitsch M. Endocrine and metabolic effects of adipose tissue in children and adolescents. Zdr Varst. 2015;54(2):131-8.
15. Unnikrishnan R, Shah VN, Mohan V. Challenges in diagnosis and management of diabetes in the young. Clin Diabetes Endocrinol. 2016;2:18.
16. Giannini C, Weiss R, Cali A, et al. Evidence for early defects in insulin sensitivity and secretion before the onset of glucose dysregulation in obese youths: a longitudinal study. Diabetes. 2012;61(3):606-14.
17. Reinehr T, Toschke AM. Onset of puberty and cardiovascular risk factors in untreated obese children and adolescents: a 1-year follow-up study. Arch Pediatr Adolesc Med. 2009;163(8):709-15.

18. Reinehr T, Wolters B, Knop C, et al. Strong effect of pubertal status on metabolic health in obese children: a longitudinal study. J Clin Endocrinol Metab. 2015;100(1):301-8.
19. Basterfield L, Adamson AJ, Frary JK, et al. Longitudinal study of physical activity and sedentary behavior in children. Pediatrics. 2011;127(1):e24-30.
20. Nadeau KJ, Zeitler PS, Bauer TA, et al. Insulin resistance in adolescents with type 2 diabetes is associated with impaired exercise capacity. J Clin Endocrinol Metab. 2009;94(10):3687-95.
21. Barata DS, Adan LF, Netto EM, et al. The effect of the menstrual cycle on glucose control in women with type 1 diabetes evaluated using a continuous glucose monitoring system. Diabetes Care. 2013;36(5):e70.
22. Rubin KH, Glintborg D, Nybo M, et al. Development and Risk Factors of Type 2 Diabetes in a Nationwide Population of Women with Polycystic Ovary Syndrome. J Clin Endocrinol Metab. 2017;102(10):3848-57.
23. Howell SL, Tyhurst M, Green IC. Direct effects of progesterone on rat islets of Langerhans in vivo and in tissue culture. Diabetologia. 1977;13(6):579-83.
24. Agbaje IM, Rogers DA, McVicar CM, et al. Insulin dependent diabetes mellitus: implications for male reproductive function. Hum Reprod. 2007;22(7):1871-7.
25. American Diabetes Association. 14. Management of Diabetes in Pregnancy: Standards of Medical Care in Diabetes-2019. Diabetes Care. 2019;42(Suppl 1):S165-S172.
26. Metzger BE, Gabbe SG, Persson B, et al. International Association of Diabetes and Pregnancy Study Groups recommendations on the diagnosis and classification of hyperglycemia in pregnancy. Diabetes Care. 2010;33(3):676-82.
27. El Hajj N, Schneider E, Lehnen H, et al. Epigenetics and life-long consequences of an adverse nutritional and diabetic intrauterine environment. Reproduction. 2014;148(6):R111-20.
28. Pettitt DJ, Baird HR, Aleck KA, et al. Excessive obesity in offspring of Pima Indian women with diabetes during pregnancy. N Engl J Med. 1983;308(5):242-5.
29. Goulet ED, Hassaine A, Dionne IJ, et al. Frailty in the elderly is associated with insulin resistance of glucose metabolism in the postabsorptive state only in the presence of increased abdominal fat. Exp Gerontol. 2009;44(11):740-4.
30. Longo M, Bellastella G, Maiorino MI, et al. Diabetes and Aging: From Treatment Goals to Pharmacologic Therapy. Front Endocrinol (Lausanne). 2019;10:45.
31. De Rekeneire N, Resnick HE, Schwartz AV, et al. Diabetes is associated with subclinical functional limitation in nondisabled older individuals: the Health, Aging, and Body Composition study. Diabetes Care. 2003;26(12):3257-63.
32. Selvin E, Steffes MW, Zhu H, et al. Glycated hemoglobin, diabetes, and cardiovascular risk in nondiabetic adults. N Engl J Med. 2010;362(9):800-11.

# SECTION 3

# Endovigilance in Diabetes

# CHAPTER 15

# Endovigilance in Refractory Hyperglycemia

*A Prem Kumar, Sanjay Kalra*

## INTRODUCTION

Pathogenesis of diabetes is multifactorial and its clinical presentations quite varied. The spectrum of hyperglycemia can extend from asymptomatic to frank osmotic symptoms, a catabolic state to a disease associated with long-term complications. Some patients may present with difficult-to-manage hyperglycemia despite intensive pharmacological therapy. Others may have significant glycemic variability and/or recurrent hypoglycemia that impedes the attainment of desired therapeutic targets. Occasional patients who present with a phenotype of type 2 diabetes mellitus (T2DM) but do not respond well to oral pharmacological agents and demonstrate rapid progression to intensive insulin treatment may have secondary cause of diabetes.

Endocrine function is a key regulator of glucose, lipid and protein metabolism and disorders of the endocrine system often manifest as obesity, hyperglycemia, hypertension, dyslipidemia and metabolic syndrome. These disorders include both hormone excess states such as acromegaly, Cushing's syndrome, hyperthyroidism, pheochromocytoma, glucagonoma, etc. and hormone deficiency states such as growth hormone deficiency, hypothyroidism and hypogonadism. An astute clinician should know when to suspect underlying endocrine disorders as a cause of refractory hyperglycemia, since targeted treatment of the endocrine disorder is associated with significant clinical improvement in metabolic disorders.

## EPIDEMIOLOGY OF SECONDARY DIABETES

While most individuals with diabetes are either type 1 diabetes mellitus (T1DM) or T2DM, approximately 3–5% of individuals have other causes of hyperglycemia.[1] Diabetes is, therefore classified into T1DM, T2DM, gestational diabetes mellitus (GDM) and other specific types.[2] The category "other specific types" is broad and includes genetic defects in insulin secretion such as maturity-onset diabetes of the young (MODY) or mitochondrial diabetes and genetic defects in insulin action (genetic syndromes of insulin resistance), lipodystrophies, pancreatic disorders, drug-induced diabetes and endocrine disorders. The classification of diabetes is summarized in Table 1. Among these causes, classic syndromes that present as refractory hyperglycemia include acromegaly, Cushing's syndrome, pheochromocytoma, glucagonoma, somatostatinoma and lipodystrophy.

In a general healthcare practitioner's clinic, these other forms of diabetes are commonly uncommon. But that may also be due an inability to adequately classify diabetes and identify secondary types and contributory factors. On the other hand, in a referral center or in an endocrine practice, secondary diabetes is commonly common. An obvious reason for this is referral bias due to clustering together of atypical and difficult-to-manage cases of diabetes. Additionally, clinicians specifically trained in diabetes and endocrinology are more likely to be vigilant of the possibility of other causes.

Several clinical indicators may point toward underlying endocrine disorders causing or contributing to hyperglycemia. Diabetes due to endocrinopathies may present in extremes of age group with other somatic and biochemical indicators of endocrine disorders and share a common platform of severe insulin resistance. A rapid increase or decrease in weight is a common presentation. There may be characteristic fat distribution as seen in Cushing's syndrome or absence of subcutaneous fat as seen in lipodystrophies. Oligo-amenorrhea or rapid virilization in females should again increase the suspicion to look for an underlying endocrinopathy. A good clinical

**TABLE 1** Classification of diabetes mellitus.

| Category | Causes | |
|---|---|---|
| Type 1 | Autoimmune or idiopathic destruction of β-cells | |
| Type 2 | Insulin resistance with relative insulin deficiency | |
| Gestational | Insulin resistance with relative insulin deficiency during pregnancy | |
| Other specific types: | | |
| Genetic | • Genetic defects of β-cell function—MODY, mitochondrial<br>• Genetic defects of insulin action—insulin receptor defects, lipodystrophy<br>• Genetic syndromes—Down's syndrome, Klinefelter syndrome, Turner's syndrome, Laurence–Moon–Biedl syndrome, etc. | |
| Pancreatic disease | • Pancreatitis<br>• Fibrocalculous pancreatopathy<br>• Pancreatic cancer | • Pancreatectomy<br>• Trauma<br>• Cystic fibrosis |
| Endocrinopathy | • Acromegaly<br>• Cushing's syndrome<br>• Hyperthyroidism<br>• Pheochromocytoma | • Glucagonoma<br>• Somatostatinoma<br>• Primary hyperaldosteronism |
| Drugs | • Glucocorticoids<br>• Immunosuppressants<br>• Antipsychotics<br>• Pentamidine | • Thiazides<br>• β-blockers<br>• Diazoxide<br>• α-interferon |

(MODY: maturity-onset diabetes of the young)

history and physical examination can avoid many costly investigations and streamline the evaluation.

Genetic forms of diabetes and lipodystrophies have been discussed in the chapter "Endocrine Syndromes in Diabetes" and pancreatogenic diabetes has been discussed in detail in the chapter "Glucocrinology of Pancreas". In addition, readers are referred to chapters 2–9 for a detailed discussion on respective endocrine disorders causing diabetes. Endocrinopathies are great masquerader in individuals with difficult-to-control diabetes and in the present chapter, the authors discuss a simplified approach in identifying and evaluating them.

## ACROMEGALY

Acromegaly is a state of chronic growth hormone (GH) excess and is an important endocrine cause of refractory diabetes. Elevated GH and insulin-like growth factor-1 (IGF-1) lead to increased hepatic glucose output and reduced skeletal muscle glucose uptake.[3] Therefore, acromegaly is associated with significant insulin resistance. In addition, GH is lipolytic and results in increased circulating free fatty acid (FFA) concentrations. Diabetes is prevalent in 16–56% of acromegaly patients and impaired glucose tolerance (IGT) may be seen in as many as one-third of them.[4] The prevalence and severity of hyperglycemia are directly proportional to the duration of disease and the magnitude of excess GH production.

Acromegaly is typically associated with bone and soft tissue overgrowth, resulting from the effects of GH and IGF-1 excess.[3] The somatic features of acromegaly appear gradually and it has been estimated that they take an average of 7–10 years to manifest and can be brought out by reviewing old photographs.[3] As GH is lipolytic, patients with acromegaly do not have abdominal obesity that is characteristic of T2DM. There are several clinical clues that can raise the suspicion of a chronic GH excess state. Clinical manifestations are noticed from head to toes but the most prominent among them are frontal bossing, coarse facies, prognathism, macroglossia, spade-like hands, greasy hands, excessive sweat, acanthosis, skin tags, enlarged shoe size and osteoarthritis. These are enlisted in Box 1.

When there is a clinical suspicion of acromegaly, focused investigations are required to establish biochemical diagnosis. These include a GH suppression test using 75 g oral glucose, similar to oral glucose tolerance test (OGTT) with evaluation of GH levels in addition to plasma glucose values. In addition, a fasting IGF-1 level is measured. A GH level >1 ng/mL after a 75 g glucose load with accompanying elevated IGF-1 establishes the diagnosis of GH excess state.

Uncontrolled hyperglycemia leads to elevated GH and variable IGF-1 levels. Therefore, it is prudent to perform a glucose-suppressed GH estimation after controlling hyperglycemia. GH response to glucose suppression is preserved in acromegaly patients with diabetes and hence GH levels can be used for diagnosis. IGF-1 level is variable and may not be that useful in assessing GH excess.[5] Diagnosis of acromegaly can be difficult in people with T1DM (T1DM) where GH hypersecretion is observed. T1DM is a state of GH resistance and IGF-1 levels tend to be lower in them. Therefore, an elevated IGF-1 level can be used reliably to establish the diagnosis of GH excess in T1DM patients.

> **BOX 1    Clinical features of acromegaly.**
>
> **Musculoskeletal**
> - Prognathism
> - Macroglossia
> - Frontal bossing
> - Coarse Facies
> - Jaw malocclusion
> - Acral enlargement and gigantism
> - Osteoarthritis and arthralgia
> - Myopathy
>
> **Skin**
> - Thick oily skin
> - Hyperhidrosis
> - Skin tags
> - Acanthosis nigricans
>
> **Cardiovascular**
> - Hypertension
> - Dilated cardiomyopathy
> - Ventricular hypertrophy
> - Congestive cardiac failure
> - Coronary artery disease
>
> **Respiratory System**
> - Obstructive sleep apnea
> - Upper airway obstruction
>
> **Metabolic**
> - Impaired glucose tolerance and diabetes
> - Dyslipidemia
> - Hypercalciuria
>
> **Others**
> - Headache
> - Carpal tunnel syndrome
> - Fatigue
> - Organomegaly
> - Sleep disturbances
>
> **Local tumor effects**
> - Headache
> - Visual field defect
> - Galactorrhea
> - Cranial nerve palsy
> - Hypopituitarism (hypogonadism, hypothyroidism, hypocortisolism)

Following biochemical diagnosis, imaging modalities are required to localize the GH-producing tumor, which is usually pituitary adenoma. A magnetic resonance imaging (MRI) of the sella will be sufficient to localize the pituitary adenoma; in acromegaly, macroadenoma (size >10 mm) is common. Surgical removal should be attempted in all cases of acromegaly and a transsphenoidal approach is preferred in a predominant sellar mass. GH should be suppressed to at least 1 µg/dL after oral glucose load after surgery.[6] Chance of cure is more in microadenoma and less than one-third of macroadenoma patients achieve desired GH suppression.

Conventional or gamma knife radiotherapy is an option in those with inadequate GH suppression and significant residual mass following surgical resection. Almost 15% patients, especially those with lacto-somatotropinoma, respond to bromocriptine or cabergoline.[7] Somatostatin analogs can be used as a primary therapy in those who are unfit for surgery, in postoperative period with residual mass, and in those who relapse after surgery.

## Acromegaly and Refractory Diabetes

There are no specific recommendations for the treatment of acromegaly-associated diabetes. All antidiabetic agents can be used in acromegaly patients and a stepwise approach that has been suggested for management of hyperglycemia in T2DM can be applied. However, there are some unique challenges in the management of secondary diabetes due to acromegaly:

- Acromegaly can be associated with significant insulin resistance and many patients may require intensive pharmacological treatment for glycemic control
- A significant proportion of acromegaly patients do not respond well to available oral antihyperglycemic agents and require insulin initiation
- The insulin requirements can be very high; often exceeding those seen in T1DM or T2DM. Multiple subcutaneous insulin injection regimen is used in many patients to optimize glycemic control prior to definitive treatment
- Following successful surgical resection of the tumor, metabolic improvement occurs within 2 hours. Therefore, careful down-titration of pharmacological agents is required to reduce the risk of hypoglycemia
- Somatostatin analogs such as octreotide and lanreotide have variable effect on glycemic control. On the one hand, they can result in reduced GH secretion from the pituitary adenoma. But on another hand, they act by reducing insulin release from the islets, and can impair glycemic control in acromegaly patients[8]
- Pasireotide, a new-generation somatostatin analog, has a significant hyperglycemic effect because it reduces insulin secretion but also increases glucagon secretion. Regular monitoring of blood glucose during pasireotide treatment is required
- Other medical therapies utilized in acromegaly management, including pegvisomant and dopamine agonists such as bromocriptine or cabergoline, have a positive impact on glycemic control

Successful treatment of acromegaly leads to remission of diabetes in 40% of patients. The longer acromegaly remains untreated, the lesser chance of diabetes remission exists.[9]

## CUSHING'S SYNDROME

Cushing's syndrome is a pathological state of chronic glucocorticoid excess, resulting from a broad range of exogenous and endogenous causes. In clinical practice, exogenous Cushing's is commonly encountered and is due to prolonged exposure to glucocorticoids in bronchial asthma, dermatological ailments, rheumatological disorders, etc. and is being surreptitiously used by quacks as parenteral or oral preparation in rural settings. Many indigenous systems of medicine do have significant concentration of natural and synthetic steroids in them and studies notice that around 30–40% of individuals with diabetes in India take concomitant native medications along with allopathic medicines.

Endogenous Cushing's syndrome due to excess cortisol secretion is relatively rare. Cushing's disease resulting from adrenocorticotropic hormone (ACTH)-secreting corticotroph adenoma is seen in 2–3 cases per 1 million per year.[10] Ectopic ACTH syndrome and cortisol-secreting adrenal tumors are the other causes for endogenous Cushing's syndrome.

Glucocorticoids increase hepatic glucose output, increase muscle proteolysis, decrease glucose uptake in muscle and increase lipolysis. Hence, both exogenous glucocorticoids as well as endogenous hypercortisolism are important causes of secondary diabetes. The effect of glucocorticoids on glucose homeostasis, the pathogenesis of glucocorticoid-induced diabetes, and its management are discussed in detail in the chapter "Glucocrinology of Adrenal Cortex".

Overt diabetes is seen in 20% patients with Cushing's disease and 40% have impaired glucose tolerance.[11] Postprandial hyperglycemia is seen in 25-90% patients receiving chronic glucocorticoid therapy and the odds ratio for developing diabetes is 1.36-2.31.[12] The severity of hyperglycemia is reflected by the type, dose, and duration of exposure to glucocorticoids.

Cushing's syndrome is associated with similar comorbidities as T2DM including obesity, hypertension, dyslipidemia, cardiovascular risk and increased fracture risk. However, there are several important clinical indicators that can point toward a state of chronic hypercortisolism, as enlisted in Box 2. These include typical pattern of body fat distribution (increased central fat with thinning of extremities), Cushingoid facial appearance, facial plethora, violaceous striae, easy bruisability and proximal myopathy. In addition, there may be menstrual irregularities, acne, hirsutism or hypertrichosis, and psychiatric disturbances. Presence of hirsutism, hyperpigmentation, alopecia, and psychiatric disturbance points toward endogenous hypercortisolism. Cushing's disease is common in females and can masquerade as polycystic ovary syndrome (PCOS). Presence of new onset or rapidly progressing hirsutism, virilisation, and muscle wasting in a patient with PCOS phenotype should entertain the possibility of underlying Cushing's syndrome.

The existence and relevance of subclinical Cushing's syndrome in patients with obesity and T2DM is controversial. Studies estimate a prevalence of subclinical Cushing's syndrome as 0-9.4% in various ethnic population. However, a recent publication by Shah et al. from India advises against routine screening for this entity in patients with T2DM.[13]

The presence of these distinct phenotypic features should evoke a suspicion of hypercortisolism. A carefully elicited history of glucocorticoid use, both obvious and surreptitious, should be taken in all individuals presenting with refractory hyperglycemia. An 8:00 AM serum cortisol must be obtained—a suppressed basal morning serum cortisol (<1.8 µg/dL) is suggestive of exogenous Cushing's syndrome. If morning cortisol is not suppressed, plasma ACTH levels are measured and screening with overnight dexamethasone suppression test is performed. A suppressed ACTH level is suggestive of cortisol-producing adrenal tumor. An elevated ACTH could result from ACTH-producing pituitary tumor or ectopic ACTH-producing tumor. Focused radiological investigations are performed after biochemical evaluation. In Cushing's disease, microadenoma on MRI image may be forthcoming and inferior petrosal sinus

| BOX 2 | Clinical features of Cushing's syndrome. |
|---|---|
| **Higher discriminatory value** | **More common but less discriminatory value** |
| • Easy bruisability | • Weight gain |
| • Facial plethora | • Prominent dorsocervical fat |
| • Proximal myopathy | • Centripetal obesity |
| • Red violaceous striae >1 cm width | • Hirsutism, acne and alopecia |
| | • Psychiatric disturbance |
| | • Recurrent fungal infections |

sampling (IPSS) is needed in those with negative imaging and when there is difficulty in localizing the exact site of ACTH overproduction (pituitary or ectopic).[14]

The first approach to management of Cushing's disease remains surgical. Remission rates vary between 65% and 85%. Within 48 hours of surgery, most patients in remission from Cushing's disease develop a glucocorticoid withdrawal syndrome associated with circulating cortisol levels of 2 µg/dL or less. Medical therapy is the standard second-line treatment if surgery is not successful or if it is not possible. Steroidogenesis inhibitors mitotane, ketoconazole, metyrapone and etomidate are used. The glucocorticoid receptor antagonist mifepristone can be used to block the peripheral effects of elevated cortisol, including hyperglycemia. Radiation therapy is an option in those whose source is not elucidated and in those who remit after surgery.[14,15] Adrenalectomy is the choice of treatment in those with cortisol-producing adrenal adenomas and ACTH-independent macronodular adrenocortical hyperplasia (AIMAH). Well localized bronchial carcinoids are amenable for surgery; but bronchogenic carcinoma producing ectopic ACTH usually have rapid progression and are usually managed with medical adrenalectomy.[15]

There are no specific guidelines for the management of diabetes associated with hypercortisolism. Many patients of Cushing's syndrome may have refractory hyperglycemia that is difficult to manage with lifestyle modification and oral antidiabetic drugs. Managing hyperglycemia in Cushing's syndrome warrants careful choosing due to multiple factors:

- Metformin forms the first-line therapy as it addresses the insulin resistance and is weight neutral
- Recent evidence suggests that incretin-based drugs including glucagon-like polypeptide-1 (GLP-1) receptor agonists and dipeptidyl peptidase-4 (DPP-4) inhibitors may be suitable in glucocorticoid-induced diabetes as they suppress glucagon levels as well; have good tolerability and can result in weight reduction
- Incretin-based drugs are particularly useful in pasireotide-induced hyperglycemia, as they improve insulin secretion as well as suppress glucagon secretion
- Acarbose may lead to gastrointestinal intolerance when used in conjunction with somatostatin analogs
- Pioglitazone is not a preferred agent in Cushing's syndrome as it can lead to weight gain, fluid retention, and osteoporosis[16]
- Sodium-glucose cotransporter-2 inhibitors may be beneficial because of their pleiotropic benefits, but are limited by their side effects such as an increased risk of genital mycotic infections, urinary tract infections and diabetic ketoacidosis. Since individuals with glucocorticoid excess are immunocompromised, they should be used sparingly and with caution
- Many patients with hypercortisolism will require insulin therapy for optimal glycemic control. There is greater postprandial hyperglycemia in Cushing's syndrome and basal-bolus therapy is the most optimal insulin regimen for the management of refractory hyperglycemia. Patients with glucocorticoid-induced diabetes usually require higher prandial insulin doses and lower basal insulin doses than individuals with T1DM or T2DM.
- Perioperative glycemic control is important to reduce the risk of complications including post-operative infections, wound dehiscence, prolonged hospital stay

and mortality. Basal-bolus insulin or even intravenous insulin infusion may be required
- Surgical resection of the tumor often results in rapid improvements in insulin sensitivity. Many patients who undergo remission of hypercortisolism may demonstrate resolution of hyperglycemia. This requires regular monitoring of blood glucose and a rapid down-titration of insulin doses
- With regards to the glycemic effects of medical therapy for hypercortisolism, different drugs may affect glycemia variably. Pasireotide worsens glycemic control while ketoconazole and mifepristone may improve glycemic control[17]
- In patients on exogenous glucocorticoids, rapid improvement in insulin sensitivity is seen following tapering of glucocorticoids or their discontinuation. Therefore, doses of antidiabetic medications need to be reduced to avoid hypoglycemia
- In patients who take glucocorticoids for therapeutic purpose, a dose reduction after consultation with concerned specialty or a pulse regimen, if appropriate, can be considered. Insulin sensitizers with DPP-4 inhibitors forms a good choice in them. Glucose levels starts rising after 6–8 hours of parenteral steroids and the hyperglycemia lasts for 2–3 days after the last dose. Timing of prandial insulin to match the postprandial glucose elevation will be a wise attempt to manage patients receiving parenteral steroids.

## PHEOCHROMOCYTOMA

Pheochromocytomas are catecholamine (epinephrine, norepinephrine and dopamine) secreting tumors of adrenal medullary origin.[18] The classical presentation of pheochromocytomas is described as the paroxysmal triad of headache, sweating and tachycardia. However, most patients do not manifest paroxysmal episodes but may present as sustained hypertension with/without postural hypotension. Pheochromocytoma is a relatively common cause of secondary hypertension in young hypertensives with normal body weight. Diagnosis is established by demonstrating elevated metanephrine levels in serum and in 24-hour urine sample. Imaging with CT/MRI localizes the tumor in adrenal or in extra adrenal location.

Epinephrine reduces insulin secretion from pancreas and activates glycogenolysis. In addition, there is increased gluconeogenesis in the liver, fueled by increased availability of substrates for gluconeogenesis (amino acids and fatty acids) due to increased muscle glycolysis and adipose tissue lipolysis.[19] Around 35–50% of patients with pheochromocytomas or other catecholamine-producing tumors (paragangliomas) have hyperglycemia.

While most patients with pheochromocytomas demonstrate only mild glucose intolerance, pheochromocytomas may present with overt diabetes in at-risk individuals or may cause worsening of glycemic control in individuals with pre-existing diabetes. In fact, some patients have been reported to present with acute hyperglycemic emergency.

Mild hyperglycemia can be managed with medical nutrition therapy, lifestyle modification and oral antidiabetic agents. However, oral hypoglycemic agents may be insufficient in some cases of pheochromocytoma and insulin therapy is the only effective way of managing hyperglycemia in them. Prior to surgery, there is a need for maintaining adequate hydration and optimal glycemic control with intensive insulin regimen. Perioperative monitoring of volume status, blood pressure and heart rate along with blood glucose values is required. After surgical resection of the tumor, there may occur a sudden improvement in insulin sensitivity, requiring down-titration of insulin doses. In many cases, there may occur complete resolution of hyperglycemia, while those with underlying diabetes (either type 1 or type 2 or other specific types) will require retitration of antidiabetic drugs.

## HYPERTHYROIDISM

Thyroid hormone excess can result in hyperglycemia due to increased hepatic glucose output, increased glucose absorption, and insulin resistance.[20] Hyperglycemia is seen in approximately one-third of patients with hyperthyroidism and around 8% have overt diabetes. Both diabetes and thyroid dysfunction are relatively common disorders and may coexist in the same individual. While one reason could be that this is a chance of co-occurrence, individuals with T1DM often manifest other autoimmune disorders, the most common being autoimmune thyroid dysfunction. In addition, T2DM and thyroid dysfunction may also have a bidirectional relationship where thyroid dysfunction affects insulin sensitivity and diabetes affects thyroid physiology. This has been discussed in the chapter "Glucocrinology of Thyroid".

Clinical presentation of hyperthyroidism may overlap with the catabolic features of hyperglycemia and its diagnosis may be delayed if adequate vigilance is not maintained. Both thyrotoxicosis and poorly controlled diabetes may present with weight loss. Increased appetite, fatigue and sarcopenia can be seen in patients with poorly controlled diabetes. Hence when they coexist, the presence of either one of them may be overlooked and the diagnosis may get delayed.[21,22]

Undetected hyperthyroidism may significantly worsen glycemic control and has been reported to even precipitate diabetic ketoacidosis in individuals with T1DM. On the other hand, hypothyroidism increases the risk of hypoglycemia. Therefore, sudden unexplained worsening of glycemic control, glycemic variability or recurrent unexplained hypoglycemia should raise the suspicion for underlying thyroid dysfunction, especially in patients with T1DM. Achieving a euthyroid state in patients with hyperthyroidism by using antithyroid drugs helps improve glycemic control. Most individuals with hyperthyroidism will require frequent self-monitoring of blood glucose and intensive insulin regimens for glycemic control and the doses may need to be titrated regularly as the thyroid dysfunction improves.

In addition, thyroid-associated ophthalmopathy (TAO) may require treatment with parenteral or oral glucocorticoids and may also impact glycemic control. Caution is needed with the use of pioglitazone in patients with TAO due to the risk of retro-orbital adipocyte proliferation associated with thiazolidinediones.[23]

## GLUCAGONOMA

Glucagonoma is a rare neuroendocrine tumor (NET) presenting with diabetes. It results from glucagon-producing tumors of the α-cells of pancreatic islets. Glucagonomas have been classically described to present with necrolytic migratory erythema, glossitis, angular cheilitis, weight loss and anemia.[24] Diagnosis is based on the presence of glucagonoma syndrome (triad of necrolytic migratory erythema, diabetes, and stomatitis/cheilitis) and elevated blood glucagon levels. Treatment remains localization and surgical resection of the lesion.

## OTHER ENDOCRINOPATHIES WITH REVERSIBLE HYPERGLYCEMIA

Around 50% patients with primary hyperaldosteronism can have hypokalemia-related reduced insulin secretion and hyperglycemia. With removal of the aldosterone-producing adenoma, hyperglycemia reverses or improves in many of them. Similarly, primary hyperparathyroidism is associated with endothelial dysfunction and insulin resistance, and surgical removal of parathyroid adenoma might reverse or improve glycemic control.

## CONCLUSION

Acromegaly, Cushing's syndrome (both endogenous and exogenous), pheochromo-cytoma, hyperthyroidism, and other hyperfunctioning endocrinopathies can contribute to refractory hyperglycemia. These disorders can cause secondary diabetes per se, and they can also worsen diabetes control in individuals with pre-existing diabetes due to other causes.

A failure to identify endocrinopathy as the underlying cause of refractory hyperglycemia can result in significant morbidity, impaired quality of life, and increase the mortality risk as well. Endovigilance is, therefore, called for in all patients with refractory hyperglycemia. We advocate an "angle of clinical endocrinology", laying focus on exhaustive, empathic history taking, and a dedicated physical examination as an essential approach for evaluation of individuals presenting with difficult-to-manage hyperglycemia. This should be followed through with specific diagnostic tests based on underlying clinical suspicion.[25,26]

Most of these individuals will require intensive insulin therapy for optimal glycemic control, and multiple subcutaneous insulin or basal-bolus regimen allows for fine titration of insulin doses. Appropriate management of underlying endocrinopathy, both medical and surgical, is likely to result in improvement in insulin sensitivity and glycemic control. This may sometimes result in complete remission of diabetes, or there may be a need to reduce the doses of insulin and/or other antidiabetic agents following improvement of underlying endocrine disorder.

## REFERENCES

1. Bullard KMK, Cowie CC, Lessem SE, et al. Prevalence of Diagnosed Diabetes in Adults by Diabetes Type-United States, 2016. MMWR Morb Mortal Wkly Rep. 2018;67(12):359-61.
2. American Diabetes Association. 2. Classification and Diagnosis of Diabetes: Standards of Medical Care in Diabetes-2018. Diabetes Care. 2018;41:S13-S27.
3. Capatina C, Wass JA. 60 years of neuroendocrinology: Acromegaly. J Endocrinol. 2015;226(2):T141-60.
4. Dreval AV, Trigolosova IV, Misnikova IV, et al. Prevalence of diabetes mellitus in patients with acromegaly. Endocr Connect. 2014;3(2):93-8.
5. Lim DJ, Kwon HS, Cho JH, et al. Acromegaly associated with type 2 diabetes showing normal IGF-1 levels under poorly controlled glycemia. Endocr J. 2007;54(7):537-41.

6. Giustina A, Chanson P, Bronstein MD, et al. A consensus on criteria for cure of acromegaly. J Clin Endocrinol Metab. 2010;95(7):3141-8.
7. Katznelson L, Laws ER Jr, Melmed S, et al. Acromegaly: an endocrine society clinical practice guideline. J Clin Endocrinol Metab. 2014;99(11):3933-51.
8. Colao A, Auriemma RS, Pivonello R. The effects of somatostatin analogue therapy on pituitary tumor volume in patients with acromegaly. Pituitary. 2016;19(2):210-21.
9. González B, Vargas G, de Los Monteros ALE, et al. Persistence of Diabetes and Hypertension After Multimodal Treatment of Acromegaly. J Clin Endocrinol Metab. 2018;103(6):2369-75.
10. Steffensen C, Bak AM, Rubeck KZ, et al. Epidemiology of Cushing's syndrome. Neuroendocrinology. 2010;92:1-5.
11. Barbot M, Ceccato F, Scaroni C. Diabetes Mellitus Secondary to Cushing's Disease. Front Endocrinol (Lausanne). 2018;9:284.
12. Kwon S, Hermayer KL, Hermayer K. Glucocorticoid-induced hyperglycemia. Am J Med Sci. 2013;345(4):274-7.
13. Budyal S, Jadhav SS, Kasaliwal R, et al. Is it worthwhile to screen patients with type 2 diabetes mellitus for subclinical Cushing's syndrome? Endocr Connect. 2015;4(4):242-8.
14. Nieman LK, Biller BM, Findling JW, et al. The diagnosis of Cushing's syndrome: an Endocrine Society Clinical Practice Guideline. J Clin Endocrinol Metab. 2008;93(5):1526-40.
15. Nieman LK, Biller BM, Findling JW, et al. Treatment of Cushing's Syndrome: An Endocrine Society Clinical Practice Guideline. J Clin Endocrinol Metab. 2015;100(8):2807-31.
16. Mazziotti G, Gazzaruso C, Giustina A. Diabetes in Cushing syndrome: basic and clinical aspects. Trends Endocrinol Metab. 2011;22(12):499-506.
17. van Raalte DH, Diamant M. Steroid diabetes: from mechanism to treatment? Neth J Med. 2014;72(2):62-72.
18. Lenders JW, Duh QY, Eisenhofer G, et al. Pheochromocytoma and paraganglioma: an endocrine society clinical practice guideline. J Clin Endocrinol Metab. 2014;99(6):1915-42.
19. Ruohonen ST, Ruohonen S, Gilsbach R, et al. Involvement of α2-Adrenoceptor Subtypes A and C in Glucose Homeostasis and Adrenaline-Induced Hyperglycaemia. Neuroendocrinology. 2012;96(1):51-9.
20. Roubsanthisuk W, Watanakejorn P, Tunlakit M, et al. Hyperthyroidism induces glucose intolerance by lowering both insulin secretion and peripheral insulin sensitivity. J Med Assoc Thai. 2006;89:S133-40.
21. Mouradian M, Abourizk N. Diabetes mellitus and thyroid disease. Diabetes Care 1983;6(5):512-20.
22. Kalra S, Khandelwal D. Thyrovigilance in diabetes; glucovigilance in thyroidology. J Pak Med Assoc. 2018;68(6):966-67.
23. Arnetz L, Lantz M, Brismar K, et al. Effect of Pioglitazone on Thyroid Hormones and IGF-I in Patients with Type 2 Diabetes. Thyroid Disorders Ther. 2013;3:139.
24. Song X, Zheng S, Yang G, et al. Glucagonoma and the glucagonoma syndrome. Oncol Lett. 2018;15(3): 2749-55.
25. Kalra S, Talwar V. Refractory diabetes: Focus on the obvious. J Pak Med Assoc. 2017;67(1):146-7.
26. Kalra S, Priya G, Gupta R. Difficult diabetes: the 7d approach. J Pak Med Assoc. 2019;69(1):130-1.

# CHAPTER 16

# Hypoglycemia in Diabetes: Endocrine Perspectives

*Akshata Desai, Andrew E Uloko*

## INTRODUCTION

Diabetes is a chronic disease that requires continuous medical care and self-management education to prevent acute complications and reduce the risk of long-term complications.[1] Iatrogenic hypoglycemia is one of the most important limiting factors in the glycemic management of diabetes, causing recurrent morbidity in people with type 1 diabetes mellitus (T1DM) and those with advanced type 2 diabetes mellitus (T2DM), sometimes being fatal. It impairs defenses against subsequent falling plasma glucose concentrations and thus causes a vicious cycle of recurrent hypoglycemia. It generally precludes maintenance of euglycemia over a lifetime of diabetes and thus full realization of the benefits of glycemic control.

Several factors contribute to hypoglycemia in diabetes including antidiabetic agents (especially insulin and sulfonylureas), diet and drug mismatch, excessive physical activity, loss of counter-regulatory mechanisms, nutrient malabsorption, long-term complications (gastroparesis, chronic kidney disease, chronic liver disease, cardiovascular disease and autonomic neuropathy), and concomitant endocrine disorders (hypothyroidism, adrenal insufficiency, hypopituitarism and celiac disease). Endocrine vigilance is needed in the evaluation of hypoglycemia in individuals with diabetes to identify the underlying factors and appropriately address them.

In addition, glycemic control should be individualized based on patient characteristics. Fasting plasma glucose (FPG), postprandial plasma glucose (PPG), and HbA1c are established therapeutic targets of glycemic control. But recently, hypoglycemia prevention and reduction of glycemic variability have been recognized as important therapeutic targets as well. Hypoglycemia prevention, in fact, has been given vital importance in various management guidelines for diabetes. It is important for us to recognize hypoglycemia risk factors, select appropriate regimens and empower treating physicians and patients with educational programs to minimize the risk of hypoglycemia, while maintaining optimal glycemic control so as to prevent long- term complications.

# FREQUENCY OF HYPOGLYCEMIA IN DIABETES

Hypoglycemia can affect people with diabetes in various ways, regardless of the type of diabetes. By far, the highest burden of hypoglycemia is borne by individuals with type 1 or type 2 diabetes mellitus.

## Type 1 Diabetes Mellitus

Patients with T1DM report an average of up to three episodes of severe hypoglycemia (episodes requiring the assistance of another person) per year.[2] Studies using continuous glucose monitoring (CGM) show much more frequent episodes of clinically important hypoglycemia [<54 mg/dL (3 mmol/L)], ranging from every 2-3 days to every 6 days.[3] Clinically important hypoglycemia detected with CGM is much more common than prior estimates based on self-reported events or fingerstick glucose assessments. Of note, CGM may over-report hypoglycemia, especially in the lower range of glycemia, which suggests that the frequency of clinically important hypoglycemia may be overstated with CGM.

## Type 2 Diabetes Mellitus

Hypoglycemia is less frequent in T2DM when compared to T1DM.[4] However, due to the greatly increased numbers of individuals with T2DM, the prevalence of hypoglycemic episodes is actually greater than in T1DM. The frequency of hypoglycemia increases over time as patients approach the insulin-deficient end of the spectrum in T2DM.

Patients with T2DM are at higher risk to develop hypoglycemia if treated with insulin, a sulfonylurea or a meglitinide than those treated with diet or other medications. Among the insulin secretagogues, hypoglycemia is more often seen with long acting agents, such as glibenclamide,[5] as compared with the shorter-acting glipizide, glimepiride and gliclazide. Unlike insulin and insulin secretagogues, agents that do not cause unregulated hyperinsulinemia, such as metformin, $\alpha$-glucosidase inhibitors, thiazolidinediones, glucagon-like peptide-1 (GLP-1) receptor agonists, dipeptidyl peptidase-4 (DPP-4) inhibitors, and sodium-glucose co-transporter-2 (SGLT-2) inhibitors do not usually cause hypoglycemia. However, they are associated with increased risk if used with insulin or an insulin secretagogue.[4]

The incidence of hypoglycemia among persons with diabetes varies based on clinical practice setting, level of patient motivation and presence of comorbidities among several other factors. In a Nigerian tertiary hospital, hypoglycemia accounted for 11.8% of all diabetes-related admissions.[6]

# GLUCOSE COUNTER-REGULATORY PHYSIOLOGY

In normal individuals, as glucose levels decline within the normal range, physiological defenses begin; with a decrement in insulin secretion followed by an increase in hepatic and renal production of glucose. As glucose levels fall below the physiologic range, increments in glucagon and epinephrine stimulate hepatic glucose production; and mobilize gluconeogenic precursors from muscle and fat; and also stimulate renal glucose production and limit glucose utilization by muscle and fat.[4]

**TABLE 1:** Physiological Responses to decrease in plasma glucose concentration below normal range.

| Plasma glucose concentration (mg/dL) | Compensatory physiological response | Clinical response |
|---|---|---|
| 80 mg/dL | Suppression of insulin secretion | None |
| 65–70 mg/dL | Increased glucagon and epinephrine secretion | Mild autonomic symptoms – sympathetic (tremors, palpitations, anxiety) and parasympathetic (hunger, sweating, paresthesia) |
| 55–60 mg/dL | • Increased glucagon and epinephrine<br>• Increase in other counter-regulatory hormones – cortisol and growth hormone | Marked autonomic symptoms |
| 50–55 mg/dL | Neuroglycopenia, decreased cognition | Neuroglycopenic symptoms (dizziness, weakness, drowsiness, delirium, confusion, seizures, altered sensorium) |

The behavioral defense against falling plasma glucose concentrations is carbohydrate ingestion, prompted largely by the perception of neurogenic (autonomic) symptoms. These include catecholamine-mediated or adrenergic symptoms such as palpitations, tremors and anxiety/arousal and acetylcholine-mediated or cholinergic symptoms such as sweating, hunger and paresthesias. The autonomic symptoms are largely sympathetic neural, rather than adrenomedullary, in origin. Table 1 summarizes the physiological responses to falling plasma glucose levels that prevent hypoglycemia. All of these defenses are compromised in T1DM and advanced T2DM.[4]

Hypoglycemia unawareness can thus be defined as the onset of neuroglycopenia before the occurrence of autonomic symptoms or a failure to sense a significant drop in plasma glucose concentration below the normal range.[7] This may be responsible for some of the cases of death-in-bed syndrome in diabetes. Several factors predispose to hypoglycemia unawareness including longer duration of diabetes, history of recent and/or recurrent hypoglycemic episodes, intensive glycemic control and advanced age.[8] Awareness of hypoglycemia can also be lost as a result of pharmacological agents that block the pathways mediating these neurogenic symptoms such as β-blockers and selective serotonin reuptake inhibitors.[8]

## PATHOPHYSIOLOGY OF HYPOGLYCEMIA IN DIABETES

Episodes of therapeutic hyperinsulinemia, produced by treatment with an insulin secretagogue (sulfonylurea or glinide) or with insulin are a prerequisite for the development of iatrogenic hypoglycemia. Absolute therapeutic insulin excess of sufficient magnitude can cause isolated episodes of hypoglycemia despite intact glucose counter-regulatory defenses against hypoglycemia. But that is an uncommon event. Iatrogenic hypoglycemia is typically the result of the interplay of mild-to-moderate absolute therapeutic insulin excess, and compromised physiological and behavioral defenses against falling plasma glucose concentrations in diabetes.[4]

In T1DM, due to β-cell failure, insulin replacement is exogenous and the levels do not decline in response to a decrease in glucose levels; the first physiological defense is lost. Endogenous insulin is secreted into portal circulation and undergoes extensive hepatic first pass metabolism. On the other hand, exogenous insulin is administered via subcutaneous route and it reaches greater systemic concentrations. The altered portosystemic gradient of insulin predisposes the individual to greater risk of hypoglycemia.

Furthermore, as glucagon levels do not increase when glucose levels are falling, the second physiological defense is lost which is possibly attributable to β-cell failure since a decrease in β-cell secretion, coupled with a low α-cell glucose concentration, normally signals α-cell glucagon secretion.[9] Finally, the increase in epinephrine levels, the third physiological defense against hypoglycemia is attenuated. The resulting defective glucose counter regulation is associated with a 25-fold increased risk of severe hypoglycemia in T1DM. The attenuated epinephrine response is a marker of the blunting of the sympathoadrenal response, including the sympathetic neural response that is responsible for the neurogenic symptoms and behavioral response of carbohydrate ingestion. This sets the stage for the clinical syndrome of "hypoglycemia unawareness", associated with a six-fold increased risk of severe hypoglycemia in T1DM.

Defenses against hypoglycemia are intact early in the course of T2DM, as against those in T1DM. However, in advanced T2DM (endogenous insulin deficiency), there is defective glucose counter regulation.[4] In addition, individuals with secondary pancreatogenic diabetes are also at increased risk of hypoglycemia due to both β-cell and α-cell dysfunction as well nutrient malabsorption.

## SYMPTOMS OF HYPOGLYCEMIA

Hypoglycemia causes neurogenic (autonomic) and neuroglycopenic symptoms. Older adults and patients with long-term diabetes may have more neuroglycopenic than neurogenic manifestations of hypoglycemia.
- *Neurogenic symptoms*: The neurogenic symptoms include tremors, palpitations, and anxiety/arousal (catecholamine-mediated, adrenergic) and sweating, hunger, and paresthesias (acetylcholine-mediated, cholinergic).[4]
- *Neuroglycopenic symptoms*: The neuroglycopenic symptoms include dizziness, weakness, drowsiness, delirium, confusion and, at lower plasma glucose concentrations, seizure and coma.[10] Prolonged hypoglycemia can cause brain death in an unobserved patient with diabetes; but the vast majority of episodes are reversed after the glucose level is raised. The rare fatal episodes are generally thought to be the result of ventricular arrhythmia.[10]

In patients with diabetes, the onset of symptoms of hypoglycemia may occur at glucose levels less than 65 mg/dL (3.6 mmol/L), although the specific value varies between and within individuals over time.

The lower limit of the normal FPG value is typically 70 mg/dL (3.9 mmol/L). The glycemic thresholds for these responses shift to higher plasma glucose concentrations in patients with poorly controlled diabetes and to lower plasma glucose concentrations in patients with repeated episodes of hypoglycemia, such as those on intensive therapy.[11] In hypoglycemia unawareness, symptoms may be absent to a given degree of hypoglycemia caused by recent antecedent hypoglycemia, prior exercise or sleep in patients with diabetes.[4]

## THE IMPACT OF HYPOGLYCEMIA IN DIABETES

Iatrogenic hypoglycemia causes recurrent physical and psychosocial morbidity and impairs defenses against subsequent hypoglycemia in patients with diabetes, precluding the maintenance of euglycemia over a lifetime of diabetes.

Hypoglycemia causes brain fuel deprivation that, if unchecked, results in functional brain failure that is typically corrected after the plasma glucose concentration is raised.[10,11] Rarely, hypoglycemia can result in sudden death as a result of cardiac arrhythmia, especially in patients with pre-existing cardiac abnormalities.[12] Sudden death has been associated with QT interval prolongation and reduced baroreflex sensitivity in patients with classic diabetic autonomic neuropathy.[12] Profound and prolonged hypoglycemia may result in permanent brain dysfunction and brain death.

Additionally, hypoglycemia has been demonstrated to be procoagulant and pro-atherothrombotic.[13] Furthermore, severe hypoglycemia has been associated with increased risk of death extending many months after the sentinel episode.[14] Up to 10% of deaths in T1DM are attributed to hypoglycemia. As many as 10% of patients with severe sulfonylurea-induced hypoglycemia die.

At the very minimum, an episode of hypoglycemia is a nuisance, impairs judgment, behavior and performance of tasks like driving. It may cause transient neurologic defects, seizure or even loss of consciousness. Recurrent hypoglycemia has also been associated with neurocognitive abnormalities. Hypoglycemia and fear of hypoglycemia are associated with significant impairment of quality of life.

## HYPOGLYCEMIA-ASSOCIATED AUTONOMIC FAILURE

Recent antecedent hypoglycemia, as well as prior exercise or sleep, cause both defective glucose counter-regulation and hypoglycemia unawareness by reducing sympathoadrenal and neurogenic symptom responses during subsequent hypoglycemia. Therefore, a vicious cycle of recurrent hypoglycemia develops.[9] This phenomenon is termed as hypoglycemia-associated autonomic failure (HAAF).

The exact mechanism of the attenuated sympathoadrenal response to falling glucose levels, the key feature of HAAF, is not known. Several explanations that have been proposed including increased blood-to-brain transport of a metabolic fuel, effects of a systemic mediator such as cortisol on the brain, altered hypothalamic mechanisms, and activation of an inhibitory cerebral network mediated through the thalamus.[9] The sequence of events leading to HAAF are depicted in Flowchart 1.

As little as 2-3 weeks of scrupulous avoidance of hypoglycemia reverses hypoglycemia unawareness and improves the attenuated epinephrine component of defective glucose counter-regulation in most affected patients. Therefore, glycemic

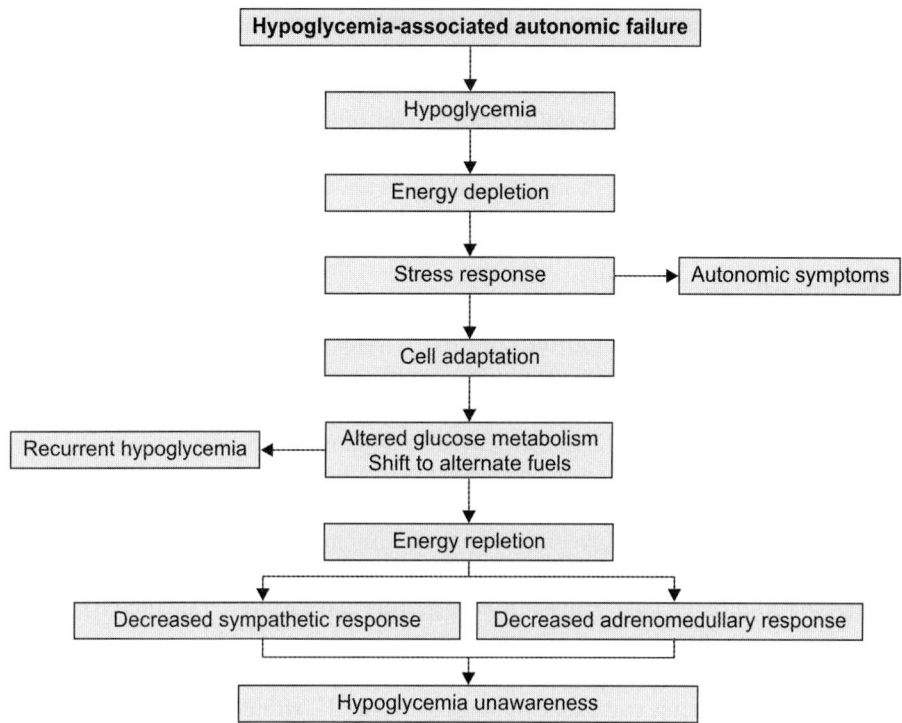

**FLOWCHART 1:** Pathogenesis of hypoglycemia-associated autonomic failure.

targets should be revised to less stringent ones in individuals with recurrent hypoglycemia and hypoglycemia unawareness till such time that hypoglycemia unawareness abates.

## ETIOLOGY OF HYPOGLYCEMIA IN DIABETES

Risk factors for iatrogenic hypoglycemia are conditions that predispose to absolute or relative insulin excess coupled with compromised physiological and behavioral defenses against falling plasma glucose concentrations. The following factors can contribute to hypoglycemia in individuals with diabetes.

### Medications

Hypoglycemia results when insulin or insulin secretagogue doses are higher than required, inappropriately timed and/or are of the wrong type causing a mismatch. Alcohol ingestion can also result in hypoglycemia due to decreased endogenous glucose production.

In addition to the above, there are a host of other drugs that have been associated with episodes of hypoglycemia such as cibenzoline, gatifloxacin, pentamidine, quinine, indomethacin and glucagon during endoscopy. Other drugs that may cause hypoglycemia (low-quality evidence) are artesunate, lithium, propoxyphene, angiotensin-converting enzyme (ACE) inhibitors, angiotensin receptor blockers (ARBs), β-adrenergic receptor antagonists, levofloxacin, mifepristone, trimethoprim sulfamethoxazole, heparin and 6-mercaptopurine.[11] Use of over-the-counter complementary medications is quite common among individuals with diabetes. The composition of active ingredients and mechanism of action of these drugs remains largely unknown and the use of such medications should be inquired into as they can increase the risk of hypoglycemia.

## Medical Conditions

Several complications and comorbid conditions associated with diabetes increase the risk of hypoglycemia by effects on glucose counter-regulatory mechanisms, altered drug clearance and pharmacokinetics (including prolongation of insulin action) and increased insulin sensitivity. These are discussed below:
- Hepatic and/or renal failure predispose to hypoglycemia due to endogenous glucose deficiency and altered drug kinetics. In individuals presenting with recurrent or severe hypoglycemia, renal and hepatic function assessment should be done. Doses of several pharmacological agents including antidiabetic drugs need to be adjusted based on estimated glomerular filtration rate (eGFR)
- Hypoglycemia has been rarely described as a clinical sign of severe sepsis. Hypoglycemia in sepsis is associated with a grave prognosis[15]
- Adrenal insufficiency can cause hypoglycemia and it should be suspected in those with hypotension, severe hypoglycemia, hyponatremia, and weight loss
- Hypoglycemia may be caused by hypothyroidism alone, or more often, by concurrent adrenal insufficiency due to autoimmune adrenal disease or hypothalamic-pituitary disease. The presumed mechanism is decreased gluconeogenesis
- Celiac disease may result in nutrient malabsorption and increase the risk of hypoglycemia
- Chronic pancreatitis is associated with reduced α-cell function and impaired glucose counter-regulation. In addition, exocrine pancreatic insufficiency furthers the risk of hypoglycemia by causing malabsorption.

## Improvement in Insulin Sensitivity

There may occur improvements in insulin sensitivity resulting from personal efforts such as improved nutritional management, dietary carbohydrate restriction, physical activity or systemic weight loss. Some of the factors resulting in improved insulin sensitivity in individuals with diabetes include:
- Physical activity and exercise result in improvement in insulin sensitivity. Increased physical activity may result in episodes of hypoglycemia in patients with diabetes due to the mismatch between endogenous/exogenous insulin and glucose especially if on insulin or insulin secretagogues
- Weight loss also results in improvement in insulin sensitivity and reduced requirement of medications for glycemic control
- In gestational diabetes mellitus and diabetes in pregnancy, insulin resistance improves rapidly after delivery of the baby and placenta. Timely adjustment of

medications in these situations helps avoid episodes of hypoglycemia. Lactation is also associated with marked improvement in insulin sensitivity
- Systemic glucocorticoids result in dose-dependent worsening of glycemic control which usually requires intensification of antihyperglycemic therapy for the duration used. The duration of hyperglycemic effects of glucocorticoids is a function of the type and mode of glucocorticoid administration. Following tapering of glucocorticoid regimens or their discontinuation, there occurs a rapid improvement in insulin sensitivity. Therefore, antidiabetic medications and/or insulin need to be adjusted accordingly to avoid episodes of hypoglycemia
- Following the successful treatment of Cushing's syndrome or acromegaly with surgery or medical management, there is improvement in insulin sensitivity and antidiabetic medications need adjustment accordingly.

## Elderly Individuals

The elderly (age ≥75 years) are particularly susceptible to develop hypoglycemia due to the coexistence of comorbidities, polypharmacy, frailty, undernutrition and cognitive dysfunction.[16] Therefore, attention should be paid to the management of undernutrition in the general elderly population by improving energy intake and maintaining muscle mass. Having a more conservative approach to glycemic targets in frail older people with diabetes may be worthwhile.

## ENDOCRINE VIGILANCE IN HYPOGLYCEMIA

"An ounce of prevention is worth a pound of cure". This is absolutely apt for hypoglycemia where efforts should be driven toward prevention of hypoglycemia episodes. This practice of hypoglycemia risk reduction requires us to acknowledge the problem first, consider the conventional risk factors as well as those indicative of HAAF in diabetes and accordingly individualize treatment targets.[4,17]

### Acknowledge the Problem

Hypoglycemia should be addressed at the very first contact with a patient and reiterated at every visit with those at risk. In addition to the patient's comments and review of the individual's self-monitoring of blood glucose (SMBG) data (as well as any CGM data), it is helpful to know the glucose level at which the patient can detect hypoglycemia and what symptoms and signs they experience at various hypoglycemic levels.

### Consider Risk Factors for Hypoglycemia and Hypoglycemia-associated Autonomic Failure

Relative or absolute hyperinsulinemia, decreased exogenous glucose delivery, decreased endogenous glucose production or increased glucose utilization due to improved sensitivity need to be considered carefully in any patient with iatrogenic hypoglycemia. Attention needs to be paid to the dose, timing, and type of the insulin or insulin secretagogues and other concomitant medications used and other illnesses that may predispose to hypoglycemia.

An episode of severe hypoglycemia begets further such episodes if no fundamental adjustments are made to the treatment regimen.

## Principles of Tactful Glycemic Control

These include careful drug selection, individualized glycemic goals, structured patient education, selective application of diabetes treatment technologies, and short-term scrupulous avoidance of hypoglycemia.[4] The International Hypoglycaemia Study Group recommends that people with diabetes treated with a sulfonylurea, a glinide or insulin should be educated about hypoglycemia, SMBG, self-titration of insulin doses, detection of hypoglycemia and its management.

Drug selection to minimize the risk of hypoglycemia includes avoidance of sulfonylureas and glinides that may increase the risk of hypoglycemia. Therefore agents with a low risk of hypoglycemia such as metformin, GLP-1 receptor agonists, SGLT-2 inhibitors, DPP-4 inhibitors or thiazolidinediones, more physiological insulin regimens with long-acting or even ultra-long-acting basal insulin analogs plus rapid-acting prandial insulin analogs should be used.[18,19] Insulin analogs reduce the frequency of nocturnal hypoglycemia including severe nocturnal hypoglycemia as compared to conventional human insulin.[18] In insulin-requiring T2DM, basal insulin preparations are associated with less hypoglycemia than prandial insulin regimens. In insulin-treated patients, hypoglycemia can occur during or shortly after or even late after exercise.[19] Measures to avoid early-onset exercise hypoglycemia include interspersing episodes of intense exercise (which tends to raise plasma glucose concentrations), adding carbohydrate ingestion, and reducing insulin doses.[19]

Diabetes treatment technologies include continuous subcutaneous insulin infusion (CSII), CGM, and combinations of CSII and CGM. Recent evidence suggests that CSII treatment improves glycemic control as compared to multiple daily injections.[20] CGM devices have been shown to improve glycemic control and decrease the time spent in hypoglycemia in patients with diabetes.[21] With improving accuracy, several CGM systems have been approved by the US FDA to even replace point of care blood glucose testing.[22] The combination of CSII and real-time CGM or the sensor-augmented pump (SAP), particularly those including an insulin pump programmed to stop insulin infusion for up to 2 hours when CGM values fall to a selected glucose level, has been reported to reduce the frequency of severe hypoglycemia in T1DM.[23] Several promising studies have investigated approaches for leading closed-loop insulin (or insulin and glucagon) replacement. The development of automated closed-loop insulin pumps represents an area of ongoing research. It is proposed that a fully closed-loop insulin or insulin and glucagon replacement or pancreatic islet transplantation will significantly reduce hypoglycemia.

## Individualized Glycemic Targets

Glycemic targets should be linked not only to the level of glycemic control (i.e. the HbA1c) but also to the risk of hypoglycemia, specifically the drugs used (a sulfonylurea, a glinide or insulin), the degree of endogenous insulin deficiency, associated comorbidities, presence of diabetes complications, and the anticipated benefit of the targeted level of glycemic control.

For the majority of the non-pregnant adults, a reasonable goal for HbA1c is <7%. For selected individuals with long life expectancy, without significant comorbidities (especially cardiovascular disease), stringent HbA1c goals (<6.5%) should be targeted, if this can be achieved without significant hypoglycemia.[24] For children and adolescents, an HbA1c of <7.5% should be the goal, although a lower target (<7%) is reasonable if it can be achieved without excessive hypoglycemia. On the other hand, much higher levels of HbA1c (7.5-8.0%) may be appropriate in elderly patients or those with renal and hepatic failure, where hypoglycemia may be harmful. Even higher targets (HbA1c <8.5%) may be appropriate in individuals with very limited life expectancy.

Of note, it needs to be underscored that severe hypoglycemia can and does occur at HbA1c levels between 8% and 10% in both T1DM or T2DM. Thus, severe hypoglycemia is not just a consequence of "low or near normal" HbA1c values. Recent data show that severe hypoglycemia occurring in individuals with T2DM above 60 years of age with elevated HbA1c may have greater serious adverse events and increased mortality as compared to individuals with improved glycemic control and lower HbA1c values.

## Structured Patient Education

The core element of hypoglycemia prevention is thorough and structured patient education (often re-education) that teaches the patient how and when their drugs can cause hypoglycemia, how to adjust their medications, meal plans and exercise to optimize glycemic control and minimize hypoglycemia, and also how to recognize and treat hypoglycemia.[4]

In patients with impaired awareness of hypoglycemia, structured patient education should be combined with 2-3 weeks of scrupulous avoidance of hypoglycemia, which may require acceptance of somewhat higher glycemic goals in the short-term since that can be expected to restore awareness of hypoglycemia in most affected patients.

## TREATMENT OF HYPOGLYCEMIA IN DIABETES

The goal of the treatment of hypoglycemia is to raise the plasma glucose concentration to normal by providing dietary or parenteral carbohydrate (specifically glucose), or in cases of severe hypoglycemia outside of a medical center, by stimulating endogenous glucose production by administering glucagon.

Hypoglycemia is classified into three categories—hypoglycemia alert value, clinically significant hypoglycemia, and severe hypoglycemia[25] for therapeutic purposes, as shown in Table 2. Pre-emptive action when hypoglycemia alert value is encountered can prevent clinically significant hypoglycemia. Most episodes of symptomatic hypoglycemia or asymptomatic hypoglycemia detected on CGM are adequately treated by consumption of glucose tablets or carbohydrates, a reasonable

**TABLE 2:** Classification of hypoglycemia.

| Level | Glycemic criteria | Description |
| --- | --- | --- |
| Hypoglycemia alert value (level 1) | <70 mg/dL (3.9 mmol/L) | Sufficiently low for treatment with fast-acting carbohydrate and adjustment of glucose-lowering therapy |
| Clinically significant hypoglycemia (level 2) | <54 mg/dL (3 mmol/L) | Sufficiently low to indicate serious and clinically important hypoglycemia |
| Severe hypoglycemia (level 3) | No specific glucose threshold | Hypoglycemia associated with severe cognitive impairment requiring external assistance for recovery |

dose being 20 g, with clinical improvement occurring within 15–20 minutes of ingestion. Patients are instructed to retest after 15 minutes and if the glucose remains <70 mg/dL, retreatment is necessary. It is advisable to eat a meal containing long-acting carbohydrate shortly after glucose level is raised to counteract ongoing hyperinsulinemia as the effect of oral glucose is usually transient, lasting about 2 hours. In patients taking insulin or an insulin secretagogue with an α-glucosidase inhibitor (acarbose, miglitol or voglibose), only pure glucose (glucose tablets) should be used to treat symptomatic hypoglycemia as table sugar (sucrose) will be less effective considering α-glucosidase inhibitors slow digestion of disaccharides.

During an episode of hypoglycemia, if the patient is unable to take carbohydrate orally (due to neuroglycopenia), parenteral therapy is essential. Glucagon can be administered by the patient's attendant either subcutaneously or intramuscularly at a dose of 1 mg in adults. Glucagon administration is lifesaving, although can cause substantial transient hyperglycemia, nausea, and even vomiting. In cases of severe hypoglycemia, patients already in the hospital can be treated promptly by administration of 25 g of 50% glucose (dextrose) intravenously.

The duration of an episode of hypoglycemia is a function of its cause. An episode caused by rapid-acting insulin or an insulin analog will be relatively brief as compared to that caused by long-acting insulin or an insulin secretagogue.

Further therapeutic decision-making involves identifying the underlying cause of hypoglycemia and its management. In cases of skipped meals, low carbohydrate intake, meal-dose mismatch or excess physical activity, appropriate nutrition education, and titration of insulin and oral antidiabetic doses is required. Readjustment of therapeutic targets to less stringent ones and down-titration of medications is needed in case of recurrent hypoglycemia and hypoglycemia unawareness.[26] In individuals at greater risk of hypoglycemia, switching from conventional insulin to insulin analogs[27] and use of antidiabetic medications with inherent lower risk of hypoglycemia is recommended.

Unexplained hypoglycemia merits further evaluation of renal and liver functions, thyroid functions, and serum cortisol assessment. Rare cases of insulinoma have also been reported in individuals with prior diabetes. Therefore, the clinician should be vigilant of the wide variety of factors that can contribute to hypoglycemia in individuals with diabetes.

## CONCLUSION

Hypoglycemia is the most limiting factor that makes optimal glycemic control elusive in diabetes care. While most commonly, hypoglycemia in individuals with diabetes results from iatrogenic causes such as medications, inappropriate dose, skipped or reduced meals, insulin dose-meal mismatch, etc., the diabetes care practitioner must be vigilant of the possibility of other endocrine factors that may be contributory. Glucose counter-regulatory mechanisms are often abnormal in both T1DM, T2DM as well as secondary pancreatic diabetes.

In addition, comorbidities and complications such as renal or hepatic impairment, autonomic neuropathy, malabsorption, gastroparesis, etc. may further increase the risk of hypoglycemia. Other endocrine factors that require exclusion include hypothyroidism, adrenal insufficiency and hypopituitarism and celiac disease. Hypoglycemia prevention remains an important therapeutic target that is an important determinant of the quality of life of individuals living with diabetes.

## REFERENCES

1. Seaquist ER, Anderson J, Childs B, et al. Hypoglycemia and diabetes: a report of a workgroup of the American Diabetes Association and the Endocrine Society. J Clin Endocrinol Metab. 2013;98(5):1845-59.
2. Pedersen-Bjergaard U, Thorsteinsson B. Reporting Severe Hypoglycemia in Type 1 Diabetes: Facts and Pitfalls. Curr Diab Rep. 2017;17(2):131.
3. Heinemann L, Freckmann G, Ehrmann D, et al. Real-time continuous glucose monitoring in adults with type 1 diabetes and impaired hypoglycaemia awareness or severe hypoglycaemia treated with multiple daily insulin injections (HypoDE): a multicentre, randomised controlled trial. Lancet. 2018;391(10128):1367-77.
4. Cryer PE. Hypoglycemia in Diabetes. Pathophysiology, Prevalence, and Prevention, 3rd edition. Alexandria: American Diabetes Association; 2016.
5. Gangji AS, Cukierman T, Gerstein HC, et al. A systematic review and meta-analysis of hypoglycemia and cardiovascular events: a comparison of glyburide with other secretagogues and with insulin. Diabetes Care. 2007;30(2):389-94.
6. Uloko AE, Adeniyi AF, Abubakar LY, et al. Pattern of diabetes admissions in a Northern Nigerian Tertiary Health Centre. Nigerian Endocrine Practice. 2013;7(1):15-20.
7. Vignesh JP, Mohan V. Hypoglycemia unawareness. J Assoc Phys India. 2004;52:727-32.
8. Moghissi E, Ismail-Beigi F, Devine RC. Hypoglycemia: minimizing its impact in type 2 diabetes. Endocr Pract. 2013;19:526-35.
9. Cryer PE. Mechanisms of hypoglycemia-associated autonomic failure in diabetes. N Engl J Med. 2013;369(4):362-72.
10. Cryer PE. Hypoglycemia, functional brain failure, and brain death. J Clin Invest. 2007;117(4):868-70.
11. Murad MH, Coto-Yglesias F, Wang AT, et al. Drug induced hypoglycaemia: A systematic review. J Clinical Endocrinol Metab. 2009;94(3):741-5.
12. Gill GV, Woodward A, Casson IF, et al. Cardiac arrhythmia and nocturnal hypoglycaemia in type 1 diabetes "dead in bed" syndrome revisited. Diabetologia. 2009;52(1):42-5.
13. Jialal I., Dhindsa S. Hypoglycemia and the predisposition to cardiovascular disease: Is the pro-inflammatory-pro-coagulant diathesis a plausible explanation? Atherosclerosis. 2016;251:504-6.
14. Lee AK, Warren B, Lee CJ, et al. The Association of Severe Hypoglycemia With Incident Cardiovascular Events and Mortality in Adults With Type 2 Diabetes. Diabetes Care. 2018;41(1):104-11.
15. Plummer MP, Deane AM. Dysglycemia and Glucose Control During Sepsis. Clin Chest Med. 2016;37(2):309-19.
16. Abdelhafiz AH, Rodríguez-Mañas L, Morley JE, et al. Hypoglycemia in older people-a less well recognized risk factor for frailty. Aging Dis. 2015;6(2):156-67.

17. International Hypoglycaemia Study Group. Minimizing Hypoglycemia in Diabetes. Diabetes Care. 2015;38(8):1583-91.
18. Garber AJ, King AB, Del Prato S, et al. Insulin degludec, an ultra-longacting basal insulin, versus insulin glargine in basal-bolus treatment with mealtime insulin aspart in type 2 diabetes (BEGIN Basal-Bolus Type 2): a phase 3, randomised, open-label, treat-to-target non-inferiority trial. Lancet. 2012;379(9825):1498-507.
19. Gallen IW. Hypoglycemia associated with exercise in people with type 1 diabetes. Diabetic Hypoglycemia.2014;7(1):3-10.
20. Benkhadra K, Alahdab F, Tamhane SU, et al. Continuous subcutaneous insulin infusion versus multiple daily injections in individuals with type 1 diabetes: a systematic review and meta-analysis. Endocrine. 2017;55(1):77-84.
21. Beck RW, Riddlesworth T, Ruedy K, et al. Effect of Continuous Glucose Monitoring on Glycemic Control in Adults With Type 1 Diabetes Using Insulin Injections: The DIAMOND Randomized Clinical Trial. JAMA. 2017;317(4):371-8.
22. US Food and Drug Administration. FDA approves first continuous glucose monitoring system for adults not requiring blood sample calibration. 2017. Available from https://www.fda.gov/news-events/press-announcements/fda-approves-first-continuous-glucose-monitoring-system-adults-not-requiring-blood-sample [Last Accessed May 2019].
23. Bergenstal RM, Klonoff DC, Garg SK, et al. Threshold-based insulin-pump interruption for reduction of hypoglycemia. N Engl J Med. 2013;369(3):224-32.
24. American Diabetes Association. 6. Glycemic Targets: Standards of Medical Care in Diabetes-2018. Diabetes Care. 2018;41:S55-S64.
25. International Hypoglycaemia Study Group. Glucose concentrations of less than 3.0 mmol/L (54 mg/dL) should be reported in clinical trials: a joint position statement of the American Diabetes Association and the European Association for the Study of Diabetes. Diabetes Care. 2017;40(1):155-7.
26. Cryer PE. Glycemic goals in diabetes: trade-off between glycemic control and iatrogenic hypoglycemia. Diabetes. 2014;63(7):2188-95.
27. Pedersen-Bjergaard U, Kristensen PL, Beck-Nielsen H, et al. Effect of insulin analogues on risk of severe hypoglycaemia in patients with type 1 diabetes prone to recurrent severe hypoglycaemia (HypoAna trial): a prospective, randomised, open-label, blinded-endpoint crossover trial. Lancet Diabetes Endocrinol. 2014;2(7):553-61.

# CHAPTER 17

# Endovigilance in Diabetes Therapy

Sameer Aggarwal, Jaikrit Bhutani, Dina Shrestha

## INTRODUCTION

Achieving optimal glycemic control in diabetes has been a challenge for clinicians since decades and requires the use of multiple drug regimens targeting various pathophysiological defects. Adverse drug events including weight gain and hypoglycemia remain formidable factors in our inability to attain glycemic targets.

The novel concept of glucocrinology emphasizes the relationship between metabolic and endocrine health.[1] While endocrine diseases are associated with alterations in glucose homeostasis, diabetes also results in significant effects on endocrine function. In addition, many antidiabetic agents have effects on endocrine health beyond glucose lowering. While some of these effects may be detrimental, others may be useful. A diabetes care practitioner should be vigilant of these endocrine effects to optimize and individualize patient care. In this chapter, we will describe the endocrine effects of diabetes therapy with a focus on need for endovigilance in diabetes care.

## INSULIN

While endogenous insulin secretion is carefully regulated in response to circulating blood glucose concentration along with the secretion of counter-regulatory hormones when glucose falls below threshold, such a fine tuning of exogenous insulin therapy is not possible. Therefore, even with more advanced insulin formulations and delivery systems, mimicking normal physiology remains a distant dream and the risk of hypoglycemia remains a significant challenge with insulin therapy. In addition, exogenous subcutaneous insulin is absorbed into systemic circulation and results in an altered portosystemic gradient of insulin with higher systemic concentrations. On the other hand, more than 80% of endogenous insulin is extracted by the liver in first pass and less amounts reach systemic circulation.[2] This further increases the risk of hypoglycemia with injectable insulin.

Hypoglycemia with insulin is more common in patients with type 1 diabetes mellitus (T1DM) as compared to type 2 diabetes mellitus (T2DM) as the former have an almost absolute deficiency of insulin and associated abnormalities in counter-regulatory hormones.[3] The risk of hypoglycemia is greater with skipped or delayed meals, insulin dose-meal mismatch, erratic absorption kinetics, excessive physical activity, comorbidities and concomitant illness such as chronic kidney disease, autonomic neuropathy, celiac disease or hypothyroidism. Various insulin formulations differ in their relative risk of hypoglycemia. Greater risk is seen with prandial insulins compared to basal insulins. Insulin analogs have a lower risk of overall and nocturnal hypoglycemia compared to conventional insulins. Hypoglycemia risk with insulin therapy may be reduced by frequent self-monitoring of blood glucose and careful titration of insulin dose. Continuous subcutaneous insulin infusion (CSII) or insulin pumps, especially when combined with continuous glucose monitoring (CGM), can minimize the risk of hypoglycemia and are useful in individuals with recurrent hypoglycemia, hypoglycemia unawareness or marked glycemic variability.

Insulin therapy is also associated with significant weight gain, with predominant increase in adipose tissue. Several factors may contribute to weight gain:
- Improved glycemic control with reduced glycosuria and calorie loss
- Catch-up weight gain in individuals with catabolic features
- Increased appetite due to central effect
- Defensive snacking due to fear of hypoglycemia
- Promotion of lipogenesis by insulin.

In the first year after insulin initiation, weight gain of as much as 3–7 kg has been reported.[4] The United Kingdom Prospective Diabetes Study (UKPDS) study reported 7 kg weight gain over a decade of insulin therapy in individuals with T2DM, with maximum weight gain soon after insulin initiation.[5] Intensive insulin regimens are associated with a greater weight gain. Less intensive therapy with either insulin or a sulfonylurea was associated with a 3.5–4.8 kg weight gain at 3 years versus no change with metformin monotherapy.[6] Weight gain is positively correlated with insulin dose. Among various insulin formulations, more weight gain occurs with prandial insulin compared to basal insulin and less weight gain has been reported with hepato-preferential insulins such as detemir. Insulin-associated weight gain can be avoided by adequate patient counseling and implementation of strict diet and exercise plans. Several antidiabetic agents such as glucagon-like polypeptide-1 receptor agonists (GLP-1RAs), sodium-glucose cotransporter-2 (SGLT-2) inhibitors and dipeptidyl peptidase-4 (DPP-4) inhibitors may limit weight gain associated with insulin.

Data on the impact of insulin on fractures in individuals with T2DM is scarce and remains controversial; with some observational studies showing an increased risk of falls and fractures. Lack of randomized controlled trials makes it difficult to draw a relationship between insulin use and fractures.[7]

## SULFONYLUREAS

With sulfonylureas, hypoglycemia remains the most bothersome side effect. The risk of hypoglycemia is inherent to their mechanism of action. Sulfonylureas lead to closure of ATP-sensitive K-channels on the cell membrane of β-cells, thereby leading to membrane depolarization and insulin secretion. However, the insulin secretion is not coupled to glucose-sensing and continues to occur even at lower blood glucose concentration. A systematic review reported a prevalence of hypoglycemia (glucose ≤56 mg/dL) in 10.1% while severe hypoglycemia was reported in 0.8% of sulfonylurea users.[8] Hypoglycemia is less common with gliclazide or glimepiride, compared to long-acting sulfonylureas (chlorpropamide or glyburide), with lowest risk being reported with gliclazide.[8] Highest incidence of hypoglycemia has been reported in those patients taking glyburide.

Endovigilance for hypoglycemia is required when using long-acting more potent sulfonylureas like glyburide and high-dose regimens. Patients must be cautioned about the risk of hypoglycemia, especially if there is missed or delayed meals and if it is taken after exercise. Individuals who are undernourished, have significant alcohol intake, those with impaired renal or cardiac function or gastrointestinal disease, or concurrent therapy with salicylates, sulfonamides, fibric acid derivatives (such as gemfibrozil), and warfarin are at greater risk.[9] Hypoglycemia may persist for several hours and require in-hospital treatment.

In addition, sulfonylureas cause significant weight gain, though it is less than that reported with insulin therapy. The mechanism of weight gain seems to be related to increased endogenous insulin secretion. Gliclazide and glimepiride have been associated with slightly less weight gain compared to other agents.

Interestingly, chlorpropamide was associated with hyponatremia as it increases the action of vasopressin. There are several case reports of the syndrome of inappropriate antidiuretic hormone (SIADH) secretion with the use of chlorpropamide.[10] Similar effect has not been reported with any of the currently used sulfonylureas.

Electrophoretic studies, especially with first-generation sulfonylureas, have shown that they competitively inhibit the binding of thyroid hormones (T3 and T4) to thyroxine-binding globulin (TBG). Reduced protein-bound iodine (PBI) and elevated resin uptake have been reported as evidence of their antithyroid property. In fact, some studies reported a higher incidence of hypothyroidism in diabetics treated with first-generation sulfonylureas compared to control group treated with diet alone or insulin.[11] An increase in thyroid volume and decrease in radioactive iodine uptake (RAIU) have been shown after sulfonylurea treatment.

## METFORMIN

Metformin has low risk of hypoglycemia and a neutral to slightly beneficial effect on body weight. There have been concerns regarding precipitation of lactic acidosis since its early use; however, the incidence is very low. Symptoms may include anorexia, nausea, vomiting, abdominal pain, lethargy, hyperventilation and hypotension. A systematic review of 347 randomized trials and prospective cohort studies representing 70,490 patient-years of metformin use, and 55,451 patient-years in the comparator group reported no cases of lactic acidosis.[12] Despite its rare incidence, metformin-associated lactic acidosis (MALA) is associated with high case fatality rate. MALA usually presents as acute or progressive renal impairment, acute or progressive heart failure, acute pulmonary decompensation, sepsis or fluid deficit. Treatment of MALA requires optimal hydration, replacement of bicarbonate and in severe cases, bicarbonate hemodialysis that removes the drug and replenishes bicarbonate.[13]

However, considering that lactic acidosis risk is largely minimal, the hitherto contraindications to the use of metformin have been revised. Metformin can be used in stage 2 and 3 chronic kidney disease. It is contraindicated when the glomerular filtration rate (GFR) is below 30 mL/min/m$^2$, there is hypersensitivity to metformin or in cases with acute or chronic metabolic acidosis. Factors that may increase the risk of lactic acidosis include concomitant use of carbonic anhydrase inhibitors, use of contrast agents, hypoxic states, excessive alcohol intake, and renal and hepatic impairment, where it should be used with caution.

Metformin is an activator of 5'-AMP activated protein kinase (AMPK), but it inhibits hypothalamic AMPK, which is involved in the regulation of hypothalamic-pituitary-thyroid axis. It may reduce thyrotropin-releasing hormone secretion with reduction in thyroid-stimulating hormone (TSH) levels in patients with treated hypothyroidism, but does not have any effect in euthyroid individuals. Moreover, metformin does not cause any change in circulating total or free thyroid hormone levels, despite a slight TSH suppression.[14] Other mechanisms involving interactions between metformin and thyroid hormones are modification of thyroid hormone receptor affinity, thyroid hormone binding and interference with the TSH assay. It is necessary to monitor TSH levels when starting metformin. A slight reduction in TSH after initiation of metformin does not warrant a reduction in levothyroxine dose. In other studies, metformin was found to reduce the volume of thyroid nodules, inhibit growth of thyroid carcinoma, and potentiate the antimitogenic effect of chemotherapeutic agents.[14] More research is needed to understand the effect of metformin on thyroid tumors.

Metformin also has varied effects on reproductive function in men and women. Metformin has beneficial effects in women with polycystic ovary syndrome (PCOS) with reduced insulin resistance and hyperinsulinemia, improved LH pulsatility, increased sex hormone binding globulin (SHBG) levels, improved cycle regularity and reduced serum androgen concentration.[15] However, the effect on serum androgen levels has not been consistent and it does not seem to have a significant effect on hyperandrogenic symptoms such as acne and hirsutism.

Metformin regulates oocyte maturation, improves oocyte quality and has been shown to improve ovulation rates and clinical pregnancy rates when added to other ovulation induction regimens. It also reduced the risk of ovarian hyperstimulation with gonadotropins. Use in early pregnancy was associated with reduced risk of miscarriages, gestational diabetes and preeclampsia. Short-term effects in gestational diabetes seem to be beneficial with no increased risk of congenital malformations, but a slight increased risk of premature birth.[15] The effects of metformin on epigenetic programing in fetus need further evaluation; an offspring follow-up study reported higher body mass index (BMI) in offspring exposed to metformin. But this was largely attributed to increased subcutaneous fat and not visceral fat.

In utero exposure to metformin was associated with reduced fetal testis size and Sertoli cell number, which has been attributed to increased lactate production. However, no effect on sperm count, morphology or motility has been reported in adult mice. In fact, metformin improved sperm count and motility in obese rats.[15] Metformin reversibly decreased testosterone production in mice and human fetal testis. On the other hand, in obese men, metformin has been reported to increase LH pulsatility and testosterone concentration. In models of testicular ischemia, metformin reduced oxidative stress and had cytoprotective effect on germ cells.[15]

In girls with precocious puberty and hyperinsulinemia, metformin was shown to delay pubertal progression and insulin-like growth factor-1 (IGF-1) increase. This correlated with decrease in adiposity and insulin concentrations.[15] Metformin may have beneficial effects in endometrial, ovarian and breast cancers.

## THIAZOLIDINEDIONES

Peroxisome proliferator-activated receptor-γ (PPAR-γ) agonists or thiazolidinediones (TZDs) are no longer considered first-choice agents due to an increased risk of weight gain, fluid retention, heart failure and fractures associated with their use. In addition, rosiglitazone was associated with an increased risk of myocardial infarction in randomized trials, while pioglitazone has been linked with bladder cancer in observational data. The overall risk of hypoglycemia with TZDs is low, as they act by improving insulin sensitivity and do not stimulate insulin secretion, per se.

All TZDs cause substantial weight gain which is both dose- and time-dependent. In a cohort of patients taking pioglitazone continuously, the average weight gain increased steadily up to 30 months but then plateaued (≈5.3 kg) by 36 months.[16] While weight gain is partly due to fluid retention and edema, TZDs also activate PPAR-γ in the adipose tissue as well as central nervous system leading to an expansion of subcutaneous adipose tissue. However, pioglitazone leads to increased differentiation of preadipocytes into insulin-sensitive adipocytes, with a more favorable adipokine secretory profile and decreased adipose tissue inflammation. In addition, there is reduction in visceral, hepatic and ectopic fat, with resultant beneficial effects on insulin sensitivity and metabolic health despite a net weight gain. Low-dose pioglitazone has been associated with less weight gain but still retains positive effects on glucose and lipid metabolism.[17] Reduction in hepatocellular fat has been associated with beneficial effects in nonalcoholic fatty liver disease (NAFLD).

Thiazolidinediones have a negative effect on bone health and are associated with a substantial increase in fracture risk. This is primarily due to reduced bone mineral density (BMD) and increased bone marrow fat content.[18] Observational studies report an annual rate of bone loss of –0.61% in postmenopausal women using pioglitazone compared to nonusers.[18] PPAR-γ regulates the differentiation of mesenchymal cells and hematopoietic cells and in the bone, it promotes adipocyte differentiation.[19] This leads to diversion of bone marrow stromal cells from osteoblast lineage into adipocyte lineage with decreased bone formation and increased adipogenesis. Also, TZDs downregulate the components of IGF-1 pathway, both in vivo and in vitro, which is essential for osteoblast proliferation and differentiation. In addition, TZDs increase bone resorption by increased osteoclast recruitment and differentiation. This may be mediated via a functional cross-talk between PPAR-γ and estrogen receptor (ER) as estrogen deficiency was associated with greater TZD-induced bone loss in animal models.[18] TZDs induce the production of receptor activator of nuclear factor-κB ligand (RANKL), which results in increased osteoclastogenesis.[19] There is also some evidence that TZDs may delay fracture healing.

Clinical trials with pioglitazone demonstrated that women taking pioglitazone were at increased risk of fractures than control group. The fracture sites included distal upper or lower extremities (forearm, hand, wrist, foot, ankle, fibula and tibia). However, a similar effect was not reported in men. On the other hand, a population-based study showed a greater risk of low-trauma fractures in women as well as men [odds ratio (OR) 2.59, 95% confidence interval (CI) 0.96–7.01].[20] Elderly individuals, women, those with longer duration of pioglitazone use and those at risk for osteoporosis are more susceptible and hence, pioglitazone should be used with caution in such individuals.

It has been suggested that lower doses may have a less detrimental effect on bone health. The possibility of developing selective modulators of PPAR-γ so that metabolic effects are retained while bone effects are minimized is an avenue for research. Combining TZDs with incretin-based drugs that stimulate osteoblast activity and reduce osteoclast activity may reduce the negative effects of TZDs on bone but requires evaluation.

Peroxisome proliferator-activated receptor-γ also plays a role in reproductive health and fertility. TZDs decrease ovarian androgen synthesis by decreasing insulin resistance and improved cycle regularity and ovulation rates as well serum androgen concentrations and hirsutism score in women with PCOS, despite an increase in body weight. However, pioglitazone has the potential for teratogenicity, requiring caution when using in reproductive age women.

Quite interestingly, it has been reported that PPAR-γ is expressed in pituitary gland and pituitary tumors. PPAR-γ agonists were found to inhibit pituitary tumor development and tumoral hypersecretion in rodents.[21] However, there is discrepancy between in vitro and human clinical data on the effect of PPAR-γ agonists on adrenocorticotropic hormone (ACTH) secretion and they do not seem to have any clinically meaningful effect in humans.

## DIPEPTIDYL PEPTIDASE-4 INHIBITORS

Dipeptidyl peptidase-4 (DPP-4) inhibitors are usually well tolerated with minimal effect on body weight or risk of hypoglycemia in the absence of concomitant treatment with insulin or sulfonylureas. Major concern has been regarding the risk of pancreatitis. Several observational studies and analysis of adverse-event reporting databases reported an increased incidence of pancreatitis with DPP-4 inhibitors. However, meta-analyses of randomized trials and large-scale cardiovascular outcome trials have not confirmed this risk, and no causal relationship has been established. In one meta-analysis, the overall incidence of pancreatitis was low (35 cases among 68,318 patients, 20 in patients taking DPP-4 inhibitors and 15 in comparator group).[22] Further studies are warranted. Meanwhile, endovigilance is required when using DPP-4 inhibitors in patients at risk of pancreatitis, such as those with gallstone disease or significant alcohol intake and they should be avoided in those with previous history of pancreatitis. Asymptomatic elevations in serum amylase and lipase have been reported but regular monitoring of their levels is not recommended. DPP-4 inhibitors should be promptly discontinued in patients who develop pancreatitis. DPP-4 inhibitors have also been related to pancreatic cancer risk, but the results have been conflicting and insignificant.[22]

The effects of DPP-4 inhibitors on bone health seem to be largely positive. They promote bone formation and decrease bone resorption through an increase in DPP-4 substrates (gastric inhibitory polypeptide or GIP, glucagon-like peptide-1 and stromal cell-derived factor-1α or SDF-1α) and have been associated with increase in BMD and improved bone quality. DPP-4 inhibitors may decrease parathyroid hormone (PTH) secretion and increase 25-hydroxyvitamin D concentration. Sitagliptin resulted in dose-dependent increase in volumetric BMD in vertebrae in animal studies.[23] On the other hand, saxagliptin and vildagliptin did not have a similar effect. In a meta-analysis of 28 randomized trials, DPP-4 inhibitors were associated with reduced risk of fractures compared to placebo or active comparators but similar effect was not demonstrated by another meta-analysis.[23]

## GLUCAGON-LIKE PEPTIDE-1 RECEPTOR AGONISTS

Glucagon-like peptide-1 receptor agonists (GLP-1RA) are associated with significant reduction in body weight and waist circumference. Weight loss occurs due to increased satiety, reduced food intake, and delayed gastric emptying, while there is no change in energy expenditure. There is reduction in subcutaneous and visceral fat, but not in lean body mass. Liraglutide and semaglutide lead to greater weight loss in comparison to exenatide, lixisenatide or dulaglutide. While weight loss is beneficial in most individuals with T2DM, endovigilance may be required in lean catabolic individuals.

Glucagon-like peptide-1 receptor agonists have been evaluated in both euglycemic and diabetic patients with moderate to severe hypothalamic obesity. Over a period of up to 51 months, 8 out of 9 patients experienced substantial weight loss ranging from 9 to 22 kg, with improved insulin sensitivity and glycemic control.[24] Liraglutide is approved for use in obesity in doses of 3 mg once daily and can result in weight loss of 6–8%. Other GLP-1RAs are currently not approved for obesity management in nondiabetic individuals.

Glucagon-like peptide-1 receptor agonists have a potential role in the management of NAFLD and initial studies have shown positive effects on hepatic enzymes, inflammation, fibrosis, and NAFLD activity scores. In the LEAN trial, 1.8 mg of liraglutide administered daily for 48 weeks reduced nonalcoholic steatohepatitis (NASH) scores with no worsening of fibrosis in 39% subjects, and reduced hepatic fat content in 82.6% subjects.[25] However, they have been linked to increased incidence of gallstone disease, probably due to obesity and subsequent significant weight loss.

The benefits of GLP-1RAs may also extend to women with PCOS and this warrants further evaluation. Small studies have reported that exenatide and liraglutide resulted in significant weight loss in obese PCOS women, along with reduction in serum androgen levels, insulin sensitivity and cycle regularity.

Glucagon-like peptide-1 receptor agonists are also associated with an increased risk of acute pancreatitis though the number of events in clinical trials has been few. Therefore, a causal relationship cannot be established. Concern has also been raised about a possible risk of pancreatic cancer, but the evidence remains inconsistent. GLP-1RAs should be avoided in individuals with a history of pancreatitis and discontinued if there is suspicion of pancreatitis. Routine monitoring of amylase and lipase levels is, however, not recommended.

The effect of liraglutide on adrenal functions has been evaluated in individuals with T2DM. There occurred a borderline significant increase in dehydroepiandrosterone sulfate (DHEAS) in 12 men with T2DM, aged 48.6 ± 10.4 years, who received 6 months of liraglutide. These patients experienced improvement in glycemic control, weight as well as waist circumference.[26] Liraglutide also reduced salivary cortisol, a marker of stress, in persons with binge-eating disorder.

All GLP-1RAs carry a box warning in package inserts related to thyroid C-cell tumors. In rodent studies, liraglutide and dulaglutide were associated with benign and malignant thyroid C-cell tumors. In addition, stimulation of calcitonin release was reported in rats and mice exposed to exenatide and liraglutide.[27] While no adverse signals have been reported in humans, the potential effect of long-acting GLP-1RAs on thyroid C-cells requires further investigation. Due unavailability of such data at present, GLP-1RAs are contraindicated in patients with a personal or family history of medullary thyroid cancer or multiple endocrine neoplasia 2A or 2B.

## SODIUM-GLUCOSE COTRANSPORTER-2 INHIBITORS

Sodium-glucose cotransporter-2 (SGLT-2) inhibitors are associated with significant weight loss due to glycosuria and calorie loss. Initial weight reduction occurs over 3–6 months and thereafter weight plateaus due to adaptive changes such as increased appetite and reduced energy expenditure. There is greater reduction in fat mass compared to lean body mass. This would be particularly useful in overweight and obese diabetic individuals but may be a cause of concern in individuals who have catabolic features.

Empagliflozin was compared to metformin in women with PCOS and resulted in significantly greater reduction in weight, BMI, waist circumference and fat mass. However, there was no difference in hormonal and metabolic parameters.[28] Initial studies have also reported beneficial effects in NAFLD, with reduction in liver fat content, hepatic transaminases, steatosis, ballooning and fibrosis.[29]

Sodium-glucose cotransporter-2 inhibitors have two key concerns requiring endovigilance—increased risk of fractures and diabetic ketoacidosis (DKA). Patients taking canagliflozin had a greater incidence of low-trauma fractures (1.4 and 1.5 fractures per 100 patient-years exposure to canagliflozin 100 mg and 300 mg, respectively, compared with 1.1 per 100 patient-years, in placebo group). These fractures are known to occur as early as 12 weeks after starting the drug. The underlying mechanism of these fractures is possibly orthostatic hypotension resulting in postural dizziness and falls. Additionally, it has been suggested that SGLT-2 inhibitors adversely affect BMD. In a trial enrolling 716 older patients, progressively greater loss of BMD over time was noted with canagliflozin (0.9–1.2% decline in BMD at hip and 0.3–0.7% decline at spine).[30] More recently, these concerns have been dispelled by a meta-analysis of randomized trials that reported no increase in fracture risk with dapagliflozin or empagliflozin and insignificant risk with canagliflozin.[31] There have also been concerns about an increased risk of amputations with canagliflozin and caution is advised in patients at high risk such as those with previous amputations and peripheral vascular disease.

Another concern with the use of SGLT-2 inhibitors is a risk of DKA. Several mechanisms by which SGLT-2 inhibitors may precipitate ketoacidosis have been proposed, including stimulation of glucagon production, reduced renal excretion of acetoacetate and inappropriate insulin dose reduction which leads to increased lipolysis and ketogenesis.[32] Factors associated with increased DKA risk include T1DM, significant insulin deficiency, concurrent infections, surgical or medical illness, insulin pump failure, and skipped insulin doses or inappropriate insulin dose reduction. A high index of suspicion for diagnosis of DKA is required in patients presenting with symptoms as blood glucose levels may not be very high (euglycemic DKA) and urine ketones may not be significantly elevated.[32] It is recommended that SGLT-2 inhibitors should be discontinued in case of acute illness and prior to elective surgery and be reinstituted only after the patient is hemodynamically stable.

## OTHER DRUGS

Bromocriptine is a dopamine agonist used in the treatment of pituitary tumors, hyperprolactinemia, Parkinson's disease and neuroleptic malignant syndrome. Bromocriptine-QR is recommended for the treatment of T2DM in a dose of 1.6–4.8 mg once daily. It may suppress prolactin secretion and interfere with lactation. This warrants vigilance and appropriate counseling.

## CONCLUSION

In recent years, appropriate diabetes management involves increasing use of guidelines and algorithms, with major orientation to numbers. This has led to neglect of basic clinical cues which may lead to serious consequences. The concept of endovigilance in diabetes therapy is to sensitize diabetes care providers about the holistic multifaceted nature of diabetes as a disorder, and ensure comprehensive management.

## REFERENCES

1. Kalra S, Priya G, Gupta Y. Glucocrinology. J Pak Med Assoc. 2018;68(6):963-5.
2. Matteucci E, Giampietro O, Covolan V, et al. Insulin administration: Present strategies and future directions for a noninvasive (possibly more physiological) delivery. Drug Des Devel Ther. 2015;9:3109-18.
3. Donnelly LA, Morris AD, Frier BM, et al. Frequency and predictors of hypoglycaemia in Type 1 and insulin-treated Type 2 diabetes: A population-based study. Diabet Med. 2005;22(6):749-55.
4. Pontiroli AE, Miele L, Morabito A. Increase of body weight during the first year of intensive insulin treatment in type 2 diabetes: Systematic review and meta-analysis. Diabetes Obes Metab. 2011;13(11):1008-19.
5. Intensive blood-glucose control with sulphonylureas or insulin compared with conventional treatment and risk of complications in patients with type 2 diabetes (UKPDS 33). UK Prospective Diabetes Study (UKPDS) Group. Lancet. 1998;352(9131):837-53.
6. United Kingdom Prospective Diabetes Study (UKPDS). 13: Relative efficacy of randomly allocated diet, sulphonylurea, insulin, or metformin in patients with newly diagnosed non-insulin dependent diabetes followed for three years. BMJ. 1995;310(6972):83-8.
7. Losada-Grande E, Hawley S, Soldevila B, et al. Insulin use and excess fracture risk in patients with type 2 diabetes: A propensity-matched cohort analysis. Sci Rep. 2017;7(1):3781.

8. Schopman JE, Simon AC, Hoefnagel SJ, et al. The incidence of mild and severe hypoglycaemia in patients with type 2 diabetes mellitus treated with sulfonylureas: A systematic review and meta-analysis. Diabetes Metab Res Rev. 2014;30(1):11-22.
9. Shorr RI, Ray WA, Daugherty JR, et al. Incidence and risk factors for serious hypoglycemia in older persons using insulin or sulfonylureas. Arch Intern Med. 1997;157(15):1681-6.
10. Kadowaki T, Hagura R, Kajinuma H, et al. Chlorpropamide-induced hyponatremia: Incidence and risk factors. Diabetes Care. 1983;6(5):468-71.
11. Belgin E, Kebap M, Emre E, et al. Effects of second generation sulfonylureas on the thyroid. Turk J Endocrinol Metab. 1999;4:173-6.
12. Salpeter SR, Greyber E, Pasternak GA, et al. Risk of fatal and nonfatal lactic acidosis with metformin use in type 2 diabetes mellitus. Cochrane Database Syst Rev. 2010;(1):CD002967
13. Heaney D, Majid A, Junor B. Bicarbonate haemodialysis as a treatment of metformin overdose. Nephrol Dial Transplant. 1997;12(5):1046-7.
14. Fournier JP, Yin H, Yu OH, et al. Metformin and low levels of thyroid-stimulating hormone in patients with type 2 diabetes mellitus. CMAJ. 2014;186(15):1138-45.
15. Faure M, Bertoldo MJ, Khoueiry R, et al. Metformin in reproductive biology. Front Endocrinol (Lausanne). 2018;9:675.
16. King A, Armstrong D, Chinnapongse S. Clinical observations of weight gain associated with pioglitazone: 3 years. Diabetes. 2003;52 (Suppl 1):A123.
17. Yanai H, Adachi H. The low-dose (7.5 mg/day) pioglitazone therapy. J Clin Med Res. 2017;9(10):821-5.
18. Pop LM, Lingvay I, Yuan Q, et al. Impact of pioglitazone on bone mineral density and bone marrow fat content. Osteoporos Int. 2017;28(11):3261-9.
19. Lecka-Czernik B. Bone loss in diabetes: Use of antidiabetic thiazolidinediones and secondary osteoporosis. Curr Osteoporos Rep. 2010;8(4):178-84.
20. Meier C, Kraenzlin ME, Bodmer M, et al. Use of thiazolidinediones and fracture risk. Arch Intern Med. 2008;168(8):820-5.
21. Emery MN, Leontiou C, Bonner SE, et al. PPAR-gamma expression in pituitary tumours and the functional activity of the glitazones: Evidence that any anti-proliferative effect of the glitazones is independent of the PPAR-gamma receptor. Clin Endocrinol (Oxf). 2006;65(3):389-95.
22. Monami M, Dicembrini I, Mannucci E. Dipeptidyl peptidase-4 inhibitors and pancreatitis risk: A meta-analysis of randomized clinical trials. Diabetes Obes Metab. 2014;16(1):48-56.
23. Yang Y, Zhao C, Liang J, et al. Effect of dipeptidyl peptidase-4 inhibitors on bone metabolism and the possible underlying mechanisms. Front Pharmacol. 2017;8:487.
24. Zoicas F, Droste M, Mayr B, et al. GLP-1 analogues as a new treatment option for hypothalamic obesity in adults: Report of nine cases. Eur J Endocrinol. 2013;168:699-706.
25. Armstrong MJ, Gaunt P, Aithal GP, et al. Liraglutide safety and efficacy in patients with non-alcoholic steatohepatitis (LEAN): A multicentre, double-blind, randomised, placebo-controlled phase 2 study. Lancet. 2016;13:387(10019):679-90.
26. Piédrola G, Cepero D, Gil C, et al. Changes in insulin sensitivity and DHEAS in type 2 diabetic men treated with liraglutide. Endocr Abstr. 2014;35:487.
27. Madsen LW, Knauf JA, Gotfredsen C, et al. GLP-1 receptor agonists and the thyroid: C-cell effects in mice are mediated via the GLP-1 receptor and not associated with RET activation. Endocrinology. 2012;153(3):1538-47.
28. Javed Z, Papageorgiou M, Deshmukh H, et al. Effects of empagliflozin on metabolic parameters in polycystic ovary syndrome: A randomised controlled study. Clin Endocrinol (Oxf). 2019;90(6): 805-13.
29. Lai LL, Vethakkan SR, Nik Mustapha NR, et al. Empagliflozin for the treatment of nonalcoholic steatohepatitis in patients with type 2 diabetes mellitus. Dig Dis Sci. 2019.
30. Watts NB, Bilezikian JP, Usiskin K, et al. Effects of canagliflozin on fracture risk in patients with type 2 diabetes mellitus. J Clin Endocrinol Metab. 2016;101(1):157-66.
31. Tang HL, Li DD, Zhang JJ, et al. Lack of evidence for a harmful effect of sodium-glucose co-transporter 2 (SGLT2) inhibitors on fracture risk among type 2 diabetes patients: A network and cumulative meta-analysis of randomized controlled trials. Diabetes Obes Metab. 2016;18(12):1199-1206.
32. Priya G, Kalra S, Bhambhri V. Sodium-glucose co-transporter 2 inhibitors in type 1 diabetes—A dangerous ally. US Endocrinol. 2017;13(2):75-9.

# CHAPTER 18

# Endovigilance in Diabetic Vasculopathy

*Soumya S, Darvin Vamadevan Das, C Jayakumari, Sanjay Kalra*

## INTRODUCTION

Diabetes is a multisystem disorder characterized by hyperglycemia. Chronic complications of diabetes include both microvascular and macrovascular disease. The endocrine system regulates energy homeostasis, glucose, protein and lipid metabolism, and in turn, metabolism may impact endocrine health. Therefore, endocrine disorders may present with dysglycemia or may result in worsening of glycemic control in pre-existing diabetes. Endocrinopathies also impact other cardiovascular risk factors and may contribute to microvascular and cardiovascular risk.

At the same time, diabetes is associated with significant alterations in various endocrine axes. Vascular complications of diabetes may also impact endocrine health. In this chapter, we discuss the need for endocrine vigilance in diabetic vasculopathies such as chronic kidney disease (CKD) and cardiovascular disease (CVD).

## ENDOVIGILANCE IN CHRONIC KIDNEY DISEASE

The kidneys are involved in the synthesis and degradation of various hormones. Therefore, CKD may affect endocrine function. Further, several coexistent conditions like metabolic acidosis, inflammation and malnutrition can alter the endocrine system. The estimation of plasma concentration of several hormones may be affected by different mechanisms enlisted in Table 1. These include altered results of hormone suppression or stimulation tests; presence of inactive hormone isoforms that may interfere with hormone assays; or the target organ response to trophic hormones may be increased or suppressed.[1] In this section, the authors have discussed the abnormalities in various endocrine axes that occur in CKD.

### Thyroid Function Abnormalities in Chronic Kidney Disease

In CKD, the hypothalamus–pituitary–thyroid (HPT) axis as well as the peripheral metabolism of thyroid hormones is affected, as discussed below and summarized in Table 2.

| TABLE 1 | Mechanism of alteration of endocrine function in chronic kidney disease. | |
|---|---|---|
| **Mechanism** | **Effects** | **Specific hormones** |
| Abnormalities of hormone catabolism | Decreased metabolic clearance | Insulin, PTH, leptin, adiponectin and gastrin |
| Abnormalities of hormone production | Reduced hormone production in endocrine organs | Testosterone, estrogen |
| | Reduced hormone production by the kidney | 1,25(OH)$_2$D$_3$, erythropoietin |
| | Reactive hypersecretion of hormone to reestablish homeostasis | PTH, FGF23 and erythropoietin |
| | Inappropriate hypersecretion due to disturbed feedback | ACTH, LH and prolactin |
| | Abnormal secretion pattern (pulsatility, circadian rhythm) | GH, LH |
| Abnormalities of hormone activity | Increased isoforms with potentially less bioactivity (because of post-transcriptional modifications) | LH |
| | Increased serum hormone-binding proteins concentration resulting in the reduced availability of free hormone | IGF |
| | Decreased serum hormone-binding proteins concentration resulting in the increased availability of free hormone | Leptin |
| | Changed receptor quantity and/or structure | Vitamin D receptor |
| | Altered postreceptor cellular signaling | Insulin, GH |
| | Altered activation of prohormones | Proinsulin, thyroxine (T4) |

[ACTH: adrenocorticotropic hormone; FGF23: fibroblast growth factor 23; GH: growth hormone; IGF: insulin-like growth factor; LH: luteinizing hormone; 1,25(OH)$_2$D$_3$: 1,25-dihydroxyvitamin D3; PTH: parathyroid hormone]

## Thyroid Hormones

Low triiodothyronine (T3) syndrome is the most common disturbance in CKD patients. It is due to impaired conversion of thyroxine (T4) to T3 caused by decreased activity of iodothyronine deiodinase, as a result of malnutrition and/or chronic metabolic acidosis and reduced clearance of inflammatory cytokines such as tumor necrosis factor-α (TNF-α) and interleukin-6 (IL-6). However, CKD patients with low serum T3 concentrations usually appear clinically euthyroid, probably because the expression of thyroid hormone receptors α and β in the mononuclear cells is increased.[2] Low serum T3 concentration in CKD patients is implicated as a contributory factor for endothelial dysfunction, atherosclerosis and cardiac abnormalities, and increased cardiovascular mortality in hemodialysis patients.

The serum concentration of T4 is usually normal or reduced. Serum concentrations of reverse triiodothyronine (rT3) are normal in spite of decreased renal clearance. This is probably caused by increased cellular uptake of rT3 and redistribution of rT3 from the vascular to extravascular space.[3]

**TABLE 2** Effect of chronic kidney disease due to diabetes on hypothalamic–pituitary–thyroid axis.

| Level of hypothalamic–pituitary–thyroid axis | Pathophysiological changes in chronic kidney disease in diabetes |
|---|---|
| Effects at the level of the hypothalamus and pituitary | • Normal or high TSH<br>• Altered TSH circadian rhythm<br>• Reduced TSH response to TRH<br>• Abnormal TSH glycosylation<br>• Altered TRH and TSH clearance |
| Effects on thyroid gland and peripheral thyroid hormone metabolism | • Increased thyroid volume<br>• High prevalence of thyroid nodules and thyroid carcinoma<br>• Low or normal total T3 and total T4<br>• Reduced or normal free T3 and free T4<br>• Reduced peripheral conversion of T4 to T3<br>• Elevation of free T4 induced by heparin in hemodialysis patients<br>• Normal total rT3 and elevated free rT3<br>• Alteration in binding proteins<br>• Reduced T4 response to exogenous TSH<br>• Reduced renal iodine excretion<br>• Elevated serum iodine |

(rT3: reverse triiodothyronine; T3: triiodothyronine; T4: thyroxine; TRH: thyrotropin-releasing hormone; TSH: thyroid-stimulating hormone)

## Thyroid-stimulating Hormone

In CKD patients, the pituitary receptor response to thyrotropin-releasing hormone (TRH) is blunted, which causes a decrease in the production of thyroid-stimulating hormone (TSH). Moreover, there is impaired renal clearance and prolonged half-life of TSH. The diurnal rhythm of TSH with a peak in late evening or early morning is diminished and the nocturnal TSH surge is reduced.[4]

## Hypothyroidism

The prevalence of hypothyroidism in CKD patients is between 0% and 9.5%. CKD is associated with decreased iodide excretion, which causes elevated serum inorganic iodide concentration and increased thyroid iodide content. The former causes enlargement of the thyroid gland and contributes to increased prevalence of goiter in CKD. Additionally, excess iodide may contribute to hypothyroidism through prolonged Wolff–Chaikoff effect. Inorganic iodine level increases and thyroxine-binding globulin (TBG) levels are decreased, especially when there is significant proteinuria. In chronic hemodialysis patients, a transient increase in serum T4 concentration may occur due to the use of heparin as an anticoagulant. Heparin competes with T4 at the binding site of thyroid-binding proteins. An increase in T4 may last for up to 24 hours; therefore, blood samples for thyroid function assessment should be collected before the dialysis session.[5]

Most CKD patients, however, are euthyroid and do not need treatment, unless there are clear symptoms and TSH is raised. Typical signs and symptoms of hypothyroidism, such as hypothermia, pallor and asthenia, may overlap the clinical picture of advanced CKD. Considering the similarity between the symptoms of hypothyroidism and uremia, it seems logical to perform thyroid function tests periodically in CKD patients.

## Gonadal Axis Abnormalities in Men with Chronic Kidney Disease

Chronic kidney disease may impact the hypothalamic–pituitary–gonadal (HPG) axis at multiple levels and can result in functional hypogonadism and decreased fertility.

### Gonadotropins

Chronic kidney disease is associated with irregular pulsatile secretion and decreased amplitude of gonadotropin-releasing hormone (GnRH), which leads to a loss of normal pulsatile release of luteinizing hormone (LH). These disturbances are caused mainly by reduced renal clearance of GnRH and LH.[6] Hyperprolactinemia further contributes to abnormal GnRH secretion. Basal plasma LH concentrations are elevated, due to decreased catabolism and lack of GnRH inhibition by testosterone (due to lower plasma testosterone concentration). Serum follicle-stimulating hormone (FSH) may either be elevated or in the upper normal range. FSH is an important factor involved in spermatogenesis. In CKD patients, spermatogenesis is usually impaired despite the elevated serum FSH, possibly due to testicular resistance to FSH or primary testicular dysfunction.

### Testosterone

Even though the daily circadian rhythm of serum testosterone, with a peak at 4–8 AM and nadir at 8–12 PM, is usually maintained in CKD, serum total and free testosterone concentrations are low in majority of men on hemodialysis. It is not yet known whether this is due to impaired synthesis or increased catabolism of testosterone, or a combination of both. The response to stimulation with human gonadotropin is blunted and delayed. Malnutrition also may be contributory as supplementation with essential amino acids and ketoanalogs is associated with increase in serum testosterone. Moreover, decreased serum androstenedione and dehydroepiandrosterone sulfate (DHEAS) have also been reported.[7]

### Reproductive Dysfunction

The onset of puberty in boys with CKD is delayed by an average of 2 years. Dysfunction of erection and decrease in libido have been seen in uremic patients. In addition, there is a decrease in number of germ cells in seminiferous tubules leading to reduced fertility. The deficiency of androgens in men with CKD may contribute to the changes in body composition such as increased adiposity and reduced lean body mass. Androgen deficiency may also contribute to CKD-associated bone disease and risk of bone fractures, anemia, decreased libido, impairment of sexual function and depression.

Low serum testosterone concentrations have been related with worse outcomes in men on hemodialysis. However, testosterone therapy is not exempted from risks; therefore, benefits of testosterone replacement need to be established in large clinical trials before it could be recommended in CKD patients with hypogonadism.

## Prolactin

In the majority of men on hemodialysis, serum prolactin (PRL) concentrations are elevated and its daily rhythm is altered. Moreover, sleep-induced secretory bursts of PRL secretion are rarely observed, although episodic PRL secretion during the daytime occurs. Both reduced renal PRL clearance and increased PRL production due to inadequate dopaminergic inhibition of PRL release contribute to hyperprolactinemia in patients with CKD. Hyperprolactinemia, in turn, impairs GnRH secretion and results in decreased testosterone production, sexual dysfunction and subfertility.[8] In some patients, correction of hyperprolactinemia by bromocriptine with concomitant improvement of sexual function has been described. Hyperprolactinemia may cause endothelial dysfunction and the association between hyperprolactinemia and negative cardiovascular outcome was also described in patients with CKD. In a small clinical study, reduction of blood pressure and hypertrophy of left ventricle were found in patients with CKD after bromocriptine administration.

## Gonadal Axis Abnormalities in Women with Chronic Kidney Disease

Females with CKD also present a variety of derangements of the HPG axis, which contribute to anovulation, irregular menstrual cycles and infertility.

### Luteinizing Hormone

In most premenopausal women with CKD, serum LH concentration is increased. The loss of pulsatile LH secretion results from disruption of cyclic GnRH release.[9] In healthy females, estradiol feedback blunts the magnitude of LH pulses; while in women with CKD, there is impaired feedback inhibition. The result is impaired ovulation and infertility.

### Follicle-stimulating Hormone

In majority of premenopausal women with CKD, the serum concentrations of FSH are normal; thus, the FSH/LH ratio is decreased. Therefore, the primary defect seems to be disturbed HPG axis at the hypothalamic level and not primary ovarian failure.

### Prolactin

Serum PRL concentrations are most often increased and the surge of plasma PRL after TRH administration is blunted. This commonly manifests as amenorrhea.

### Estrogen

Serum concentrations of estradiol may either be normal, or low and are consistently lower if hyperprolactinemia occurs. In the second half of menstrual cycle, serum progesterone concentrations are decreased due to defective follicle luteinization.

### Reproductive Dysfunction

Therefore, women with CKD may have functional hypothalamic amenorrhea or menstrual irregularities. Functional hypothalamic amenorrhea is associated with a hypoestrogenic state. This significantly contributes to impaired bone health in women with CKD.[10] In women who are on maintenance renal replacement therapy (dialysis), women with hypoestrogenism and amenorrhea have lower bone mineral density (BMD) as compared to women who have regular menstruation. Few small interventional studies have evaluated the use of transdermal estradiol and raloxifene in postmenopausal women on maintenance hemodialysis and reported an increase in BMD. However, there are no long-term studies that have evaluated the effects of hormone replacement therapy or selective estrogen receptor modulators (SERMs) in women with CKD. The cardiovascular safety of such an approach must be assessed as CKD is associated with significant cardiovascular morbidity and mortality.

## Abnormalities in the Growth Hormone Axis

The somatotropic axis in humans is orchestrated by several hormones and growth factors including growth hormone (GH), insulin-like growth factor-1 and -2 (IGF-1 and -2), insulin-like growth factor-binding proteins (IGFBPs) and the IGFBP proteases, the physiological function of which is somatic growth and cellular proliferation. Disruptions in somatotropic axis have been reported in children as well as in adults with CKD and may have substantial clinical consequences.

### Growth Hormone

In uremic patients, GH levels increase due to about 50% reduction in renal clearance; on the other hand, coexistent metabolic acidosis suppresses GH secretion. In both children and adults with CKD, serum GH levels are normal or elevated depending on the extent of the glomerular filtration rate (GFR) impairment. Hyperglycemia induced by glucose infusion suppresses GH secretion in individuals with no kidney disease, but fails to do so in CKD patients.[11] There occurs exaggerated GH secretion after stimulation with exogenous growth hormone-releasing hormone (GHRH).

This suggests that terminal CKD is a state of GH resistance, resulting from reduced expression of GH receptors in target organs or impaired postreceptor signal transduction via Janus kinase 2 (JAK2) and signal transducer and activator of transcription (STAT) signal transduction pathways. Further, there is increased expression of suppressor of cytokine signaling (*SOCS2* and *SOCS3*) genes that contributes to impaired GH action. Other factors contributing to the GH resistance in CKD include: metabolic acidosis, inflammation and hyperparathyroidism.

### Insulin-like Growth Factors

Growth hormone acts in the liver to increase the secretion of IGF-1 that in turn promotes growth at the growth plate of long bones. However, not all effects of GH are mediated by IGF-1. While liver is the main source of circulating IGF-1, IGF-1 and IGF-2 can be synthesized locally by most tissues, including the growth plate. Most circulating IGF-1 is bound to IGFBP-3 and the acid-labile subunit (ALS), although IGF-1 can also form complexes with other IGF-binding proteins (IGFBP-1 to 6).

Concentration of IGF-1, the most important factor determining rapid growth during puberty, tends to be normal in preterminal kidney disease (CKD stages 1–4). Serum-free IGF-1 concentration decreases with the stages of CKD. In CKD stage 5, such a decrease is mostly due to elevated IGFBPs that results in lower levels of free

IGF-1 that is bioactive. In addition, there is increased proteolysis of IGFBP-3 that further reduces bioavailable IGF-1. Some studies have documented the presence of a small molecule inhibitor of IGF-1 in the sera of individuals with CKD. Furthermore, there are defects in the intracellular signaling of IGF-1 that adds to the resistance to IGF-1 action in CKD. While serum levels of IGF-2 are within the normal range in CKD stages 1–4, the levels of IGF-2 have been reported to be elevated in CKD stage 5.

### Clinical Manifestations

In children with CKD, impairment of GH/IGF-1 axis is an important cause of growth retardation and short stature. The final adult height may be compromised in these children in the absence of appropriate treatment. In fact, growth retardation may be sometimes the first clinical manifestation of previously undiagnosed kidney disease and renal function evaluation should be included in the routine biochemistry panel for evaluation of short stature. In adults, impaired GH secretion is also associated with increased morbidity and mortality as GH has important metabolic effects.

### Growth Hormone Therapy

In spite of normal or increased serum GH concentration and target organ resistance/insensitivity to GH, there is a role of recombinant human growth hormone (rhGH) in the treatment of short stature related to CKD. CKD is an approved indication for GH therapy. GH therapy was found to be both efficacious and safe and resulted in catch-up growth in children with short stature and CKD. About 65% of children treated with rhGH may reach almost normal height in the adulthood.

The best response to rhGH treatment was found in patients in predialysis stages of CKD, probably due to better GH sensitivity. The treatment with rhGH has been proven to be also effective in treatment of growth retardation in children after kidney transplantation; the growth retardation being mainly attributed to chronic glucocorticoid administration.[12] On one hand, rhGH replacement extends certain benefits such as improved protein-energy balance and increase in skeletal muscle mass. However, the safety profile of rhGH replacement in CKD has not been well-documented and there is a need to assess efficacy and safety of GH replacement therapy in CKD.

## Alterations in Insulin/Glucagon Homeostasis

Glucose metabolism is altered in CKD via several mechanisms. Renal impairment affects insulin secretion and action as discussed below. In addition, impaired GFR also alters the pharmacokinetics of several antidiabetic agents including insulin.

### Insulin Secretion and Clearance

Insulin secretion is impaired in CKD; this effect seems to result from decreased availability of active vitamin D and elevated parathyroid hormone (PTH). The kidney has important role in metabolic clearance of insulin. Insulin is filtered at the glomerulus and is then reabsorbed from the proximal tubule. The renal clearance of insulin has been estimated to be 200 mL/min in healthy individuals. Since this is in excess of GFR, there is significant peritubular uptake of insulin. Almost 6–8 units of insulin are removed from the circulation daily by the kidneys, thereby contributing to about 25–40% of the total clearance of endogenous insulin. A decline in GFR below 40 mL/min is associated with reduced metabolic clearance of insulin. This may result in decreased insulin requirements with a progressive decline in GFR in individuals who are on exogenous insulin therapy and also contributes to increased risk of hypoglycemia.[13]

## Insulin Resistance

Peripheral insulin sensitivity begins to decline early during the course of CKD; insulin resistance worsens as the decline in kidney function progresses. There is reduced skeletal muscle glucose uptake due to reduced insulin receptor expression as well as impaired postreceptor signaling. Impairment of phosphatidylinositol 3-kinase (PI3K) activity has been documented in CKD patients.

After initiating renal replacement therapy, peripheral insulin resistance markedly decreases; however, this occurs only after several weeks of treatment. Presumably, unidentified dialyzable uremic "toxins" are involved in the pathogenesis of insulin resistance. Some studies have documented the presence of small compounds, almost 1–2 kDa in molecular weight, in individuals with uremia.

Renal impairment is associated with several modifiable factors that contribute to insulin resistance. Dietary protein restriction has been reported to partially ameliorate insulin resistance in individuals who are not on renal replacement therapy. In addition, treatment with erythropoietin and 1,25-dihydroxyvitamin D3 [$1,25(OH)_2D_3$] may also improve insulin sensitivity in those on hemodialysis. Elevated levels of serum GH and glucagon have also been implicated in the causation of insulin resistance. Renal impairment may be associated with chronic metabolic acidosis, inflammation and increased renin–angiotensin–aldosterone system (RAAS) activity. All of these may exacerbate insulin resistance.[14]

## Clinical Implications

Renal impairment is associated with increased risk of hypoglycemia, on one hand and insulin resistance and hyperglycemia, on the other. While many patients require a reduction in insulin doses, others may require intensive insulin therapy with relatively high doses for glycemic control. There is an increased risk of salt-sensitive hypertension resulting from enhanced sodium reabsorption from the renal tubules. This further exacerbates the progression of renal failure. CKD is strongly associated with increased cardiovascular risk. Decreased insulin sensitivity may both be a cause and consequence of malnutrition and sarcopenia associated with CKD. There is increased muscle catabolism through the activation of a common proteolytic pathway via the ubiquitin-proteasome system.[14]

In addition, individuals with diabetes and CKD require modification of doses of most antidiabetic medications and titration of insulin dose requirements based on estimated glomerular filtration rate (eGFR). This is especially true for medications which have a primarily renal route of excretion. In addition, sodium-glucose cotransporter-2 (SGLT-2) inhibitors have reduced glucose-lowering efficacy at lower eGFR and are currently not recommended at eGFR <45 mL/min/1.73 m$^2$ even though they have documented nephroprotective effect.

## Abnormalities in Bone Mineral Homeostasis

### Abnormal Vitamin D Metabolism

The prevalence of 25-hydroxyvitamin D3 or 25(OH)$D_3$ deficiency increases with the progression of CKD and reaches 80% in patients with CKD stage 5. Additionally, in patients with nephrotic syndrome, the urinary excretion of 25(OH)$D_3$ is increased. Moreover, in patients on peritoneal dialysis, vitamin D is washed out with the peritoneal dialysis fluid. The amount of 25(OH)$D_3$ delivered to the kidney (via receptor-mediated mechanism involving megalin) is also decreased.

25-hydroxyvitamin D3 is hydroxylated in the kidney by 1α-hydroxylase to its active metabolite—1,25-dihydroxyvitamin D3 or 1,25(OH)$_2D_3$. With decline in GFR, the activity of 1α-hydroxylase decreases resulting in reduced activation of vitamin D. 1α-hydroxylation may also be inhibited by increased plasma concentration of fibroblast growth factor 23 (FGF23). Therefore, in CKD, the serum concentration of 1,25(OH)$_2D_3$ is often reduced while there is increase in inactive metabolites such as 24,25(OH)$_2D_3$. A decrease in the density of 1,25(OH)$_2D_3$ receptors [vitamin D receptor (VDR)] has also been described, leading to target organ resistance.

Supplementation with ergocalciferol in CKD patients is considered to be safe and is recommended when serum 25(OH)$D_3$ concentration is below 30 ng/mL.

### Secondary and Tertiary Hyperparathyroidism

Calcitriol deficiency plays an important role in the development of secondary and tertiary hyperparathyroidism in CKD. It results in decreased absorption of calcium from the intestine, defective bone mineralization, myopathy, skeletal resistance to the calcemic action of PTH as well as impaired longitudinal growth in children. 1,25(OH)$_2D_3$ deficiency may be responsible for the increase in cardiovascular and all-cause mortality in CKD patients.[15]

Small interventional studies suggest that treatment with calcitriol or other VDR agonists may reduce mortality. Recent studies demonstrated that 1,25(OH)$_2D_3$ deficiency increases proteinuria in CKD and paricalcitol treatment seemed to ameliorate this pathology. Cinacalcet may be beneficial as it decreases plasma FGF23 levels resulting in less vitamin D3 degradation. Cinacalcet may reduce cardiovascular risk, but large prospective studies are required to establish this.

### Bone Health in Chronic Kidney Disease

Disturbances in calcium and phosphorus homeostasis occur early in the course of CKD and progress as kidney function declines. If left untreated, these alterations can result in significant consequences. Disorders of bone mineral metabolism in CKD not only affect skeletal health, but also result in alterations at extraskeletal sites, including vasculature. The metabolic bone disease in CKD can be classified into high-turnover bone disease or osteitis fibrosa and adynamic bone disease with an extremely low bone turnover.

### High-turnover Bone Disease

High-turnover bone disease is the result of secondary hyperparathyroidism. Etiological factors leading to hyperparathyroidism include—retention of phosphorus, calcitriol deficiency, intrinsic alterations within the parathyroid gland that give rise to increased PTH secretion as well as increased parathyroid growth, skeletal resistance to the actions of PTH and hypocalcemia.

## Low-turnover Bone Disease

End-stage renal failure is associated with extremely low rates of bone formation and low-turnover bone disease. Impaired bone mineralization and osteomalacia may result from vitamin D deficiency in some patients. In the past, aluminum-based phosphate binders were commonly used and accumulation of aluminum in the bone was implicated as the cause of osteomalacic lesions. The use of aluminum-based phosphate binders is now rare.

Adynamic bone disease, on the other hand, is being found with increasing frequency and has been described in some cases even before dialysis. The pathogenesis of adynamic bone is not well-defined but a number of factors contributing to a relative state of hypoparathyroidism have been implicated. A high calcium load may result from the use of calcium-containing phosphate binders, potent activated vitamin D preparations and calcium-containing dialysates. This has been described as one of the causative factors in adynamic bone disease. Bone turnover also declines with aging and may be associated with osteopenia or osteoporosis. Metabolic acidosis, malnutrition, uremic toxins, abnormal cytokine profile, altered growth factors, osteoprotegerin, N-terminally truncated PTH fragments and corticosteroid therapy in some patients may be some of the factors that contribute to low-turnover bone disease in renal impairment.[16]

## Abnormalities in Adrenal Axis

The morning serum cortisol and aldosterone as well as plasma adrenocorticotropic hormone (ACTH) levels are normal in patients with uremia, while dehydro-epiandrosterone (DHEA) levels are decreased. However, the counterregulatory response to hypoglycemia mediated via corticotropin-releasing hormone (CRH)-ACTH-cortisol axis is blunted in CKD. Adrenal insufficiency may occur due to treatment with steroids, amyloidosis, or coagulation disorders in CKD patients. Due to the similarity of the clinical symptoms of adrenal insufficiency (hyperkalemia and hyponatremia or anemia), diagnosis of adrenal insufficiency may be missed. There is a need for endocrine vigilance and appropriate testing of adrenal function should be done in case of clinical suspicion.[17]

Renin–angiotensin–aldosterone system mediates multiple effects in the heart vasculature and kidneys and regulates blood pressure, fluid and electrolyte balance. Diabetes is associated with a hyperactive RAAS and this is a major determinant of target organ damage, especially CKD and CVD. Angiotensin II is a potent vasoconstrictor that acts predominantly on postglomerular arterioles. Increased RAAS activity results in increased glomerular filtration pressure, resulting in enhanced ultrafiltration of proteins. Glomerular hyperfiltration, proteinuria and the resultant damage to nephrons result in progressive nephron loss and progression of renal damage. In addition, RAAS also may accelerate kidney damage by contributing to inflammation, interstitial fibrosis and tubular atrophy. Inhibitors of RAAS such as angiotensin-converting enzyme (ACE) inhibitors and angiotensin receptor blockers (ARBs) have been shown to retard the progression of renal damage and have renoprotective effects. ACE inhibitors and ARBs can reduce proteinuria and retard GFR decline in diabetic and nondiabetic renal disease.[18]

## SECONDARY DIABETES DUE TO ENDOCRINOPATHIES: EFFECT ON CHRONIC KIDNEY DISEASE

Several endocrinopathies are associated with secondary diabetes. The risk of microvascular complications and CKD in these disorders may be increased due to several factors.

### Acromegaly

Chronic GH excess can result in increased blood flow to the kidneys and GFR, possibly mediated by IGF-1. In addition, kidney size has been reported to be increased. There was an increased prevalence of microalbuminuria in acromegaly patients, especially if there was impaired glucose tolerance or secondary diabetes. There existed a positive correlation between urinary albumin excretion and duration of GH excess as well as insulin resistance. However, albuminuria did not correlate with serum GH concentration.[19]

### Cushing's Syndrome

Chronic exposure to glucocorticoids, both endogenous and exogenous, has been associated with a decrease in GFR and increased cardiovascular risk. In addition, hyperglycemia may further enhance the risk of renal impairment. There is increased risk of proteinuria and albuminuria in Cushing's syndrome resulting from glomerular dysfunction. Renal biopsy may demonstrate evidence of glomerulosclerosis in some individuals. In addition, tubular dysfunction has also been documented with resultant impairment of urinary concentrating ability, increased renal sodium reabsorption, increased renal calcium excretion and increased risk of urolithiasis.[20]

### Thyroid Dysfunction

There is a high prevalence of thyroid dysfunction in individuals with diabetes. Thyroid hormone status affects the functioning renal mass (measured as the kidney to body mass ratio); in hypothyroidism, the functioning renal mass is reduced while it is increased in hyperthyroidism.

Hyperthyroidism may be associated with type 1 diabetes mellitus. GFR increases by about 18–25% in hyperthyroid patients.[3] In addition, there is increased sensitivity of macula densa leading to RAAS activation. Increased renal plasma flow results in osmotic diuresis and impaired urinary concentrating ability. Total body water may be reduced in hyperthyroidism; while exchangeable potassium is also reduced, sodium pool does not seem to be altered. In most individuals, serum electrolytes remain within normal range. Severe hyperthyroidism may result in increased protein breakdown and eventual renal atrophy.

Hypothyroidism is more commonly associated with both type 1 and type 2 diabetes mellitus. GFR is reversibly reduced (by about 40%) in more than 55% of adults with hypothyroidism.[3] There is decreased sensitivity to β-adrenergic stimulus and decreased renin release along with decreased angiotensin II and impaired RAAS activity, resulting in loss of GFR. In addition, the reabsorption of sodium, chloride and water from the proximal tubule is decreased. This results in decreased chloride delivery to distal tubule, thereby increasing tubule glomerular feedback at the macula densa and decreasing the activity of RAAS.[3]

The activity of sodium-potassium ATPase is diminished only in the proximal tubule early on, but later there is reduced $Na^+/K^+$-ATPase activity in all segments of the nephron. Tubular transport capacity is, thus, impaired and this contributes to reduced sodium and bicarbonate reabsorption from renal tubules. Increased sodium and bicarbonate excretion from the tubules result in impaired urinary acidification and decreased urinary concentrating ability due to impaired ability to maintain medullary hypertonicity. However, hypothyroidism causes a reversible increase in vasopressin sensitivity of the collecting ducts, thus increasing free water reabsorption.[3]

Studies have demonstrated that both overt and subclinical hypothyroidism are associated with greater risk of microvascular disease in diabetes, including diabetic nephropathy.[3] However, whether T4 supplementation affects renal outcomes or has not been established.

## Primary Hyperparathyroidism

Primary hyperparathyroidism (PHPT) is associated with hypercalciuria, nephrolithiasis, and nephrocalcinosis. PHPT is also associated with declining renal function. Therefore, in case of asymptomatic mild PHPT, annual renal functional assessment is advised and parathyroid surgery is indicated if eGFR is <60 mL/min/1.73 $m^2$.[21]

## Primary Hyperaldosteronism

In hyperaldosteronism, there occurs an increase in renal tubular sodium reabsorption mediated due to the effects of aldosterone on the renal tubule. This leads to an expansion of extracellular fluid volume and hypertension. Renal perfusion pressure is elevated and renin secretion is suppressed. In addition, since the intrarenal vascular resistance is decreased, aldosterone excess results in glomerular hyperfiltration. Persistent hypertension and direct effect of aldosterone in the kidneys may mediate structural damage, primarily in the intrarenal vessels. This may culminate in nephron loss and progression of CKD.[22]

## ENDOVIGILANCE IN CARDIOVASCULAR DISEASE

Diabetic macrovascular disease may affect various vascular beds including cardiovascular, cerebrovascular and peripheral vascular beds. Diabetes is associated with a significant burden of cardiovascular morbidity and mortality. In addition, certain conditions like hemochromatosis can cause cardiomyopathy and multiple endocrine dysfunctions including diabetes. The effects of diabetic vasculopathy on the endocrine system include:

- *Antepartum pituitary necrosis*: The anterior pituitary enlarges during pregnancy with an increase in its blood flow. Diabetic vasculopathy and hypercoagulability increase the risk of ischemia and necrosis of the pituitary.[23] Diabetic vasculopathy may cause antepartum pituitary necrosis and hypopituitarism. This has been described in pregnant women with pre-existing type 1 diabetes mellitus, most frequently in the 3rd trimester. Most common signs and symptoms were intractable headaches and the Houssay phenomenon—frequent episodes of hypoglycemia caused by GH or ACTH deficiency, resulting in a sudden decrease in insulin requirement
- *Cardiovascular disease and thyroid dysfunction*: Subclinical hypothyroidism may be associated with CVD. Presence of CVD can be considered as a relative indication for levothyroxine (LT4) replacement in diabetics with subclinical hypothyroidism. Patients with known coronary artery disease (CAD) and hypothyroidism should always be started on a low LT4 dose (12.5–25 µg/day), with gradual uptitration based on symptoms and serum TSH levels, for fear of precipitating cardiac events.[24]

Triiodothyronine levels are reduced in patients with advanced congestive heart failure. In certain selected circumstances, liothyronine may be useful as an adjunctive therapy in patients with congestive heart failure because of its effect of relaxing vascular smooth muscle.

Several drugs used for the treatment of CVD may have endocrine effects as enlisted in Table 3. Endocrine vigilance is particularly required when using amiodarone. Amiodarone-induced thyroid dysfunction may occur in approximately 15–20% of individuals and can include a spectrum of thyroid disorders ranging from both overt hypothyroidism to overt thyrotoxicosis. Persistent iodine excess may inhibit thyroid gland function resulting in amiodarone-induced hypothyroidism (AIH). AIH is more

**TABLE 3** Endocrine effects of drugs used for the treatment of cardiovascular disease.

| Drug category/specific drug | Endocrine effects |
|---|---|
| Thiazide diuretics | • Hypokalemia<br>• Hypercalcemia<br>• Hypomagnesemia<br>• Hyperglycemia<br>• Hyperuricemia |
| Angiotensin-converting enzyme inhibitors/angiotensin receptor blockers | • Hyperkalemia<br>• Mild glucose-lowering effect |
| Beta-blockers | • Insulin resistance—hyperglycemia<br>• Inhibit normal counterregulatory response to hypoglycemia—hypoglycemia unawareness<br>• Can worsen erectile dysfunction |
| Amiodarone | • Amiodarone-induced hypothyroidism<br>• Amiodarone-induced thyroiditis types 1 and 2 |
| Statins | • Hyperglycemia<br>• Increase bone density<br>• Improve erectile dysfunction |

common in those individuals who have underlying thyroid autoimmunity. Persistent hypothyroidism requires treatment with LT4, often in high doses since amiodarone inhibits deiodinase activity and peripheral conversion of T4 to T3.

The other end of spectrum involves two distinct forms of amiodarone-induced thyrotoxicosis (AIT)—(1) type 1 AIT and (2) type 2 AIT. Type 1 AIT is characterized by increased production and secretion of thyroid hormones from an overactive gland. Type 1 AIT is a hyperthyroid state and requires treatment with antithyroidal drugs. On the other hand, type 2 AIT occurs due to secretion of preformed thyroid hormones from an inflamed thyroid tissue and is a form of destructive thyroiditis. Management of type 2 AIT is more symptomatic, with glucocorticoids and beta-blockers and supportive symptomatic care. Differentiation of these forms of AIT can sometimes be challenging and thyroid scintigraphy may be required.[25]

# SECONDARY DIABETES DUE TO ENDOCRINOPATHIES: EFFECT ON CARDIOVASCULAR DISEASE

Acromegaly, Cushing's syndrome, pheochromocytoma, hyperthyroidism, hyperparathyroidism and hyperaldosteronism are associated with insulin resistance and diabetes. They may impact cardiovascular risk through multiple mechanisms.

## Acromegaly and Cardiovascular Risk

Acromegaly is commonly associated with acromegalic cardiomyopathy. Almost two-thirds of acromegaly patients meet echocardiographic criteria for left ventricular hypertrophy (LVH), even those who are normotensive. Patients with severe cardiomyopathy may progress to heart failure, seen in 3–10% of patients. Cardiac valve disease, aortic and mitral regurgitation are also frequent and the risk increases with duration of GH excess.[26]

Acromegaly is associated with an increased incidence of abnormalities in cardiac rhythm. Electrocardiogram (ECG) may demonstrate left-axis deviation, prolongation of QT interval, presence of septal Q waves, or depression of ST-T segment. Over 50% of individuals with acromegaly may demonstrate late potentials on ECG and are at increased risk of arrhythmias. Rhythm alterations may be exacerbated during exercise; there may occur atrial or ventricular ectopic beats, paroxysmal supraventricular tachycardia (PSVT), paroxysmal atrial fibrillation or ventricular tachycardia (VT) in some individuals. Sick sinus syndrome and bundle branch block have also been documented.

Several characteristic abnormalities have been reported in cardiac tissue on histopathology, including cardiomyocyte hypertrophy, inflammation and interstitial fibrosis, increased extracellular collagen deposition and decreased capillary density. These alterations involve both myocardium and valvular tissue and their severity increases proportionate to the duration and degree of GH/IGF-1 excess. Early stages of acromegaly are characterized by increased myocardial contractility, reduced systemic vascular resistance, increased cardiac performance and an increase in cardiac output. As acromegaly progresses, biventricular hypertrophy, impaired exercise tolerance and diastolic dysfunction may appear after almost 5 years of active disease. In later stages, a characteristic pattern of acromegalic cardiomyopathy emerges with systolic as well as diastolic dysfunction, cardiomegaly, dilatation of ventricles and an increase in systemic vascular resistance.[26]

## Cushing's Syndrome and Cardiovascular Risk

Hypercortisolism is associated with significant cardiovascular risk due to hypertension, central obesity, insulin resistance, dyslipidemia and abnormal coagulation. On echocardiography, LVH with concentric remodeling of the ventricles, subclinical systolic dysfunction, and diastolic dysfunction have been reported.[27] There may be increased thickness of the interventricular septum and posterior wall. Left ventricular (LV) mass index has also been reported to be increased. Diastolic dysfunction in Cushing's syndrome is characterized by impairment of early LV relaxation as well as global myocardial relaxation. Many of these parameters improve at least partially with treatment of hypercortisolism.

## Pheochromocytoma and Cardiovascular Risk

Pheochromocytoma is associated with episodic or sustained hypertension. High blood pressure variability due to catecholamine excess has been linked to a higher incidence of target organ damage as compared to essential hypertension. Resolution of hypertension has been reported in about 50% of patients after successful surgical treatment of pheochromocytoma. There is also endothelial dysfunction and increased carotid intima-media thickness (IMT). Normalization of catecholamine levels after surgical removal of pheochromocytoma has been shown to improve carotid IMT and reduce carotid wall fibrosis.[28]

Catecholamine excess is associated with an increased incidence of cardiomyopathy, affecting almost one-fourth of pheochromocytoma patients. Both dilated cardiomyopathy (DCMP) and hypertrophic obstructive cardiomyopathy (HOCM) may occur. Findings reported on echocardiography include left atrial dilatation, LV dilatation with decreased contractility, septal hypertrophy and reduced ejection fraction. Since pheochromocytoma may present with depleted intravascular volume, diastolic filling may be impaired. LVH may occur due to persistent hypertension. Some individuals with cardiomyopathy may present with acute pulmonary edema. In addition, there is increased incidence of ischemic heart disease and the individual may present to the emergency room with acute chest pain and acute coronary syndrome.

Catecholamine-induced cardiomyopathy may be partially reversible, if the diagnosis and treatment are prompt. Catecholamine-induced cardiomyopathy improves after surgery. However, when significant myocardial damage has occurred and there is acute heart failure, the prognosis is poor. ECG may demonstrate right-axis deviation, prolonged QT interval, inverted T waves and poor R wave progression across chest leads. In severe cases with cardiomyopathy or irreversible myocardial damage, ECG may demonstrate features of LVH and myocardial ischemia. Approximately 20% of individuals with catecholamine-producing tumors may have cardiac rhythm abnormalities including sinus tachycardia, supraventricular tachycardia, sick sinus syndrome and ventricular tachycardia.

## Hyperthyroidism and Cardiovascular Risk

Overt hyperthyroidism is associated with reduced systemic vascular resistance, tachycardia, increased preload, and increased cardiac output. Reduced systemic vascular resistance results in activation of RAAS and increased preload.[25] Cardiac output is raised due to increased preload, reduced systemic vascular resistance, increased cardiac contractility and increased heart rate. Approximately one-third of patients with hyperthyroidism demonstrate systolic hypertension. Persistent thyrotoxicosis can result in LVH and LV diastolic dysfunction. In addition, thyrotoxicosis may be associated with myopathy involving skeletal musculature and respiratory muscles, which is associated with diminished exercise tolerance.

Approximately 40% of patients with overt hyperthyroidism manifest sinus tachycardia that improves with resolution of thyrotoxicosis.[29] Atrial fibrillation is the second most common arrhythmia in overt hyperthyroidism and occurs in 10–15% of patients, its prevalence increasing with age. Subclinical hyperthyroidism is also associated with an increased heart rate, reduced exercise tolerance and risk of atrial fibrillation. Treatment of hyperthyroidism reverses these hemodynamic changes.[30] Sinus rhythm can be restored in up to two-thirds of patients with overt hyperthyroidism; however, increased age and duration of atrial fibrillation correspond with higher rates of persistent arrhythmia.[31]

## Primary Hyperparathyroidism and Cardiovascular Risk

The cardiovascular risk associated with PHPT is attributable in large part to an increased prevalence of hypertension, obesity, glucose intolerance and insulin resistance. Increased calcium deposition leads to arterial stiffness; PTH also stimulates RAAS and sympathetic activity and contributes to endothelial dysfunction. Carotid artery stiffness is increased in correlation to the severity of PTH rise and the patients may have increased carotid IMT. In addition, patients may also have diastolic dysfunction.[32] In patients who have significant hypercalcemia, there may occur calcification of the aortic and mitral valves and myocardium.

Hypercalcemia can lead to cardiac conduction abnormalities, particularly when serum calcium is significantly high ($\geq 12$ mg/dL). High calcium can result in diminished plateau phase of ventricular action potential and effective refractory period. Characteristic abnormalities on ECG include short QT interval and QTc interval, increased amplitude of the QRS complex, early peak and then gradual downsloping of the descending limb of T wave, biphasic T wave or short ST segment.

Surgical excision of the parathyroid lesion may result in some improvement in blood pressure but complete resolution of hypertension may not occur.[33] ECG abnormalities usually resolve after correction of hypercalcemia and parathyroidectomy. Insulin sensitivity significantly improves, especially in those who had more severe disease.

## Primary Hyperaldosteronism and Cardiovascular Risk

Primary hyperaldosteronism is characterized by hypertension, hypokalemia, insulin resistance and impaired glucose tolerance or diabetes. Hypertension results from sodium and fluid retention resulting in volume expansion and potassium depletion resulting in vasoconstriction. In addition, aldosterone decreases the bioavailability of nitric oxide and hyperaldosteronism is characterized by reduced endothelium-dependent relaxation and endothelial dysfunction.[34]

Aldosterone has also been implicated in the causation of perivascular fibrosis and decreased vascular compliance. Hyperaldosteronism can cause impaired cardiac remodeling and LVH, diastolic dysfunction and cardiac fibrosis. In fact, the degree of LVH reported in individuals with primary hyperaldosteronism is disproportionate to that explained by hypertension alone. Aldosterone has also been shown to promote collagen deposition, activation of inflammatory cells and stimulation of fibroblast proliferation.

Surgical and medical treatments may be effective in reducing LV mass, with decrease in blood pressure and plasma aldosterone levels predictive of response to therapy. Successful resection of the aldosterone-producing adrenal lesion often results in correction of hypokalemia and at least partial amelioration of hypertension. However, individuals who have bilateral adrenal hyperplasia may be managed with mineralocorticoid receptor antagonists in the long term.

## CONCLUSION

Several endocrine axis abnormalities may be seen in individuals with diabetic vasculopathy, especially in CKD. Some of these such as abnormal bone mineral metabolism in CKD may result in significant morbidity and may affect long-term outcomes and survival. Similarly, impaired GH axis results in significant short stature in children with CKD. Other abnormalities such as altered insulin and glucose homeostasis would require titration of antidiabetic medications and insulin therapy and increase the risk of hypoglycemia. Abnormalities of thyroid, adrenal, and gonadal axis may also be seen. In addition, secondary diabetes due to endocrine disorders is also associated with increased risk of diabetic vasculopathy. Therefore, endocrine vigilance is required when managing individuals with diabetes and micro- and/or macrovascular disease.

## REFERENCES

1. Kuczera P, Adamczak M, Wiecek A. Endocrine Abnormalities in Patients with Chronic Kidney Disease. Pril (Makedon Akad Nauk Umet Odd Med Nauki). 2015;36(2):109-18.
2. Iglesias P, Díez JJ. Thyroid dysfunction and kidney disease. Eur J Endocrinol. 2009;160(4):503-15.
3. Basu G, Mohapatra A. Interactions between thyroid disorders and kidney disease. Indian J Endocrinol Metab. 2012;16(2):204-13.
4. Mohamedali M, Maddika SR, Vyas A, et al. Thyroid Disorders and Chronic Kidney Disease. Int J Nephrol. 2014;2014:520281.
5. Zoccali C, Mallamaci F, Tripepi G, et al. Low triiodothyronine and survival in end-stage renal disease. Kidney Int. 2006;70(3):523-8.
6. Iglesias P, Carrero JJ, Díez JJ. Gonadal dysfunction in men with chronic kidney disease: clinical features, prognostic implications and therapeutic options. J Nephrol. 2012;25(1):31-42.
7. Ros S, Carrero JJ. Endocrine alterations and cardiovascular risk in CKD: is there a link? Nefrologia. 2013;33(2):181-7.
8. Carrero JJ, Stenvinkel P. The vulnerable man: impact of testosterone deficiency on the uraemic phenotype. Nephrol Dial Transplant. 2012;27(11):4030-41.
9. Holley JL. The hypothalamic-pituitary axis in men and women with chronic kidney disease. Adv Chronic Kidney Dis. 2004;11(4):337-41.

10. Sugiya N, Nakashima A, Takasugi N, et al. Endogenous estrogen may prevent bone loss in postmenopausal hemodialysis patients throughout life. Osteoporos Int. 2011;22(5):1573-9.
11. Haffner D, Schaefer F, Nissel R, et al. Effect of growth hormone treatment on the adult height of children with chronic renal failure. German Study Group for Growth Hormone Treatment in Chronic Renal Failure. N Engl J Med. 2000;343(13):923-30.
12. Mehls O, Lindberg A, Nissel R, et al. Predicting the response to growth hormone treatment in short children with chronic kidney disease. J Clin Endocrinol Metab. 2010;95(2):686-92.
13. Liao MT, Sung CC, Hung KC, et al. Insulin Resistance in Patients with Chronic Kidney Disease. J Biomed Biotechnol. 2012;2012:691369.
14. Siew ED, Ikizler TA. Insulin resistance and protein energy metabolism in patients with advanced chronic kidney disease. Semin Dial. 2010;23(4):378-82.
15. Dusso A, González EA, Martin KJ. Vitamin D in chronic kidney disease. Best Pract Res Clin Endocrinol Metab. 2011;25(4):647-55.
16. Martin KJ, González EA. Metabolic bone disease in chronic kidney disease. J Am Soc Nephrol. 2007;18(3):875-85.
17. Asao T, Oki K, Yoneda M, et al. Hypothalamic-pituitary-adrenal axis activity is associated with the prevalence of chronic kidney disease in diabetic patients. Endocr J. 2016;63(2):119-26.
18. Remuzzi G, Perico N, Macia M, et al. The role of renin-angiotensin-aldosterone system in the progression of chronic kidney disease. Kidney Int Suppl. 2005;99:S57-65.
19. Baldelli R, De Marinis L, Bianchi A, et al. Microalbuminuria in insulin sensitivity in patients with growth hormone-secreting pituitary tumor. J Clin Endocrinol Metab. 2008;93(3):710-4.
20. Smets P, Meyer E, Maddens B, et al. Cushing's syndrome, glucocorticoids and the kidney. Gen Comp Endocrinol. 2010;169(1):1-10.
21. Lila AR, Sarathi V, Jagtap V, et al. Renal manifestations of primary hyperparathyroidism. Indian J Endocrinol Metab. 2012;16(2):258-62.
22. Sechi LA, Colussi G, Di Fabio A, et al. Cardiovascular and renal damage in primary aldosteronism: outcomes after treatment. Am J Hypertens. 2010;23(12):1253-60.
23. Park HJ, Kim J, Rhee Y, et al. Antepartum pituitary necrosis occurring in pregnancy with uncontrolled gestational diabetes mellitus: a case report. J Korean Med Sci. 2010;25(5):794-7.
24. Jonklaas J, Bianco AC, Bauer AJ, et al. Guidelines for the treatment of hypothyroidism: prepared by the american thyroid association task force on thyroid hormone replacement. Thyroid. 2014;24(12):1670-751.
25. Rhee SS, Pearce EN. Update: Systemic Diseases and the Cardiovascular System (II). The endocrine system and the heart: a review. Rev Esp Cardiol. 2011;64(3):220-31.
26. Castellano G, Affuso F, Conza PD, et al. The GH/IGF-1 Axis and Heart Failure. Curr Cardiol Rev. 2009;5(3):203-15.
27. Magiakou MA, Smyrnaki P, Chrousos GP. Hypertension in Cushing's syndrome. Best Pract Res Clin Endocrinol Metab. 2006;20(3):467-82.
28. Bernini G, Galetta F, Franzoni F, et al. Normalization of catecholamine production following resection of phaeochromocytoma positively influences carotid vascular remodelling. Eur J Endocrinol. 2008;159(2):137-43.
29. Northcote RJ, MacFarlane P, Kesson CM, et al. Continuous 24-hour electrocardiography in thyrotoxicosis before and after treatment. Am Heart J. 1986;112(2):339-44.
30. Osman F, Franklyn JA, Holder RL, et al. Cardiovascular manifestations of hyperthyroidism before and after antithyroid therapy: a matched case-control study. J Am Coll Cardiol. 2007;49(1):71-81.
31. Surks MI, Ortiz E, Daniels GH, et al. Subclinical thyroid disease: scientific review and guidelines for diagnosis and management. JAMA. 2004;291(2):228-38.
32. Andersson P, Rydberg E, Willenheimer R. Primary hyperparathyroidism and heart disease—a review. Eur Heart J. 2004;25(20):1776-87.
33. Bollerslev J, Rosen T, Mollerup CL, et al. Effect of surgery on cardiovascular risk factors in mild primary hyperparathyroidism. J Clin Endocrinol Metab. 2009;94(7):2255-61.
34. Young MJ, Funder JW. Mineralocorticoid receptors and pathophysiological roles for aldosterone in the cardiovascular system. J Hypertens. 2002;20(8):1465-8.

# SECTION 4

# Specific Issues in Glucocrinology

# CHAPTER 19

# Adipose Tissue Health in Diabetes

*Indira Maisnam, Nikhil Gupta, Gagan Priya*

## INTRODUCTION

Adipose tissue is an important organ involved in the maintenance of body weight, energy homeostasis and metabolic health. While earlier adipose tissue was considered as simply an inert storage organ of fat, it is now known that it is an active immune-endocrine organ that orchestrates myriad complicated functions. It is capable of calorie sensing, storing and expending energy. Excess nutrients are stored in adipose tissue and these can be mobilized during energy deficit states. It has the unique ability to sense body's nutrient status and communicate with brain and other organ systems in a bidirectional manner. Adipose tissue secretes numerous adipocytokines that are involved in an extensive crosstalk with other organs involved in energy homeostasis and also regulates inflammation.

When adipose tissue health is adversely affected in obesity and diabetes, this fine balance of metabolic homeostasis is disturbed and the dysfunctional adipose tissue becomes a propagator of metabolic insult. Indeed, adipose tissue dysfunction or adiposopathy is an important contributor to the pathogenesis of type 2 diabetes mellitus (T2DM) and metabolic syndrome. The term "diabesity" has been proposed to describe this close association between adipose tissue dysfunction and diabetes.[1] Such adipose tissue dysfunction may occur even at lower body mass index (BMI) such as seen in Asian Indians.

While lifestyle modification and weight reduction remain the cornerstone of diabetes management, long-term sustenance of these measures is a formidable challenge. In addition, existing pharmacological therapies in diabetes fail to address adipose tissue dysfunction. In recent times, adipose tissue is an area of active interest for research into newer and novel targets for management of metabolic diseases. This chapter focuses on adipose tissue health in diabetes and discusses the various approaches that target adiposopathy.

# ADIPOSE TISSUE IN HEALTH

Adipose tissue comprises a heterogeneous group of cells: adipocytes, preadipocytes, fibroblasts, myoblasts, mesenchymal stem cells (MSCs), endothelial and inflammatory cells. These cells are embedded in an extracellular matrix (ECM).[2] During adipogenesis, MSCs differentiate into preadipocytes and finally to adipocytes. Peroxisome proliferator activated receptor gamma (PPAR-γ), transcription factor CCAAT/enhancer-binding protein α (C/EBPα), sterol regulatory element-binding protein 1 (SREBP1) and other factors are required for the differentiation of preadipocytes into adipocytes. A mature adipocyte is insulin-sensitive, expressing glucose transporter-4 (GLUT-4) on the cell surface, in addition to fatty acid-binding protein (FABP) and lipoprotein lipase (LPL).[2]

## Adipose Tissue Deposits and their Physiological Function

Several morphologically and functionally distinct fat depots exist throughout the body. These include white adipose tissue (WAT) and brown adipose tissue (BAT). WAT is present in the subcutaneous and visceral sites as subcutaneous adipose tissue (SCAT) and visceral adipose tissue (VAT) respectively.

White adipose tissue, especially SCAT, stores excess energy/nutrients as triglycerides and provides for a readily-available source of fuel for mobilization during periods of increased demands. WAT is a dynamic tissue that can respond to nutritional status by changing adipocyte number and size, distribution, secretory and metabolic function and inflammatory state. Thus, during periods of energy surplus, it can act as a storehouse of surplus calories, thereby trapping free fatty acids (FFAs), the metabolites of which are otherwise toxic to most cells.[2] Adequate SCAT therefore minimizes free fatty acid-induced insulin resistance. VAT provides mechanical protection and insulation; maintains membrane function and is involved in second messenger signaling. It is not a dedicated site for fat storage. BAT is present in supraclavicular, suprarenal and paravertebral areas in adults and plays a role in thermogenesis. BAT adipocytes are enriched in mitochondria and readily oxidize fatty acids with generation of uncoupling protein 1 (UCP1) to generate heat.[2]

## White, Brown and Beige Adipocytes

Based on morphology and function, adipocytes can be divided into white and brown adipocytes, present predominantly but not exclusively, in WAT and BAT, respectively. The differences between white and brown adipocytes are given in Table 1.

### Adipocytes Population is Dynamic

Adipose tissue exhibits inherent plasticity in the phenotype of adipocytes. Browning of white adipocytes can form brite or beige adipocytes. These beige adipocytes are scattered in WAT and function similar to brown adipocytes.[3] Exposure to cold and β3-adrenergic agonists promotes beiging of white adipocytes in the SCAT. Circadian clock, hormones, and food intake also play a role. Glucagon-like polypeptide-1 (GLP-1) signaling also activates BAT and promotes beiging.[3] Time-restricted feeding

**TABLE 1** Important differences between white and brown adipocytes.

| Characteristics | White adipocytes | Brown adipocytes |
|---|---|---|
| Location | Present in white adipose tissue | Present in brown adipose tissue |
| Appearance | White | Brown |
| Morphology | Unilocular | Multilocular |
| Shape | Round | Polygonal |
| Nucleus | Periphery of cytoplasm | Centrally placed |
| Mitochondria with UCP1 | Scanty | Abundant |
| Primary function | Fat storage as triglyceride | Dissipation of energy as heat |
| Origin | Mesenchymal stem Cells | Mesenchymal stem cells |
| Progenitor cells | Myf negative | Myf positive |

(UCP1: uncoupling protein 1)

of high-fat diet (HFD) for 8 hours/day increased BAT activity and reduced adipocyte hypertrophy and inflammation in WAT compared with ad libitum HFD-fed mice.[4] However, visceral white adipocytes cannot become beige due to zinc finger protein 423 in VAT.[5]

Beige adipocytes when dormant for long can reconvert to white adipocytes. At the same time, inactive brown adipocytes can accumulate lipids like white adipocytes. Sympathetic denervation of BAT produces a "whitened" appearance of brown adipocytes.[3]

The phenotypic appearance of adipocytes and their function seem to be dynamic depending on factors that continue to be unraveled. Their phenotypic character determines whether calories are stored or released as heat. An understanding of this constant remodeling of adipose tissue offers new opportunities for the management of obesity.

## Adipokines and Enzymes

Adipose tissue secretes several adipokines that mediate an extensive crosstalk with other metabolic tissues. Additionally, several key enzymes of energy homeostasis are expressed in adipose tissue. In a way, adipose tissue can be regarded as a "master-regulator" of energy homeostasis.[6] Leptin is secreted by adipocytes and acts on the hypothalamus to promote satiety, reduce food intake and increase energy expenditure. Leptin deficiency as well as leptin resistance is associated with obesity. Adiponectin, on the other hand, improves insulin sensitivity and glucose metabolism. While adiponectin, secreted frizzled-related protein 5 (SFRP5) and interleukin-10 (IL-10) have anti-inflammatory effects, adipocytes secrete several proinflammatory molecules including leptin, resistin, retinol-binding protein 4 (RBP4), IL-6, IL-8, tumor necrosis factor-α (TNF-α), plasminogen activator inhibitor-1 (PAI-1), monocyte chemoattractant protein-1 (MCP-1) and visfatin.[6] The various adipokines and their physiological roles are summarized in Table 2.

| TABLE 2 | Adipokines and their physiological functions. |
|---|---|
| Adipocytokines | Physiological effects |
| Adiponectin | • Improves insulin sensitivity—increases peripheral glucose uptake and reduces liver glucose output<br>• Modulates appetite and energy expenditure<br>• Anti-inflammatory effect<br>• Antithrombotic<br>• Improves endothelial function |
| Leptin | • Promotes satiety—reduced food intake<br>• Increased energy expenditure<br>• Permissive role in signaling puberty, maintains reproductive function<br>• Proinflammatory effects |
| SFRP5 | Reduces inflammatory signaling |
| IL-4 and IL-10 | Anti-inflammatory effects |
| Visfatin | Insulin mimetic effects |
| IL-1 and IL-6 | • Early mediator of inflammation<br>• Impairs insulin sensitivity<br>• Acute phase reactant |
| TNF-α | • Impairs insulin sensitivity<br>• Proinflammatory—contributes to chronic inflammation<br>• Promotes atherosclerosis |
| RBP4 | Impairs insulin sensitivity—increases liver glucose output and reduces peripheral glucose uptake |
| Resistin | • Impairs insulin sensitivity<br>• Proinflammatory effect |
| Lipocalin 2 | Contributes to insulin resistance and inflammation |
| Adipsin | Promotes fat storage, reduces lipolysis |
| VEGF | Promotes angiogenesis and production of proinflammatory cytokines |
| PAI-1 | Prothrombotic and proinflammatory effects |

(IL: interleukin; PAI-1: plasminogen activator inhibitor-1; RBP4: retinol-binding protein 4; SFRP5: secreted frizzled-related protein 5; TNF-α; tumor necrosis factor-α; VEGF: vascular endothelial growth factor)

## Adipose Tissue as Energy Homeostat

Adipose tissue is an important "peripheral energy homeostat". It adapts to homeostatic challenge by adopting morphological and functional changes and releasing adipocytokines. When energy stores are adequate, adipose tissue releases leptin, a long-term calorie-status signal that acts centrally on the hypothalamus to promote energy expenditure and decrease calorie intake. Hyperleptinemia of obesity is a consequence of increased fat mass and leptin resistance.

In energy excess states, SCAT increases its fat storage capacity by increase in size and/or number of adipocytes so that FFAs do not overflow to ectopic sites. However, when the metabolic challenge is excessive, prolonged, and unabated, these adaptive mechanisms fail resulting in increased circulating FFAs, ectopic fat deposition and inflammation. This maladaptation plays a central role in the generation and propagation of insulin resistance, linking adiposity with T2DM.

## Adipose Tissue Circadian Rhythm

The circadian clock at the hypothalamic suprachiasmatic nucleus regulates metabolism and energy homeostasis. In addition, peripheral circadian rhythms exist in different tissues; adipose tissue circadian rhythm ensures proper accumulation of fat during periods of excess energy and fat mobilization in energy deficit times. Adipocytokine secretion also follows a circadian rhythm. Leptin levels peak in early dark phase and adiponectin expression is the highest in the morning.[7] Chronodisruption is defined as the chronic desynchronization of 24-hour rhythms, resulting in adverse health effects. Circadian disturbances in metabolically active tissues including adipose tissue play a role in the pathogenesis of obesity and T2DM.[7]

## ADIPOSE TISSUE HEALTH IN DIABETES

Obesity and adipose tissue dysfunction are strong risk factors for the development of T2DM, hypertension, dyslipidemia, cardiovascular disease and other metabolic disorders. Overweight and obesity are clearly associated with increased risk of diabetes, cardiovascular disease and mortality. A BMI >25 kg/m$^2$ has been related to a 30% increase in all-cause mortality and 40% increase in cardiovascular mortality.[8] The term "diabesity" aptly describes this modern epidemic of obesity and T2DM.[1] In addition, obesity is also associated with multiple comorbidities including cancer risk, chronic kidney disease, obstructive sleep apnea, gallstone disease and nonalcoholic fatty liver disease (NAFLD).[8] However, not all obese individuals are metabolically unhealthy. Almost 80% obese individuals have insulin resistance; but 10–40% of nonobese individuals are also insulin resistant.[8] Therefore, it is proposed that adipose tissue dysfunction (rather than simply adipose tissue excess) drives cardiometabolic risk.

Adipose tissue dysfunction can occur as a result of multiple factors including sustained nutrient overload, insulin resistance, chronic stress, genetic predisposition, endocrine disruptors or endocrinopathies.[9] Dysfunctional adipose tissue fails to expand in response to energy surplus and results in lipotoxicity, causing:
- Increased circulating FFAs
- Overflow of fat into ectopic sites
- Altered adipokine profile
- Chronic inflammation
- Fibrosis
- Hypoxia, and
- Mitochondrial dysfunction.

Lipotoxicity and adipose tissue dysfunction contribute to systemic insulin resistance, impaired insulin secretion, hypertension, dyslipidemia, endothelial dysfunction, chronic inflammation, hypercoagulability and atherosclerosis. There exists a vicious circle where insulin resistance impairs adipose tissue health and adipose tissue dysfunction in turn contributes to the pathogenesis of T2DM, its

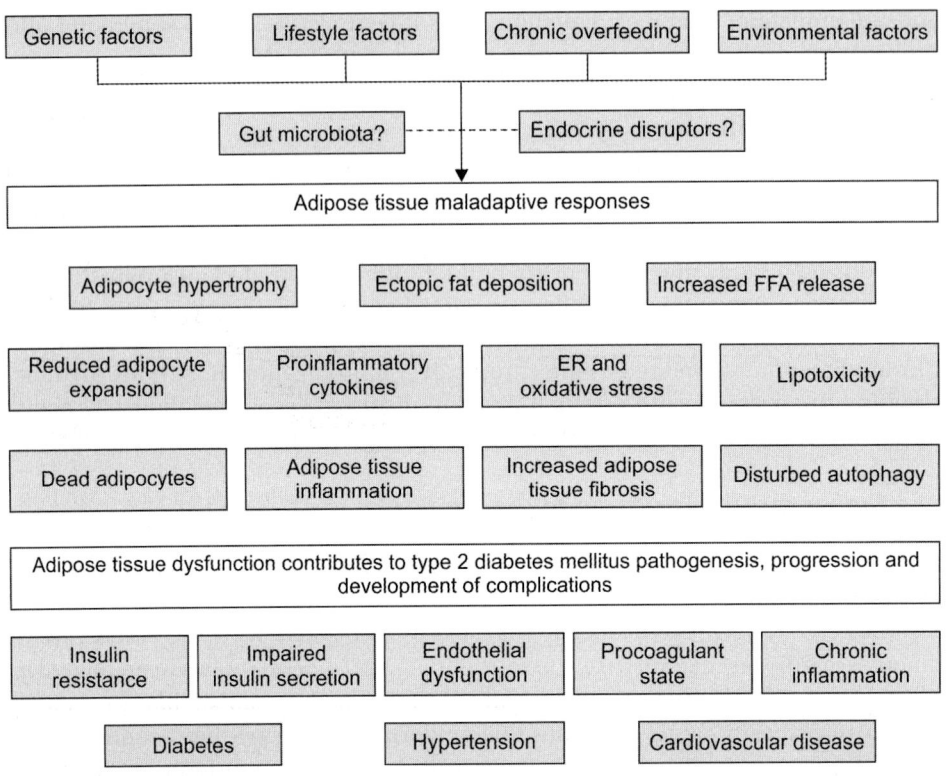

**FLOWCHART 1:** Adipose tissue in the pathogenesis of insulin resistance and type 2 diabetes mellitus.

progression and development of long-term complications.[9] The complex role of adipose tissue in diabesity is depicted in Flowchart 1 and discussed here.

## Adipose Tissue Insulin Resistance

### In Type 2 Diabetes Mellitus, Adipose Tissue is a Source and Site of Insulin Resistance

A normally functioning adipocyte is highly insulin-sensitive, where insulin promotes glucose uptake and lipogenesis and suppresses lipolysis. Insulin-resistant adipocytes release FFAs due to unsuppressed lipolysis. Insulin resistance-associated hyperinsulinemia and increased FFAs further promote adipogenesis at visceral and ectopic sites.

Elevated FFAs lower whole-body insulin sensitivity as shown in euglycemic-hyperinsulinemic clamps, enhance postabsorptive hepatic glucose production and decrease β-cell insulin secretion.[10] Lipotoxicity is associated with insulin resistance, endoplasmic reticulum stress, oxidative stress, inflammation and endothelial dysfunction.[11] In addition, FFA excess results in intracellular accumulation of toxic lipid metabolites (ceramides, diacylglycerol and others) that have been implicated in impaired β-cell function and also in nonalcoholic steatohepatitis.[11]

Adipose tissue insulin resistance was found to increase across the spectrum of glucose intolerance in obese children and adolescents.[12] Worsening insulin resistance paralleled with the progressive decline of β-cell function and β-cell failure.[13]

## Ectopic Fat Deposition

Dysfunctional WAT fails to store surplus energy, leading to overflow of fat into other tissues involved in metabolism. Such ectopic fat deposition occurs in liver, muscles, pancreas and other visceral organs and contributes to insulin resistance. In addition, it has also been implicated in impaired cellular function such as impaired β-cell function (pancreatic fat), sarcopenia (myocellular fat), diastolic dysfunction (myocardial steatosis) and liver injury (hepatic steatosis).[14]

## Structural and Functional Changes of Adipose Tissue in Diabetes

Type 2 diabetes mellitus is characterized by significant changes in adipose tissue morphology, distribution, and function. These include hyperplasia and hypertrophy of adipocytes, increased and altered macrophages, increased proinflammatory adipocytokines, increased ECM and fibrosis, decreased capillary density, increased autophagy markers and increased adipocyte apoptosis.[15] These are discussed below:

### Adipocyte Turnover: Hyperplasia, Hypertrophy, Apoptosis and Dedifferentiation
*Hypertrophic and dead adipocytes promote insulin resistance*

To increase triglyceride storage capacity, the size and/or number of triglyceride-storing adipocytes should increase and ECM supporting the expanding adipose tissue should remodel. A limited inflammation ensures healthy remodeling of adipose tissue, akin to limited inflammation that is essential for wound healing.

Adipocytes can expand by hypertrophy (increase in size) or by hyperplasia (increase in numbers). Chronic overfeeding is associated with adipocyte hypertrophy, especially in upper body fat and an unfavorable adipokine profile. Enlarged adipocytes are insulin resistant and secrete MCP-1, a chemoattractant for inflammatory cells, in addition to TNF-α, IL-6, IL-8 and resistin.[15] This is accompanied by reduced secretion of IL-10 and adiponectin. These chemotactic signals recruit inflammatory cells to the adipose tissue. Prospective studies confirmed that adipocyte hypertrophy is associated with increased risk for developing T2DM independent of BMI.[16]

Adipocyte hypertrophy induces the death receptor Fas, causing accelerated apoptosis. Fas expression is higher in obese individuals and it interferes with insulin-stimulated glucose uptake and enhanced basal lipolysis in adipocytes.[15] Indeed, adipocyte apoptosis, an important aspect of adipocyte turnover is accelerated in obesity. In addition, death adipocytes are chemoattractant for proinflammatory cells and further contribute to chronic inflammation.

*Limited hyperplastic potential contributes to insulin resistance*

At the same time, a limited hyperplastic potential of adipocytes has been linked to insulin resistance. Adipocytes with decreased hyperplastic features were insulin resistant as demonstrated by lower expression of FABP4 and GLUT-4, responsible for reduced FFA and glucose uptake in the adipose tissue.[17]

The association between limited SCAT expandability and insulin resistance is exemplified in two important phenotypes associated with abnormal metabolism without frank obesity:

SECTION 4: Specific Issues in Glucocrinology

1. *Lipodystrophy:* It is a condition associated with complete or partial absence of adipose tissue. It can be congenital or acquired; and generalized or partial. Acquired lipodystrophy is seen in HIV-infected patients treated with highly active antiretroviral treatment. Lack of adipose tissue causes insulin resistance and diabetes due to ectopic fat accumulation in liver, muscles, pancreas; reduced glucose uptake in the organs due to FFA flux; increased hepatic glucose output; and increased proinflammatory cytokines.[18] Lipodystrophy is associated with severe insulin resistance, diabetes, dyslipidemia, reproductive dysfunction and NAFLD. Unlike generalized obesity which is characterized by leptin resistance, the role of leptin in lipodystrophy seems to be important as these individuals benefit with metreleptin therapy
2. *Asian Indian phenotype:* A phenotype, less severe and more common than lipodystrophy, is the "Asian Indian" phenotype, the characteristics of which are described in Table 3. Maternal malnutrition promotes the development of a thrifty phenotype where genes vital for fetal survival are favorably expressed. This phenotype promotes the expression of genes programmed for "metabolic economy" by inducing epigenetic changes.[19] This results in compromised development of organs like adipose tissue, skeletal muscles, kidney, liver and pancreas to promote growth of organs considered immediately important for survival like the brain. Thus, at birth, the functions of metabolic organs are already compromised. When faced with calorie surplus in later life, the metabolic economy and low SCAT volume and muscle mass promote ectopic/visceral fat deposition, insulin resistance, and development of T2DM even at lower BMI.[19]

**TABLE 3** Characteristics of Asian Indian phenotype.

| | Asian Indian population | Caucasian population |
| --- | --- | --- |
| Percentage body fat | Higher body fat | Lower body fat |
| Lean body mass | Lower | Higher |
| Adipose tissue distribution | Greater visceral and ectopic fat | Less visceral and ectopic fat |
| Waist circumference | Lower | Higher |
| Waist-to-hip ratio | Higher | Lower |
| Mid arm circumference | Lower | Higher |
| Frank obesity | Less common | More common |
| Insulin resistance | Greater | Less |
| Adiponectin | Lower | Higher |
| Inflammatory cytokines | More | Less |
| C-reactive protein | Higher levels | Lower levels |
| Atherogenic dyslipidemia | More atherogenic dyslipidemia | Less marked |
| Onset of diabetes | Occurs a decade earlier | Young-to-middle age |
| Cardiovascular risk | More marked | Less |

There is a need to further understand the factors leading to adipocyte hypertrophy and explore strategies to improve adipose tissue health in diabetes.

## Adipose Tissue Extracellular Matrix Expansion

### Impaired adipose tissue extracellular matrix expansion is linked to insulin resistance

For adipose tissue expansion, the surrounding ECM has to remodel to provide adequate support and vascularity. Preservation of adipose tissue architecture during its expansion is metabolically favorable. In obesity accumulation of ECM can be excessive and aberrant.[15] Adipocytes and endothelial cells from obese adipose tissue samples showed disorganization of the basement membranes and these positively correlated with markers of insulin resistance.

## Proinflammatory Cytokines and Adipose Tissue Inflammation

Obesity is characterized by dysfunctional adipose tissue that releases proinflammatory cytokines leading to worsening of systemic insulin resistance.

### Adipose tissue inflammation and proinflammatory cytokines are increased in obesity and diabetes

Adipose tissue secretes many proinflammatory adipokines such as TNF-α, IL-6, RBP4, resistin, visfastin, MCP-1 and PAI-1.[20] Stress signals from hypertrophic adipocytes are also chemoattractant for inflammatory cells.

The adipose tissue macrophages of lean individuals are of the anti-inflammatory M2 phenotype. In obesity, proinflammatory M1 phenotype predominates. The gut microbiota, whose character is altered in obesity, is associated with insulin resistance. High fat diet and inflammation destroy gut mucosal lining making it leaky and permeable to lipopolysaccharides (from altered gut microbiota) and fatty acids.[21] These induce adipose tissue inflammation with change in macrophage phenotype to proinflammatory M1; increase proinflammatory CD8+ T-lymphocytes and reduce CD4+ regulatory T-lymphocytes. This is termed as "metabolic endotoxemia".[21]

## Fibrosis and Hypoxia

### Inadequate vascularization of adipose tissue promotes hypoxia-induced inflammation

Rapid expansion of WAT causes it to outgrow its own neovascularization. When vascularization is inadequate for expansion, hypoxia ensues. Hypoxia induces the release of hypoxia inducible factor-1α (HIF-1α) which is proinflammatory and promotes fibrosis of ECM.[15] There occurs a greater degree of fibrosis in dysfunctional adipose tissue, further limiting its remodeling capacity.

## Adipose Tissue Handling of Acute Nutrient Flux

### Impaired adipose tissue capacity to handle nutrient flux occurs in diabetes

Excess dietary fat is buffered in SCAT postprandially under the influence of insulin, preventing FFA overflow into circulation and ectopic sites. SCAT blood flow increases markedly in the postprandial period in lean individuals, but this effect is impaired in obese individuals. Glucose-dependent insulinotropic peptide (GIP) is postulated to mediate the meal-induced rise in adipose tissue blood flow (ATBF) and stimulates adipose tissue triglyceride deposition. In patients with impaired glucose tolerance, GIP infusion neither increased ATBF nor adipose tissue triglyceride uptake, exposing individuals to postprandial hypertriglyceridemia and ectopic fat deposition.[22]

## Autophagy and Metabolism

### Disordered adipose tissue autophagy contributes to insulin resistance

Autophagy is a process by which diseased cytosolic substrates are degraded by autophagosomes, prolonging cell survival. Autophagy breakdown products may be recycled as macromolecular constituents, generate energy and protect against cellular stress. In metabolism, autophagy involves fuel (glucose, lipids) breakdown and removal of organelles damaged by reactive oxygen species (ROS).[23] Autophagy, therefore, protects against glucotoxicity, lipotoxicity and ROS damage and impaired autophagy leads to inflammation and insulin resistance.

At the same time, if autophagy is disordered and prolonged, cellular harm rather than benefit ensues. It may result in increased lipolysis due to the effect of lysosomal lipase.[23] In insulin resistance, FOXOs are activated and these stimulate autophagy genes to increase WAT lipolysis.[24] Autophagosomes are indeed, increased in adipocytes derived from obese and diabetic humans. Increased autophagy in adipocytes downregulates insulin receptors and further worsens insulin resistance.[23] Dysfunctional autophagy of adipose tissue macrophages in obesity promotes a proinflammatory phenotype.

In addition, autophagy plays an important role in adipogenesis and adipose tissue differentiation. Autophagy-deficient mice adipocytes grown in culture had reduced adipogenesis.[25] AMPK activators like adiponectin induce autophagy in animal models of obesity; thereby promoting adipogenesis in SCAT and decreasing lipid accumulation in nonadipose tissues.[25] However, autophagy may favor the production of white over brown adipocytes due to selective loss of organelles, especially mitochondria during adipogenesis.

The science of autophagy is complex and needs further research. Adipose tissue autophagy in diabetes is disordered, and may be increased or decreased. Unlike autophagy inhibitors that are proposed as therapeutic option in malignancies, diabetes management would require autophagy modulation.

## ASSESSMENT OF ADIPOSE TISSUE HEALTH IN DIABETES

A clinical measure of adipose tissue dysfunction can help stratify diabetic patients for cardiovascular risk and also provide therapeutic targets for management. Several strategies have been proposed for the clinical evaluation of adipose tissue health in diabetes and include anthropometry, radiological and laboratory evaluation.

## Anthropometric Measures

Several anthropometric indices have been evaluated as indicators of obesity and more importantly central adiposity. These include:

- Body weight and BMI are a measure of adipose tissue quantity.[26] Obesity is traditionally defined as per BMI as depicted in Table 4. It is important to note that lower BMI cutoffs are suggested for Asian Indians as Asian Indian phenotype is characterized by greater insulin resistance at lower BMI levels.[27] However, BMI does not correlate well with cardiometabolic risk, as it does not reflect adipose tissue dysfunction
- Waist circumference is a good clinical measure of dysfunctional adipose tissue and is positively correlated with the levels of proinflammatory cytokines (IL-6, IL-8, TNF-α, PAI-1 and leptin) and negatively correlated with adiponectin. Waist circumference has a stronger association with insulin resistance and cardiovascular risk than BMI and reflects VAT.[26] Again, waist circumference criteria are lower for Asian Indians than Caucasians,[27] as depicted in Table 4
- Waist-to-hip ratio (WHR) is calculated using waist circumference and hip circumference. It is regarded as a measure of abdominal obesity and correlates with metabolic risk. A WHR of ≥0.9 in men and ≥0.85 in women indicates abdominal obesity.[26] In studies, waist circumference was found to correlate better with cardiovascular risk, hypertension and body fat distribution than WHR.[26]

The limitations of BMI as a measure of adiposity are increasingly being realized. Increased adiposity and more specifically abnormal fat distribution (at ectopic and visceral sites) are stronger determinants of metabolic complications than BMI. The importance of this is emphasized by the recommendations of American Association of Clinical Endocrinologists that obesity be more appropriately termed "adiposity-based chronic disease" and that the staging of obesity be "complications-centric" rather than "BMI centric".[28] Clinically, the limitations of BMI may be addressed and supplemented by measuring waist circumference which gives a measure of visceral obesity.

**TABLE 4** Diagnostic thresholds for obesity and central obesity.

| Caucasians | | Asian Indians | |
|---|---|---|---|
| **Body mass index (kg/m²)** | | | |
| <18.5 | Underweight | | |
| 18.5–24.9 | Normal weight | 18.5–22.9 | Normal weight |
| 25–29.9 | Overweight | 23–24.9 | Overweight |
| 30–34.9 | Class 1 obesity | 25–29.9 | Class 1 obesity |
| 35–39.9 | Class 2 obesity | ≥30 | Class 2 obesity |
| ≥40 | Class 3 obesity | | |
| **Waist circumference (cm)** | | | |
| Men | • >94 (IDF)<br>• >102 (NCEP-ATP III) | Men | >90 |
| Women | • >80 (IDF)<br>• >88 (NCEP-ATP III) | Women | >80 |

(IDF: International Diabetes Federation; NCEP-ATP III: National Cholesterol Education Program Adult Treatment Panel III)

## Radiological Assessment of Adipose Tissue Health

Radiological approaches allow for the quantitative assessment of body fat and adipose tissue distribution. Bioimpedance absorptiometry gives some estimate about body composition and has been used; but its clinical utility is limited. Dual-energy X-ray absorptiometry (DEXA) can measure body composition including percentage body fat, muscle mass and bone mass, but it cannot differentiate between visceral and subcutaneous fat.[29] Volumetric computed tomography (CT) and magnetic resonance imaging (MRI) can provide an accurate measure of SCAT and VAT. Quantity of VAT, but not SCAT, correlates well with proinflammatory adipokine levels and cardiometabolic risk.[29] Proton magnetic resonance spectroscopy further allows for a functional imaging of adipose tissue. But these modalities cannot be used in routine diabetes care and their use is limited to research settings.

## Clinical Markers of Adipose Tissue Health

Other markers of cardiometabolic risk combine anthropometric information with laboratory measures of dysmetabolism:
- Metabolic syndrome is defined by the occurrence of three or more of the following: elevated waist circumference, dysglycemia, hypertension, elevated triglycerides and reduced high-density lipoprotein cholesterol (HDL-C).[26] The criteria for metabolic syndrome, as enlisted in Table 5, provide a clinically meaningful assessment of cardiometabolic risk
- Visceral adiposity index is estimated using waist circumference, BMI, triglycerides and HDL-C.[26] It correlates well with metabolic syndrome and cardiovascular risk.

## Adipokine Levels

Adipokines reflect the inflammatory state of adipose tissue. There is a negative correlation between insulin resistance, metabolic syndrome, and adiponectin levels,

**TABLE 5** Diagnostic criteria of metabolic syndrome (International Diabetes Federation).

| Parameter | Diagnostic threshold | |
|---|---|---|
| Elevated waist circumference | Europids, Sub-Saharan Africans, Eastern Mediterranean and Middle East | • Men ≥94 cm<br>• Women ≥80 cm |
| | South Asians, Ethnic South and Central Americans, Chinese and Japanese | • Men ≥90 cm<br>• Women ≥80 cm |
| Elevated plasma glucose | FPG ≥100 mg/dL or treatment for hyperglycemia | |
| Elevated blood pressure | Systolic BP ≥130 mm Hg and/or diastolic BP ≥85 mm Hg, or on antihypertensive treatment | |
| Elevated triglycerides | ≥150 mg/dL or treatment for hypertriglyceridemia | |
| Reduced HDL cholesterol | <40 mg/dL in males, <50 mg/dL in females, or treatment for low HDL cholesterol | |

(BP: blood pressure; FPG: fasting plasma glucose; HDL: high-density lipoprotein)

while there is a positive correlation with proinflammatory adipokines such as leptin, resistin, visfatin and TNF-α levels.[29] But at present, adipokine profiling is not routinely available and is not applicable to routine care.

### Adipose Tissue Biopsy

Adipose tissue biopsy allows for morphological evaluation of the adipose tissue including adipocyte size, macrophage infiltration and inflammation, but is not a practical approach in routine care.

## THERAPEUTIC STRATEGIES TARGETING ADIPOSE TISSUE HEALTH IN DIABETES

It is abundantly clear that diabetes and metabolic disorders have significant adipose tissue dysfunction that contributes to the pathogenesis and progression of diabetes and its complications. Current pharmacological therapies fail to adequately address AT dysfunction and there is a compelling need to focus research in this area.

### Lifestyle Modification

Lifestyle modification and weight management cannot be overemphasized in diabetes care. However, weight management in diabetes should focus on improvement in body composition rather than just decrease of BMI.

Diet, increased physical activity and lifestyle modification can reduce adiposity and result in weight loss of 5–7%. It is associated with favorable changes in fat distribution, reduced ectopic fat, reduced adipocyte size, reduced inflammation and improved insulin sensitivity.[30] Reduction in ectopic fat has been associated with improved organ function—reduced hepatic fat content is associated with a decline in hepatic glucose output; decrease in intramyocellular fat with improved muscle glucose uptake; and decrease in myocardial and epicardial fat with improved diastolic function.[31] Liver fat content is the most responsive to weight reduction with moderately hypocaloric diets. More severe energy restriction with substantial weight reduction is needed to demonstrate improvements in skeletal muscle insulin sensitivity.

Low carbohydrate, high fat and adequate protein diet or ketogenic diet has generated a lot of interest in recent times. Ketogenic diets create carbohydrate deprivation with a shift in metabolism to utilizing fat as a source of fuel. They have been associated with greater satiety, reduced hunger and increased energy expenditure. There is increased lipolysis and gluconeogenesis while glycolysis and lipogenesis are reduced.[32] Ketogenic diets are associated with significant and sustained weight reduction, but need further evaluation to assess their long-term impact and safety.

Exercise is associated with improvements in adipose tissue plasticity and metabolism independent of weight reduction. While exercise may lead to increased intramyocellular fat, this is accompanied by increased fatty acid oxidation and improved insulin sensitivity.[31] Exercise also improves cardiovascular health. However, weight reduction by lifestyle modification is difficult to sustain in the long-term and more research is needed to assess the optimal dietary approaches that improve adipose tissue health in diabetes.

## Effect of Antidiabetic Agents on Adipose Tissue Health

Many antidiabetic agents are limited by side-effect of weight gain, including insulin, sulfonylureas, glinides and thiazolidinediones (TZDs). Two antidiabetic agents, glucagon-like polypeptide-1 receptor (GLP-1R) agonists and sodium glucose cotransporter-2 (SGLT-2) inhibitors, promote weight loss and have also demonstrated cardioprotective benefits.

The GLP-1R agonists like liraglutide not only decrease body weight but improve body composition by decreasing fat mass and visceral fat. While weight loss is largely attributed to central effects with promotion of satiety, reduced caloric intake and delayed gastric emptying, GLP-1Rs are present on adipocytes and it is likely that GLP-1R agonists have a direct effect on adipose tissue.[33]

SGLT-2 inhibitors results in glycosuria with resultant weight loss and are currently preferred as therapy in individuals where adiposity is a concern. There is a greater reduction in fat mass than lean body mass. However, initial weight reduction plateaus after 3–6 months due to increased appetite and reduced energy expenditure.

An important concern raised with the use of TZDs is that they cause weight gain. However, TZDs improve insulin sensitivity despite net weight gain and are associated with a more favorable fat distribution. This apparent paradox is because TZDs increases SCAT adipogenesis by acting on PPAR-γ, resulting in the formation of small adipocytes that avidly take up FFA.[30] This promotes postprandial "fatty acid trap"; the absence of which could raise serum triglyceride by 10-fold postprandially. Thus, TZDs prevent the overflow of fatty acids into the circulation and at ectopic sites including liver.

## Obesity Drugs

Current obesity drugs act by suppressing appetite, reducing caloric intake and increasing energy expenditure. These include—GLP-1R agonist (liraglutide), intestinal lipase inhibitor (orlistat), 5-hydroxytryptamine (5-HT) receptor 2C agonist (lorcaserin) and dual noradrenaline agonist-carbonic anhydrase inhibitor combinations (phentermine-topiramate extended release and naltrexone-bupropion sustained-release).[30] Other than GLP-1R agonists, which have a significant impact on weight and glycemia, most of these drugs achieve 3–5% reduction in body weight and have only mild beneficial effects in diabetes.

## Bariatric Surgery

Simple removal of adipose tissue through liposuction has not shown benefits in improving metabolic health. On the other hand, bariatric surgery not only causes significant weight reduction, it improves insulin sensitivity and whole-body metabolism.

Bariatric surgery causes a reduction of adipose tissue mass by almost half within the first year after surgery. However, the metabolic improvements do not correlate with reduction of adipose tissue mass alone, but with the extent to which various fat deposits are reduced.[34] Within few years of surgery, more SCAT is lost than VAT. On longer follow-up, decline in VAT continues but SCAT remains constant, suggesting that later weight loss is due to reduction in VAT. Long-term benefits occur due to reduction in total fat mass as well as a more favorable fat redistribution.

One of the ways in which these effects on metabolism are mediated includes reduction in total body fat, redistribution of fat from VAT to SCAT, favorable adipokine profile, increased sensitivity to insulin and catecholamine-induced lipolysis and reduced adipose tissue and systemic inflammation. Other effects are mediated via central regulation of metabolism and changes in gut microbiota.

Bariatric surgery can lead to significant improvements in metabolic health, with higher rates of diabetes remission, lower need of antidiabetic and antihypertensive medications and improved long-term survival. More benefits are seen with biliopancreatic diversion (BPD) and Roux-en-Y gastric bypass (RYGB) surgery than sleeve gastrectomy (SG) and results of laparoscopic adjustable gastric banding (LAGB) have been the least encouraging. RYGB seems to have the most favorable risk-benefit profile while BPD carries high morbidity.[34] Mid- and long-term effects including remission of diabetes are predominantly driven by weight loss.

## NOVEL STRATEGIES

Pharmacological approaches to reduce weight using strategies targeting central nervous system to reduce energy intake and increase energy expenditure (such as rimonabant) were limited by unwanted side-effects. Therefore, focus has shifted to directly targeting adipose tissue and improving adipose tissue health. This provides an attractive strategy for the management of diabesity. The current strategies under exploration are summarized in Table 6.

Coagonists of GLP-1 and GIP are under development and may result in more significant weight reduction and glycemic control. Promising results in animal studies were shown with a tri-agonist of GLP-1, GIP and glucagon.[30]

Adipokines provide an attractive area of research for the development of both diagnostic tools and therapeutic choices. Adiponectin levels correlate well with insulin sensitivity and can be a useful marker of insulin resistance and metabolic dysfunction. Direct administration of adiponectin has not been found to be useful and is problematic. However, an oral synthetic adiponectin receptor activator improved glucose tolerance in mice.

Leptin has been considered in the management of obesity, but obese individuals have leptin resistance. It is suggested that leptin sensitivity may improve following weight loss and human recombinant leptin or metreleptin is being tested in such individuals, especially in combination with other weight loss drugs such as pramlintide that may restore leptin sensitivity.[30] At present, metreleptin is recommended in rare monogenic obesity caused by leptin deficiency and in generalized lipodystrophy.

Fibroblast growth factor 21 (FGF21) is another interesting molecule that improves glucose and lipid metabolism and promotes beiging of WAT. FGF21 analogs improved insulin sensitivity and glucose and lipid parameters, increased energy expenditure and promoted weight loss in animal studies.[30] Two FGF21 analogs have advanced into clinical trials but there are important safety concerns as FGF21 reduces bone mass and may have other systemic effects.

Another viable option could be inhibition of IL-1β signaling. Anakinra (recombinant human IL-1 receptor antagonist) improved insulin secretion and sensitivity and reduced inflammation. Anti-IL-1β antibody, Canakinumab, has also

**TABLE 6** Novel therapeutic strategies to target adipose tissue dysfunction in diabetes.

| Novel approaches | Mechanism of benefit |
|---|---|
| GLP-1 and GIP coagonists | • Robust glucose-lowering effect, increase insulin secretion, and reduce glucagon secretion<br>• Significant weight reduction, increase satiety, delay gastric emptying, increase beiging of fat cells and increase energy expenditure |
| Selective modulators of PPAR-γ | • Promote fat redistribution and beiging of fat cells<br>• Avoid side effects related to thiazolidinediones including edema and congestive heart failure |
| β3-adrenergic receptor agonists | Promote beiging of adipocytes and increase energy expenditure |
| Thyroid hormone analogs | • Increase energy expenditure<br>• Can cause tachycardia and bone mineral loss |
| Leptin (metreleptin) | • Useful in leptin deficiency and generalized lipodystrophy<br>• Obesity associated with leptin resistance |
| FGF21 analogs | • Increase energy expenditure and promote weight loss<br>• Reduce bone mass |
| Inhibitors of IL-1β signaling | Improve insulin sensitivity and reduce inflammation |
| PAHSA | Increase insulin and GLP-1 secretion and reduce inflammation |
| FXR agonists | Reduce weight and liver glucose output |

(FGF21: fibroblast growth factor 21; FXR: farnesoid X receptor; IL-1β: interleukin-1β; GIP: gastric inhibitory polypeptide; GLP-1: glucagon-like polypeptide-1; PAHSA: palmitic acid-9-hydroxy stearic acid; PPAR-γ: peroxisome proliferator activated receptor gamma)

been shown to improve glucose tolerance.[30] Adipose-derived stem cells (ASCs) have immune-modulatory properties. Delivery of ASCs from lean mice to diet-induced obese mice reduced adipose tissue inflammation and improved insulin sensitivity.[30]

Certain adipose-derived fatty acid derivatives such as PAHSA (palmitic acid-9-hydroxy stearic acid) are promising candidates in diabesity and may be superior to omega-3-fatty acids as they augment insulin and GLP-1 secretion and reduce adipose tissue inflammation.[30]

Strategies to promote beiging of WAT may increase energy expenditure by uncoupling mitochondrial respiration and increasing thermogenesis.[30] This would in turn improve insulin sensitivity and metabolic health. Cold exposure and exercise are known to promote beiging of white adipocytes. Repeated intermittent exposure to mild cold results in reduction in fat mass. Several agents are under evaluation:

- *Catecholamine derivatives*: The β3-adrenergic receptor agonists increased beiging in WAT and ameliorated obesity and insulin resistance in rodents. Mirabegron is a selective β3-adrenergic receptor agonist that increases energy expenditure. But it also increases heart rate and blood pressure, raising concerns about cardiovascular safety
- *Farnesoid X receptor agonists*: Fexaramine reduces weight and hepatic glucose output and warrants further study
- Thyroid hormone analogs have also been explored but results have not been encouraging

- FGF21 analogs
- Brown adipose tissue transplants.

Among existing therapeutic agents, TZDs promote beige adipocyte formation. Another avenue of research is development of selective modulators of PPAR-γ that are devoid of the side-effects that limit TZDs.[30] Sirtuin 1 (SIRT1) activator, resveratrol, that acts to increase lipolysis and reduce inflammation is under phase II clinical trials.

Pharmacological approaches to block the immune pathway and reduce inflammatory activity, such as amlexanox (increases IL-6 secretion), infliximab (anti-TNF monoclonal antibody) or salsalate (suppresses production of TNF and C-reactive protein) have not yielded promising results. An oral C-C chemokine receptor antagonist that inhibits macrophage migration, however, has shown glucose-lowering efficacy and is in phase II trials. Research into novel strategies to reduce adipose tissue hypoxia and fibrosis is in its initial stages.

## CONCLUSION

In any organized system, adaptations take place in the form of remodeling, repair and regeneration so as to prolong the life of the system in a healthy way. In metabolism, adipose tissue functions as an important energy homeostat. During evolution, energy deficit states represented a threat to metabolic homeostasis as opposed to the energy surplus which is prevalent today. The adipose tissue served as a storehouse of energy to be released in times of need. In energy surplus states, adipose tissue adapts and remodels to protect the system. Important players in this remodeling are adipose tissue constituents like adipocytes, ECM, capillaries, inflammatory cells; basic cellular systems like autophagy; crosstalk with organs involved in energy homeostasis; and gene-metabolism interaction. In diabetes, these adaptations turn maladaptive when calorie intake is excessive and persistent, especially in the backdrop of a phenotype that promotes adiposity in unfavorable locations which could be determined by genetic and epigenetic factors. Adipose tissue health in diabetes is a classic example of an adaptation gone immensely wrong due to incessant assault on the system. Antidiabetic agents, which promote favorable body mass composition and fat distribution are limited. Adipose tissue targeted therapy, including specific dietary interventions and pharmacological approaches, should be the novel focus of diabetes therapy.

## REFERENCES

1. Kalra S. Diabesity. J Pak Med Assoc. 2013;63(4):532-4.
2. Booth A, Magnuson A, Fouts J, et al. Adipose tissue: an endocrine organ playing a role in metabolic regulation. Horm Mol Biol Clin Investig. 2016;26(1):25-42.
3. Pellegrinelli V, Carobbio S, Vidal-Puig A. Adipose tissue plasticity: how fat depots respond differently to pathophysiological cues. Diabetologia. 2016;59(6):1075-88.
4. Hatori M, Vollmers C, Zarrinpar A, et al. Time-restricted feeding without reducing caloric intake prevents metabolic diseases in mice fed a high-fat diet. Cell Metab. 2012;15(6):848-60.
5. Shao M, Ishibashi J, Kusminski CM, et al. Zfp423 maintains white adipocyte identity through suppression of the beige cell thermogenic gene program. Cell Metab. 2016;23(6):1167-84.
6. Giralt M, Cereijo R, Villarroya F. Adipokines and the Endocrine Role of Adipose Tissues. Handb Exp Pharmacol. 2016;233:265-82.
7. Kiehn JT, Tsang AH, Heyde I, et al. Circadian Rhythms in Adipose Tissue Physiology. Compr Physiol. 2017;7(2):383-427.

8. Abdelaal M, le Roux CW, Docherty NG. Morbidity and mortality associated with obesity. Ann Transl Med. 2017;5(7):161.
9. Yang J, Kang J, Guan Y. The mechanisms linking adiposopathy to type 2 diabetes. Front Med. 2013;7(4):433-44.
10. Boden G. Effects of free fatty acids (FFA) on glucose metabolism: Significance for insulin resistance and type 2 diabetes. Exp Clin Endocrinol Diabetes. 2003;111(3):121-4.
11. Yazıcı D, Sezer H. Insulin Resistance, Obesity and Lipotoxicity. Adv Exp Med Biol. 2017;960:277-304.
12. Hershkop K, Besor O, Santoro N, et al. Adipose insulin resistance in obese adolescents across the spectrum of glucose tolerance. J Clin Endocrinol Metab. 2016;101(6):2423-31.
13. Gastaldelli A, Gaggini M, DeFronzo RA. Role of adipose tissue insulin resistance in the natural history of type 2 diabetes: results from the San Antonio metabolism study. Diabetes. 2017;66(4):815-22.
14. Snel M, Jonker JT, Schoones J, et al. Ectopic fat and insulin resistance: pathophysiology and effect of diet and lifestyle interventions. Int J Endocrinol. 2012;2012:983814.
15. Crewe C, An YA, Scherer PE. The ominous triad of adipose tissue dysfunction: inflammation, fibrosis, and impaired angiogenesis. J Clin Invest. 2017;127(1):74-82.
16. Lönn M, Mehlig K, Bengtsson C, et al. Adipocyte size predicts incidence of type 2 diabetes in women. FASEB J. 2010;24(1):326-31.
17. Oliva-Olivera W, Coín-Aragüez L, Lhamyani S, et al.. Adipogenic impairment of adipose tissue-derived mesenchymal stem cells in subjects with metabolic syndrome: possible protective role of FGF2. J Clin Endocrinol Metab. 2017;102(2):478-87.
18. Garg A, Agarwal AK. Lipodystrophies: disorders of adipose tissue biology. Biochim Biophys Acta. 2009;1791(6):507-13.
19. Misra A, Jayawardena R, Anoop S. Obesity in South Asia: Phenotype, Morbidities, and Mitigation. Curr Obes Rep. 2019;8(1):43-52.
20. Rasouli N, Kern PA. Adipocytokines and the Metabolic Complications of Obesity. J Clin Endocrinol Metab. 2008;93(11 Suppl 1):S64-73.
21. Ramos-Molina B, Queipo-Ortuño MI, Lambertos A, et al. Dietary and Gut Microbiota Polyamines in Obesity- and Age-Related Diseases. Front Nutr. 2019;6:24.
22. Asmar M, Simonsen L, Arngrim N, et al. Glucose- dependent insulinotropic polypeptide has impaired effect on abdominal, subcutaneous adipose tissue metabolism in obese subjects. Int J Obes (Lond). 2014;38(2):259-65.
23. Barlow AD, Thomas DC. Autophagy in diabetes: β-cell dysfunction, insulin resistance, and complications. DNA Cell Biol. 2015;34(4):252-60.
24. Lettieri Barbato D, Tatulli G, Aquilano K, et al. FoxO1 controls lysosomal acid lipase in adipocytes: implication of lipophagy during nutrient restriction and metformin treatment. Cell Death Dis. 2013;4:e861.
25. Sarparanta J, García-Macia M, Singh R. Autophagy and Mitochondria in Obesity and Type 2 Diabetes. Curr Diabetes Rev. 2017;13(4):352-69.
26. Schrover IM, Spiering W, Leiner T, et al. Adipose Tissue Dysfunction: Clinical Relevance and Diagnostic Possibilities. Horm Metab Res. 2016;48(4):213-25.
27. Misra A, Chowbey P, Makkar BM, et al. Consensus statement for diagnosis of obesity, abdominal obesity and the metabolic syndrome for Asian Indians and recommendations for physical activity, medical and surgical management. J Assoc Physicians India. 2009;57:163-70.
28. Mechanick JI, Hurley DL, Garvey WT. Adiposity-based chronic disease as a new diagnostic term: the American Association of Clinical Endocrinologists and American College of Endocrinology position statement. Endocr Pract. 2017;23(3):372-8.
29. Shuster A, Patlas M, Pinthus JH, et al. The clinical importance of visceral adiposity: a critical review of methods for visceral adipose tissue analysis. Br J Radiol. 2012;85(1009):1-10.
30. Kusminski CM, Bickel PE, Scherer PE. Targeting adipose tissue in the treatment of obesity-associated diabetes. Nat Rev Drug Discov. 2016;15(9):639-60.
31. Gadde KM, Martin CK, Berthoud HR, et al. Obesity: Pathophysiology and Management. J Am Coll Cardiol. 2018;71(1):69-84.
32. Kalra S, Singla R, Rosha R, et al. The ketogenic diet. US Endocrinology. 2018;14(2):62-4.
33. Santilli F, Simeone PG, Guagnano MT, et al. Effects of liraglutide on weight loss, fat distribution, and β-cell function in obese subjects with prediabetes or early type 2 diabetes. Diabetes Care 2017;40(11):1556-64.
34. Frikke-Schmidt H, O'Rourke RW, Lumeng CN, et al. Does bariatric surgery improve adipose tissue function? Obes Rev. 2016;17(9):795-809.

# CHAPTER 20

# Bone Health in Diabetes

*Deep Dutta, Mohammad Wali Naseri, Indira Maisnam, Gagan Priya*

## INTRODUCTION

Bone is no longer regarded as an organ that provides structural support alone; it is a complex endocrine organ that plays a crucial role in mineral (calcium and phosphate) metabolism and energy homeostasis. In addition, vitamin D and parathyroid hormone (PTH) play a role in the regulation of energy metabolism and vitamin D also has immunomodulatory effects. Recent research has focused on the role of osteokines, which are bone-specific proteins, secreted by osteoblasts and osteocytes. Osteokines, including osteocalcin, osteoprotegerin, sclerostin, lipocalin 2, and bone morphogenetic protein 7 (BMP 7) have myriad effects on central energy regulation and insulin sensitivity. These aspects have been discussed in the chapter "Glucocrinology of Parathyroid and Bone Mineral Metabolism".

While the focus of diabetes care remains optimization of glucose and energy metabolism and prevention of micro- and macrovascular complications, diabetes also has a significant impact on bone health through multiple mechanisms related to the effects of hyperglycemia per se, insulin deficiency, obesity, long-term complications of diabetes, and the impact of antidiabetic drugs on bone. Diabetic bone disease with increased skeletal fragility and fracture risk remains a poorly understood complication of diabetes.[1]

Bone health, though important, is an often neglected aspect of diabetes care. Both lower bone mineral density (BMD) as well as poor bone quality has been documented in individuals with diabetes. Clinically, this translates to an increased risk of skeletal fractures. Whether diabetic osteopathy should be classified as a microvascular complication of diabetes remains a topic for debate and clearly more research is needed.[1] This chapter summarizes available literature pertaining to bone health in diabetes, with the intention of developing a better understanding of metabolic bone disorders in relation to diabetes.

# BONE HEALTH IN TYPE 1 DIABETES MELLITUS

Studies on type 1 diabetes mellitus (T1DM) have shown a 6- to 9-fold increase in the relative risk for hip fractures;[2] the relative risk for any other non-vertebral fracture is 1.3–3;[3] with no increase in the risk of vertebral fractures.[4]

Both skeletal and extra-skeletal factors may be responsible for this increased fracture risk. Almost all studies have found decreased BMD in T1DM.[5] Lower BMD partly explains the increased risk of fractures in T1DM. However, the risk of fractures is much higher than would be explained by the relatively small decrease in BMD. It has been suggested that individuals with T1DM have alterations in bone microarchitecture, and these are more important indicators of bone strength than bone density.[5]

Microarchitecture of bone includes bone geometry, distribution of trabeculae, porosity of bone, collagen content, and it's cross-linking. Reductions in volumetric BMD at both trabecular and cortical sites have been reported in children with T1DM.[5] Other studies using high-resolution peripheral quantitative computed tomography (HR-pQCT) have reported greater cortical porosity, and reduced trabecular thickness and trabecular bone volume/total bone volume ratio in individuals with T1DM.[5] Changes in bone microarchitecture are more pronounced in those with microvascular complications, especially retinopathy, than those without complications.

## Factors Leading to Impaired Bone Health in Type 1 Diabetes Mellitus

In T1DM, bone quality and microarchitecture may be affected by hyperglycemia, insulin deficiency, and vascular disease.[5] Persistent hyperglycemia adversely affects bone health through the formation of advanced glycation end-products (AGEs) that increase the apoptosis of mesenchymal stem cells (MSCs) with reduced osteoblast differentiation. High glucose levels also inhibit the secretion of osteocalcin from osteoblasts and downregulate the expression of matrix metallopeptidase-13 (MMP-13), vascular endothelial growth factor (VEGF), and glyceraldehyde-3-phosphate dehydrogenase (GAPDH).[6] AGEs also increase osteoclastic activity.

Peak bone mass may be negatively affected in children with T1DM due to several factors including suboptimal control. Insulin has a trophic effect on bone and T1DM is characterized by a near-absolute deficiency of insulin. Exogenous insulin is delivered into systemic circulation with resultant lower portosystemic gradient; this is associated with reduced hepatic insulin-like growth factor 1 (IGF-1) synthesis that stimulates bone formation.[5]

Several extraskeletal factors also explain the increased propensity for fractures. Vascular complications have been consistently associated with impaired skeletal health in T1DM. VEGF plays an important role in diabetic retinopathy and diabetic kidney disease. VEGF also determines bone vascularization, osteoblast differentiation, and bone repair.[1,5] Diabetic kidney disease is also associated with impaired bone mineral metabolism. Adynamic bone disease is characterized by low bone turnover, reduced bone volume, and reduced cellularity. At the other end of the spectrum, chronic kidney disease may be associated with secondary or tertiary hyperparathyroidism with increased bone turnover. Vitamin D deficiency may also play a contributory role.

In addition, peripheral neuropathy, foot deformities, gait instability, postural hypotension, visual impairment, and hypoglycemia unawareness result in increased tendency to fall and sustain injury. Sympathetic and parasympathetic dysfunction may also directly affect bone health as α- and β-adrenergic receptors modulate osteoblast gene expression.[1] In addition, chronic inflammation, oxidative stress, vitamin D deficiency, and altered osteokine profile may be the link between cardiovascular disease (CVD) and bone fragility.[5]

## BONE HEALTH IN TYPE 2 DIABETES MELLITUS

In contrast to T1DM, bone health interpretation in type 2 diabetes mellitus (T2DM) is more complex and subject to myriad factors. While T2DM has been associated with increased fracture risk, the evidence pertaining to changes in BMD has been heterogeneous with different studies documenting increased, decreased or similar BMD compared to the general population.

### Increased Fracture Risk in Type 2 Diabetes Mellitus

Studies in T2DM have shown an increased risk in hip, vertebral, and other non-vertebral fractures, in both men (RR 2.8; 95% CI 1.2–6.6) and women (RR 2.1; 95% CI 1.6–2.7).[7,8] The Health, Aging, and Body Composition (Health ABC) study found T2DM to be associated with increased fracture risk (RR 1.64; 95% CI: 1.07–2.5).[9] In the Women's Health Initiative study, women with diabetes had a higher relative risk (RR 1.2, 95% CI: 1.1–1.3) of fractures at 7 year follow-up, inspite of having higher BMD.[10] The Nurses' Health Study found that women with diabetes had a higher relative risk of fractures and the risk was higher in women with longer disease duration (RR 2.2, 95% CI: 1.8–2.7).[11]

### Bone Mineral Density in Type 2 Diabetes Mellitus

The Rotterdam Study (2005) which is a prospective population-based cohort study of men and women aged 55 years and over, found that after adjusting for confounding variables, the BMD at both lumbar spine and femoral neck was substantially higher in individuals with T2DM than in those without diabetes. However, subjects with diabetes had an increased risk of overall nonvertebral fractures, despite higher BMD values. In the study, subjects with newly diagnosed diabetes did not have increased fracture risk and subjects with impaired glucose tolerance had a reduced risk by 20–40%.[12] A meta-analysis by Lili Ma et al. found that diabetic individuals had higher BMD than nondiabetics independent of the skeletal site of measurement, gender, age, BMI or medication use.[12] Insulin resistance with hyperinsulinemia and increased IGF-1 and the confounding effects of obesity may explain the increased BMD in T2DM.

On the other hand, in a study by Dutta et al., BMD was lower in diabetic patients as compared to controls.[13] Schwartz et al. found that after adjustment for covariates, women with T2DM lost more BMD per year compared to women without.[14] The Health ABC Study found ethnicity to be a significant predictor of total hip BMD in older adults with T2DM.[15]

## Impaired Bone Quality in Type 2 Diabetes Mellitus

The expression of bone turnover markers including osteocalcin, type 1 cross-linked C-telopeptide (CTX-1), and type 1 cross-linked N-telopeptide (NTX) is reduced in individuals with T2DM, especially in those with longer disease duration.[6] This low bone turnover may result in inadequate repair of microfractures and poor bone quality.[16]

Studies assessing bone microarchitecture in T2DM using HR-pQCT report an increase in tibial and radial BMD and trabecular volumetric BMD and trabecular thickness in distal tibia. However, the porosity of cortical bone in radius was significantly increased.[6] This imbalance of increased trabecular bone but decreased intracortical bone likely results in compromised bending load and poor biomechanical quality of bone in T2DM.[16] In contrast, postmenopausal and senile osteoporosis are characterized by increased bone resorption and decrease in both trabecular and cortical bone.

## Factors Leading to Impaired Bone Health in Type 2 Diabetes Mellitus

While there exists heterogeneity in studies reporting changes in BMD in T2DM, diabetes has been consistently associated with poor bone quality. Diabetes adversely affects bone health via several plausible mechanisms, as depicted in Flowchart 1 and discussed further.

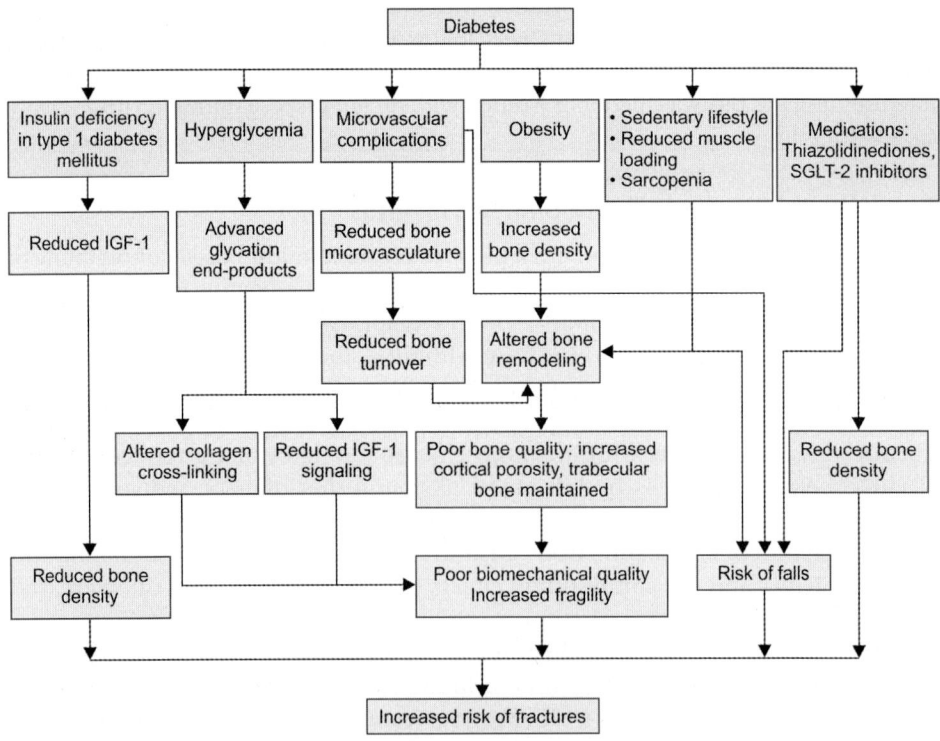

(IGF-1: insulin-like growth factor 1; SGLT-2: sodium-glucose cotransporter-2)

**FLOWCHART 1:** Mechanisms of increased fracture risk in diabetes.

Formation of AGEs from the nonenzymatic glycation of proteins may have a role in the pathogenesis of poor bone health in diabetes. AGEs accumulate in bone tissue and inhibit the synthesis of type 1 collagen and osteocalcin and mature bone formation by osteoblasts.[17] A combination of high glucose and AGEs inhibit the mineralization of osteoblastic cells, through glucose-induced increase in expression of RAGE.[18] In addition, AGEs also increased osteoclastic activity. Collagen cross-links play an important role in bone strength. Physiological (enzymatic) cross-links strengthen the links of collagen fibers, thereby increasing bone strength; however, AGE type cross-links, formed by nonenzymatic glycation and oxidation reactions, are believed to be associated with brittleness of collagen fibers.[19]

Insulin-like growth factors (IGFs) synthesized in osteoblasts are among the most important local regulators of bone mass due to their anabolic effects on the skeleton.[20] Locally produced IGFs have a significant role in bone formation and experimental studies have shown that 50% of bone formation can be blocked by inhibiting the action of IGF. Circulating IGF-1 produced by the liver also has bone anabolic effect. The stimulatory actions of IGF-1 on osteoblasts are blunted by high glucose concentrations or AGEs. AGEs also significantly decreased IGF-1 secretion in osteoblastic MC3T3-E1 cells.[20] Thus, high glucose concentrations or AGEs could cause resistance of osteoblasts to IGF-1 actions and decrease locally produced IGF-1 levels.

Studies have found an inverse association between BMD and microvascular complications. The Blue Mountain Eye Study in Australia found an association between diabetic retinopathy and fractures.[21] It has been suggested that diabetic bone disease may result from insufficient bone microvasculature resulting in impaired bone remodeling and should be classified as a microvascular complication of diabetes.[16] Diabetes is also associated with increased risk of falls due to hypoglycemia, peripheral neuropathy and foot deformities, gait instability, visual impairment, sarcopenia, frailty, and postural hypotension.

Hypercalciuria, a potential risk factor for osteoporosis, is seen in poorly controlled diabetes. T2DM is associated with reduced testosterone levels in men and this may also play a role. Some antidiabetic drugs like thiazolidinediones (TZDs) acting via peroxisome proliferator-activated receptor γ (PPAR-γ), may interfere with bone regulation.[21] The effects of antidiabetic medications on bone health are discussed later.

In addition to increased fracture risk, fracture healing may be delayed in diabetes. The rates of delayed fracture union and nonunion are reported to be higher than nondiabetic individuals.[6] This has been attributed to deficient production of collagen and growth factors and the effect of AGEs. Hyperglycemia is also associated with greater risk of postoperative infections following orthopedic surgical procedures.

## Obesity: Major Confounding Factor Affecting Bone Health Interpretation

Obesity has been linked with increased BMD, even though the bone quality may be poor.[22] Mechanisms responsible for increased BMD in obesity and diabetes include:
- Hyperinsulinemia may have bone anabolic effects through actions mediated via IGF-1 receptor present on osteoblasts;

- Obesity, by imparting a greater mechanical load on bone, stimulates an increase in bone mass;
- Reduced adiponectin and increased leptin levels are associated with increased osteoblastogenesis and reduced osteoclastogenesis; and
- Greater production of estrogen from adipose tissue increases BMD due to the antiresorptive properties of estrogen.[6]

However certain factors associated with diabetes and obesity like aortic calcification and osteoarthritis of the spine may give falsely inflated BMD values.[22]

## Body Composition and Bone Health in Type 2 Diabetes Mellitus

Recently it has been realized that the link between obesity and BMD is not so simplistic. Obesity is constituted by an increase in fat mass as well as muscle mass. A greater percentage of fat mass compared to lean mass contributed to a greater impairment of bone health. Among the various adipose tissue depots, increased visceral fat has a greater negative impact on bone health as compared to increased peripheral fat. Fat mass inversely correlated with bone mass when the mechanical loading effects of body weight on bone mass were controlled.[22] In fact, visceral adipose tissue was a negative predictor of spine BMD, whole body BMD, and bone mineral content/height in obese girls after controlling for subcutaneous adipose tissue.[23]

This inverse relationship between fat and bone could arise from the fact that they share some common genetic and molecular pathways. Adipocytes and osteoblasts arise from common MSCs and their differentiation is regulated through the PPAR-γ pathway, among others. Activation of PPAR-γ promotes the differentiation of MSCs to adipocytes instead of osteoblasts.[24] Such increased bone marrow adipogenesis has been demonstrated in both T1DM and T2DM.

With increasing age, fat mass increases and lean or skeletal muscle mass declines. Individuals increase muscle mass over the first two decades of life; begin to lose muscle mass and strength between the third and fourth decade; and the decline accelerates during the sixth decade. However, there is heterogeneity in the gain and decline of muscle mass with factors like genetic make-up, physical activity, and comorbid conditions making major contributions. Sedentary lifestyle is a very strong predictor of the loss of lean mass with aging. It is already known that certain diseases like chronic obstructive pulmonary disease, congestive heart failure, chronic kidney disease, arthritis, and cancer are associated with decrease in lean mass. Studies have shown that T2DM accelerates the age-associated loss of lean mass.[25]

Lean mass, which is predominantly skeletal muscle mass, is a primary target of insulin action, and increased muscle mass is associated with improved insulin sensitivity. Thus, low lean mass can worsen the insulin resistance already present in T2DM.[25] Insulin resistance may also result in reduced synthesis of whole-body proteins. Lower bioavailable testosterone in diabetes might contribute to lower protein synthesis; and increased proinflammatory cytokines might contribute to increased muscle breakdown, resulting in loss of muscle mass.[25]

Lean mass seems to be a strong predictor of improved bone health in many studies. The authors themselves in different cohort of patients (diabetes, hyperthyroidism, rheumatoid arthritis, HIV) and normal individuals have consistently demonstrated the positive and beneficial impact of increased lean mass on BMD and health.[26-30] One explanation could be that more lean mass would convey more frequent and higher mechanical loading to the skeleton. Skeletal muscle induces muscle and gravitational forces influencing bone mass via mechanical loading. Also, increased lean mass decreases fracture risk by not only improving BMD but also by preventing falls as a result of improved muscle strength.

In addition, exercise has a positive impact on bone health through biomechanical stimulation (direct force applied to the bone) as well as the production of myokines including irisin, that has a positive effect on bone. Sedentary lifestyle and limited exercise may further contribute to impaired bone health.[16]

## Effect of Vitamin D on Bone Health in Diabetes

Vitamin D deficiency is a global pandemic. India has a high prevalence of vitamin D deficiency ranging from 70–80% in the general population. The high prevalence of vitamin D deficiency is likely to have an adverse impact on bone health in the general population, including individuals with diabetes.[31] In fact, the peak bone mass in Indians is much lower than what is reported in Caucasians and Afro-Americans.[27-29]

However, it must be highlighted that Afro-Americans inspite of having persistently lower serum vitamin D levels have higher BMD than Caucasians.[32] This dichotomy is explained by the presence of comparable free serum vitamin D levels in both Caucasians and Afro-Americans, but lower serum total vitamin D levels in Afro-Americans due to lower circulating levels of vitamin D binding proteins (VDBP), a result of certain polymorphisms in the VDBP genes.[32] However similar data is lacking for Asian Indian population.

## Effect of Antidiabetes Medications on Bone Health

Glucose-lowering drugs used in the pharmacological management of T2DM also have effects on bone health and may affect fracture risk, as summarized in Table 1. Insulin has bone anabolic effects and stimulates bone formation. Intensive insulin therapy seems to have neutral effect on BMD in T1DM. There is lack of adequate studies assessing the impact of insulin therapy on bone health in T2DM and results have been conflicting. While insulin possibly increases BMD, it may increase the risk of falls due to hypoglycemia and its initiation often parallels longer disease duration and comorbidities, that may confound its positive effects on bone.[33]

Observational data are strongly suggestive of a protective effect of metformin on bone health as it promotes osteogenesis.[34] Metformin had a stimulatory effect on osteoblast differentiation and inhibitory effect on osteoclast differentiation, and was associated with increased bone mineral content and density in animal studies. While the risk of fractures has not been documented to be decreased with metformin in clinical trials, it reduced the levels of bone turnover markers (CTX and amino-terminal propeptide of procollagen type 1 or P1NP).[33] Sulfonylureas are largely believed to have a beneficial to neutral impact on bone health, with no change reported in BMD.[33] However, indirectly, the increased risk of falls due to hypoglycemia with sulfonylureas may increase the risk of fractures.[34]

**TABLE 1** Effect of antidiabetic medications on bone health.

| Drug class | Effect on bone turnover markers | Effect on BMD | Effect on fracture risk |
|---|---|---|---|
| Insulin | No data | Increased | May be increased—risk of falls, longer disease duration, comorbidities |
| Metformin | Reduced | Neutral or increased | Neutral or beneficial |
| Sulfonylureas | Neutral | Neutral | Conflicting; risk of falls |
| GLP-1R agonists | Resorption markers decreased; formation markers increased | No data | No data |
| DPP-4 inhibitors | Neutral | Neutral | Neutral |
| Thiazolidinediones | Resorption markers increased; formation markers decreased | Decreased | • Significantly increased<br>• Risk factors—postmenopausal females, elderly, long-term use, history of fracture |
| SGLT-2 inhibitors | Increased resorption and formation markers | Decreased or neutral | • Increased—canagliflozin in some studies; no effect of dapagliflozin or empagliflozin<br>• Risk factors—elderly, renal impairment, CVD |

(BMD: bone mineral density; CVD: cardiovascular disease, DPP-4: dipeptidyl peptidase-4, GLP-1R: glucagon-like peptide-1 receptor; SGLT-2: sodium-glucose cotransporter-2)

Glucagon-like polypeptide 1 (GLP-1) receptor agonists improved bone microarchitecture and trabecular bone mass in animal studies, but there is insufficient data of its effect on bone health in humans.[6] Receptors for gastric inhibitory polypeptide (GIP) and GLP-1 have been demonstrated on osteoblasts, and they have positive effect on bone remodeling. GLP-1 may also induce calcitonin release from thyroid C-cells, thus inhibiting bone resorption.[33] However, in clinical trials, no effects have been documented on bone markers, BMD or fracture risk. Dipeptidyl peptidase-4 (DPP-4) inhibitors are believed to be largely bone neutral.[34] In animal studies, DPP-4 inhibitors improved trabecular architecture and vertebral BMD, but in clinical trials, there was no effect on fracture risk.

In contrast, TZDs including pioglitazone have been consistently linked with increased risk of fractures. TZD use was associated with reduced BMD along with reduction in markers of bone formation (bone alkaline phosphatase and P1NP) while bone resorption markers (CTX) were increased. Increased fracture risk is especially noted with prolonged treatment and in postmenopausal women, elderly, and those with previous history of fracture.[33] Discontinuation of TZDs was associated with amelioration of the increase in fracture risk.[6] The preferential impact of PPAR-γ agonists on MSCs promoting their differentiation into an adipocyte instead of an osteoblast and suppression of osteoblast activity may explain their adverse impact on bone health.[34]

Sodium-glucose cotransporter 2 (SGLT-2) inhibitors is another class of drugs, which has been linked with impaired bone health, increased markers of bone resorption, and increased risk of fractures. Increase in bone turnover markers (CTX and osteocalcin) and a reduction in total hip BMD has been reported with canagliflozin but not dapagliflozin.[33] While the fractures were more common in the distal part of upper and lower extremities with canagliflozin in the CANVAS trial, the plausible explanation for the same was increased propensity to falls and other studies have not reported similar risk.[35] In addition, increased fracture risk has not been reported in long-term cardiovascular outcome studies of empagliflozin and dapagliflozin. SGLT-2 inhibitors act at the proximal convoluted tubules in the kidney and result in increased phosphate reabsorption. Increased phosphorus levels in blood are a potent stimulus for PTH release from the parathyroid, which in turn leads to increased bone dissolution, reduced BMD, and increased fracture risk.[36]

The rapid weight loss associated with metabolic/bariatric surgery has been linked to increased bone mineral loss and increased fracture risk. In addition, bariatric surgery may be associated with nutritional deficiencies, altered adipokine profile and central signaling pathways; and sarcopenia may accompany loss of fat mass.

## MANAGEMENT OF OSTEOPOROSIS AND REDUCTION OF FRACTURE RISK IN DIABETES

There are no diabetes-specific guidelines focusing on management of diabetic bone disease. Most of the evidence is extrapolated from studies in the general population with subgroup analysis of individuals with diabetes. Clinical evaluation should include assessment for factors that increase the risk of fractures, as enlisted in Table 2. In the absence of specific guidelines for diagnosis and management of bone fragility in diabetes, general osteoporosis guidelines can be adapted for diabetes, as depicted in Flowchart 2.

Lifestyle modification should include optimization of body weight while ensuring adequate protein, calcium and vitamin D intake and cessation of smoking. Nutrition modification should be accompanied by physical activity including weight-bearing exercises and resistance training. Prevention of falls is important. Both hyperglycemia and hypoglycemia increase the risk of falls and fractures; therefore, glycemic targets should be individualized. In individuals at risk of fractures, TZDs and SGLT-2 inhibitors should be preferably avoided and bone-neutral antidiabetic agents should be given preference.

### Assessment of Fracture Risk in Diabetes

While BMD is considered the gold-standard method for diagnosis of osteoporosis, it must be remembered that it may not correlate well with fracture risk in diabetes.[37] Fracture risk assessment tool (FRAX) is the most commonly used risk score for predicting fracture risk and incorporates multiple risk factors—age, sex, BMI, previous history of fracture, history of fracture in parents, current smoking status, alcohol intake, glucocorticoid use, and rheumatoid arthritis along with femoral neck BMD T-score. However, diabetes is not regarded as a risk factor and the FRAX score

| TABLE 2 | Factors contributing to increased risk of fractures in diabetes. |
|---|---|
| **Category** | **Contributing factors** |
| Bone specific factors | • Low BMD • Elderly<br>• History of previous fracture • Postmenopausal women<br>• Family history of hip fracture |
| Diabetes specific factors | • Diabetes duration >5 years • Persistent poor glycemic control<br>• Microvascular complications |
| Lifestyle factors | • Current smoking • Sedentary lifestyle<br>• Alcohol intake |
| Comorbidities | • Rheumatoid arthritis • Congestive heart failure<br>• Chronic kidney disease • Cardiovascular disease<br>• Chronic liver disease |
| Medications | • Glucocorticoids • SGLT-2 inhibitors<br>• Thiazolidinediones |
| Increased propensity to falls | • Visual impairment • Gait instability<br>• Peripheral neuropathy • Foot deformities<br>• Autonomic neuropathy, postural hypotension • Hypoglycemia |

(BMD: bone mineral density; SGLT-2: sodium-glucose cotransporter-2)

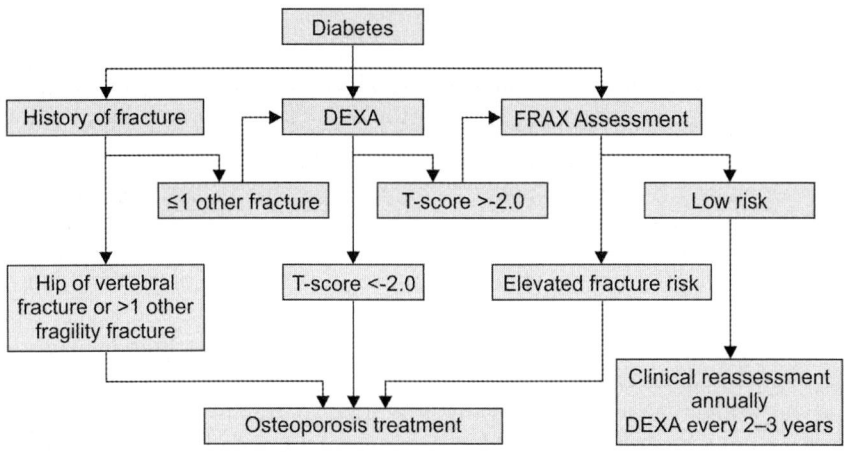

(FRAX: fracture risk assessment tool; DEXA: dual energy x-ray absorptiometry)
**FLOWCHART 2:** Algorithm for management of osteoporosis in diabetes.

may also underestimate the fracture risk in individuals with diabetes.[33] Markers of bone resorption (CTX) and bone formation (P1NP) may be useful but are not used in routine.

## Pharmacological Management of Osteoporosis

Consider pharmacological treatment when BMD T-score <-2.5 at spine or hip in postmenopausal women or men >50 years. Since BMD may underestimate the risk,

T-score cut-off of <-2.0 has been suggested.[37] Decline in BMD in subsequent visits (>5% over 2 years) should also be considered. Trabecular bone score (TBS) measured in DEXA may provide more information of fracture risk in individuals with diabetes.

Trials have not specifically evaluated the efficacy of antiosteoporotic medications in individuals with diabetes. Subgroup analysis of individuals with diabetes from intervention trials for osteoporosis suggests that the effects of antiosteoporotic drugs are not different in individuals with diabetes compared to those without diabetes.[37] Bisphosphonates remain the first-choice agents for osteoporosis management. Denosumab may be preferred in elderly and those with renal impairment. However, as bone turnover is low in diabetes, it is uncertain if antiresorptive therapies have less efficacy. Teriparatide is a bone-forming agent and may be more useful.

## Impact of Antiosteoporosis Drugs on Glycemic Control

Bisphosphonates are believed to be largely neutral with regards to their impact on glycemic control.[34] Small studies have not documented any impact of denosumab on insulin resistance and HbA1c.[34] Teriparatide is also believed to be largely glycemic neutral. Raloxifene has been linked to mild increase in insulin resistance without any impact on glycemic parameters.

## CONCLUSION

Fractures are consistently increased in both T1DM and T2DM. Several mechanisms contribute to increased fracture risk in diabetes including the effect of hyperglycemia, microvascular complications, reduced muscle mass, effect of medications, and increased risk of falls. Diabetes is associated with reduced bone quality with microarchitectural deterioration that is disproportionate to the change in BMD. Presence of comorbidities like chronic kidney disease, chronic liver disease, coronary artery disease, heart failure, and cerebrovascular disease compound this risk through direct and indirect effects on BMD, bone quality, and extraskeletal factors. Data is extremely scant on the long-term impact of optimal glycemic control on bone health. In the absence of specific studies, general guidelines for osteoporosis management are suggested when treating individuals with diabetes, with the understanding that BMD and FRAX scores may somewhat underestimate the risk in them. There is an urgent need for long-term studies focusing on evaluation and changes in bone mineral quality rather than an isolated focus on BMD in people living with diabetes. Future research should also focus on the development of glucose-lowering drugs that may have positive effects on bone health.

## REFERENCES

1. Shanbhogue VV, Hansen S, Frost M, et al. Bone disease in diabetes: another manifestation of microvascular disease? Lancet Diabetes Endocrinol. 2017;5(10):827-38.
2. Vestergaard P, Rejnmark L, Mosekilde L. Relative fracture risk in patients with diabetes mellitus, and the impact of insulin and oral antidiabetic medication on relative fracture risk. Diabetologia. 2005;48(7):1292-9.
3. Ahmed LA, Joakimsen RM, Berntsen GK, et al. Diabetes mellitus and the risk of non-vertebral fractures. the Tromsø study. Osteoporos Int. 2006;17(4):495-500.

4. Seeley DG, Kelsey J, Jergas M, et al. Predictors of ankle and foot fractures in older women: the Study of Osteoporotic Fractures Research Group. J Bone Miner Res. 1996;11(9):1347-55.
5. Keenan HA, Maddaloni E. Bone Microarchitecture in Type 1 Diabetes: It Is Complicated. Curr Osteoporos Rep. 2016;14(6):351-8.
6. Sundararaghavan V, Mazur MM, Evans B, et al. Diabetes and bone health: latest evidence and clinical implications. Ther Adv Musculoskelet Dis. 2017;9(3):67-74.
7. Vestergaard P. Discrepancies in bone mineral density and fracture risk in patients with type 1 and type 2 diabetes: a meta-analysis. Osteoporos Int. 2007;18(4):427-44.
8. Janghorbani M, Van Dam RM, Willett WC, et al. Systematic review of type 1 and type 2 diabetes mellitus and risk of fracture. Am J Epidemiol. 2007;166(5):495-505.
9. Strotmeyer ES, Cauley JA, Schwartz AV, et al. Nontraumatic fracture risk in type 2 diabetes mellitus and impaired fasting glucose in older white and black adults: the health, aging and body composition study. Arch Intern Med. 2005;165(14):1612-7.
10. Bonds DE, Larson JC, Schwartz AV, et al. Risk of fracture in women with type 2 diabetes mellitus: the Women's Health Initiative observational study. J Clin Endocrinol Metab. 2006;91(9):3404-10.
11. Janghorbani M, Feskanich D, Willett WC, et al. Prospective study of diabetes and risk of hip fracture. The Nurses' Health Study. Diabetes Care. 2006;29(7):1573-8.
12. Ma L, Oei L, Jiang L, et al. Association between bone mineral density and type 2 diabetes mellitus: a meta-analysis of observational studies. Eur J Epidemiol 2012;27(5):319-32.
13. Dutta MK, Pakhetra R, Garg MK. Evaluation of BMD in type 2 diabetes mellitus before and after treatment. Medical Journal of Armed Forces India. 2012;68(1):48-52.
14. Schwartz AV, Sellmeyer DE, Strotmeyer ES, et al. Diabetes and bone loss at the hip in older black and white adults. J Bone Miner Res. 2005;20(4):596-603.
15. Strotmeyer ES, Cauley JA, Schwartz AV, et al. Diabetes is associated independently of body composition with BMD and bone volume in older white and black men and women: the Health, Aging, and Body Composition Study. J Bone Miner Res. 2004;19(7):1084-91.
16. Lecka-Czernik B. Diabetes, bone and glucose-lowering agents: basic biology. Diabetologia. 2017;60(7):1163-9.
17. Katayama Y, Akatsu T, Yamamoto M, et al. Role of nonenzymatic glycosylation of type I collagen in diabetic osteopenia. J Bone Miner Res 1996;11(7):921-37.
18. Ogawa N, Yamaguchi T, Yano S, et al. The combination of high glucose and advanced glycation end-products (AGEs) inhibits the mineralization of osteoblastic MC3T3-E1 cells through glucose-induced increase in the receptor for AGEs. Horm Metab Res. 2007;39(12):871-5.
19. Saito M, Marumo K. Collagen cross-links as a determinant of bone quality: a possible explanation for bone fragility in aging, osteoporosis, and diabetes mellitus. Osteoporos Int. 2010;21(2):195-214.
20. McCarthy AD, Etcheverry SB, Cortizo AM. Effect of advanced glycation end products on the secretion of insulin-like growth factor-I and its binding proteins: role in osteoblast development. Acta Diabetol. 2001;38(3):113-22.
21. Ivers RQ, Cumming RG, Mitchell P, et al. Diabetes and risk of fracture: The Blue Mountains Eye Study. Diabetes Care 2001;24(7):1198-203.
22. Lan-Juan Zhao, Yong-Jun Liu, Peng-Yuan Liu, et al. Relationship of Obesity with Osteoporosis. J Clin Endocrinol Metab. 2007;92(5):1640-6.
23. Russell M, Mendes N, Miller KK, et al. Visceral Fat Is a Negative Predictor of Bone Density Measures in Obese Adolescent Girls. J Clin Endocrinol Metab. 2010;95(3):1247-55.
24. Akune T, Ohba S, Kamekura S, et al. PPAR-γ insufficiency enhances osteogenesis through osteoblast formation from bone marrow progenitors. J Clin Invest. 2004;113(6):846-55.
25. Rolland Y, Czerwinski S, Abellan Van Kan C, et al. Sarcopenia: its assessment, etiology, pathogenesis, consequences and future perspectives. J Nutr Health Aging. 2008;12(7):433-50.
26. Maisnam I, Dutta D, Mukhopadhyay S, et al. Lean mass is the strongest predictor of bone mineral content in type-2 diabetes and normal individuals: an eastern India perspective. J Diabetes Metab Disord. 2014;13(1):90.
27. Biswas D, Dutta D, Maisnam I, et al. Occurrence of osteoporosis & factors determining bone mineral loss in young adults with Graves' disease. Indian J Med Res. 2015;141(3):322-9.
28. Dutta D, Sharma M, Bansal R, et al. Low skeletal mass is an important predictor of osteoporosis in HIV-infected men in India. Endokrynol Pol. 2017;68(6):642-51.

29. Sharma M, Dhakad U, Wakhlu A, et al. Lean Mass and Disease Activity are the Best Predictors of Bone Mineral Loss in the Premenopausal Women with Rheumatoid Arthritis. Indian J Endocrinol Metab. 2018;22(2):236-43.
30. Dutta D, Garga UC, Gadpayle AK, et al. Occurrence & predictors of osteoporosis & impact of body composition alterations on bone mineral health in asymptomatic pre-menopausal women with HIV infection. Indian J Med Res. 2018;147(5):484-95.
31. Dutta D, Maisnam I, Shrivastava A, et al. Serum vitamin-D predicts insulin resistance in individuals with prediabetes. Indian J Med Res. 2013;138(6):853-60.
32. Powe CE, Evans MK, Wenger J, et al. Vitamin D-binding protein and vitamin D status of black Americans and white Americans. N Engl J Med. 2013;369(21):1991-2000.
33. Vianna AGD, Sanches CP, Barreto FC. Review article: effects of type 2 diabetes therapies on bone metabolism. Diabetol Metab Syndr. 2017;9:75.
34. Paschou SA, Dede AD, Anagnostis PG, et al. Type 2 Diabetes and Osteoporosis: A Guide to Optimal Management. J Clin Endocrinol Metab. 2017;102(10):3621-34.
35. Blevins TC, Farooki A. Bone effects of canagliflozin, a sodium glucose cotransporter 2 inhibitor, in patients with type 2 diabetes mellitus. Postgrad Med. 2017;129(1):159-68.
36. Dutta D, Khandelwal D. Sodium glucose transporter 2 inhibition, euglycemic ketosis and bone mineral loss: Refining clinical practices. Indian J Endocrinol Metab. 2015;19(6):854-5.
37. Ferrari SL, Abrahamsen B, Napoli N, et al. Bone and Diabetes Working Group of IOF. Diagnosis and management of bone fragility in diabetes: an emerging challenge. Osteoporos Int. 2018;29(12): 2585-96.

# CHAPTER 21

# Sexual Dysfunction in Diabetes

*Sunil K Kota, Sambit Das, S Abbas Raza*

## INTRODUCTION

Diabetes has a significant impact on an individual's biopsychosocial health. While the focus of diabetes care remains optimal glycemic and metabolic control and the reduction of microvascular and macrovascular complications, diabetes has ramifications on the endocrine health of an individual. In particular, diabetes and its comorbidities affect reproductive function and sexual health.

Diabetes mellitus is one of the most common chronic diseases growing at epidemic proportions, with an expected rise to 552 million by 2030.[1] Overweight, obesity, physical inactivity and increased caloric consumption are all responsible for this rising trend of type 2 diabetes mellitus (T2DM). Both men and women face disruptions in their sexual function as a comorbidity in diabetes, which are often attributed both to psychological stress and end organ damage.[2]

Sexual health is important both in males and females. A normal sex life is an important contributor to physical, mental, emotional and psychosocial well-being, and interpersonal relationships. Hyperglycemia in diabetes and its associated comorbidities, including overweight and obesity, smoking, hypertension, and atherogenic dyslipidemia, are major risk factors for sexual dysfunction in diabetes.[2] With increasing age and longer duration of disease, sexual dysfunction manifests in a large majority of individuals with diabetes. It has far-reaching impact on psychological health and interpersonal relationships and can result in significantly impaired quality of life.[2] Various types of sexual disorders are encountered in individuals with diabetes including disorders in desire, arousal, orgasm and pain. Men with diabetes have a 3-fold increased risk of erectile dysfunction (ED) compared with nondiabetic men. Sometimes ED may be the presenting symptom for diabetes and may be a marker of underlying cardiovascular disease (CVD) and a predictor of later onset of neurologic sequelae. In women, the association between diabetes and sexual dysfunction is less evident, but equally important.

In this chapter, we discuss facets of endovigilance in diabetes care, pertaining to sexual health and sexual dysfunction.

## SEXUAL RESPONSE CYCLE

The normal sexual response cycle has four phases including desire, arousal, orgasm and resolution.[3] Both men and women experience these phases, although with different timing. There is interpersonal variation in terms of intensity of the response and the duration each phase.

### Phase 1 (Desire/Excitement)

It consists of three components: (1) sexual drive, (2) sexual motivation, and (3) sexual wish. These are reflective of biological, psychological and social aspects of desire, respectively. It lasts from a few minutes to several hours; sexual drive is produced through psychoneuroendocrine mechanisms via the limbic system and the preoptic area of the anterior-medial hypothalamus. It consists of several changes like increase in muscle tone, heart rate and breathing, flushed skin (red blotches on chest and back), hard nipples, increased blood flow to genitals leading to erection of penis and swelling of woman's clitoris, vaginal wall and labia minora, fuller breasts in females with vaginal lubrication, swelling of testicles with tight scrotum, and secretion of a lubricating fluid. The sexual drive is also influenced by hormones, medications (e.g. increased by dopaminergic medications and decreased by certain antihypertensive drugs like methyldopa and clonidine, nonselective beta-adrenergic blockers, thiazide and potassium-sparing diuretics, medications used to treat Parkinson's disease), and substance abuse drugs (e.g. cocaine, alcohol).

### Phase 2 (Arousal/Plateau)

It is mediated by both physiological and psychological stimulation. This is a phase of vasocongestion preparing individuals for orgasm. The changes in phase 1 are intensified. In men, increased blood flow causes erection, penile color changes and testicular elevation. Vasocongestion in women leads to swollen and dark purple vaginal wall, vaginal lubrication, clitoral tumescence and hypersensitivity to touch, and labial color changes. In general, heart rate, blood pressure and respiratory rate as well as myotonia of many muscle groups in hands, feet and face are noted with muscle spasms.

### Phase 3 (Orgasm)

It is the climax of the sexual response cycle and it lasts only a few seconds. It manifests in the form of ongoing increase in respiratory rate, heart rate, blood pressure and muscle tone with rapid intake of oxygen, and appearance of sex flush or rash over entire body. There is voluntary and involuntary contraction of many muscle groups. In men, ejaculation is perpetuated by the contraction of the muscles at base of penis, urethra, vas deferens, seminal vesicles and prostate. In women, the uterus and lower third of the vagina contract involuntarily. Ultimately there is a forceful and sudden release of tension.

## Phase 4 (Resolution)

It is purely dependent on the achievement of orgasm. If orgasm is not achieved, irritability and discomfort can result, potentially lasting for several hours. If orgasm is achieved, resolution may last 10–15 minutes with a sense of calm and relaxation. The body slowly returns to its normal level of functioning. Respiratory rate, heart rate, blood pressure and muscle tone return to baseline. There is diminution of vasocongestion with swollen and erect body parts returning to their previous size and color. Men need recovery time after orgasm, labeled as refractory period, during which they cannot reach orgasm again. The duration of the refractory period varies among men and usually lengthens with advancing age. Women can have multiple successive orgasms secondary to a lack of a refractory period.

## SEXUAL DYSFUNCTION IN MEN WITH DIABETES

Diabetes is one of the most important causes of sexual dysfunction in men. The main types of male sexual dysfunction include:[4]
- Low libido (diminished sexual desire/interest)
- Erectile dysfunction (difficulty in achieving or maintaining an erection)
- Premature ejaculation (reaching sexual climax or orgasm too quickly)
- Delayed or inhibited orgasm
- Physical abnormalities of the penis.

### Low Libido/Sexual Desire

There are two types of sexual desire disorders—hypoactive sexual desire disorder (HSDD) and sexual aversion disorder (SAD). Diagnostic and Statistical Manual of Mental Disorders—4th Edition (DSM-IV)-TR defines HSDD as "persistently or recurrently deficient (or absent) sexual fantasies and desire for sexual activity." The clinician can make an assessment of deficiency or absence based on factors affecting sexual functioning including age and the context of the person's life. On the other hand, SAD is defined as "persistent or recurrent extreme aversion to, and avoidance of, all (or almost all) genital sexual contact with a sexual partner."[3]

### Epidemiology

The prevalence of low libido is underestimated. The National Health and Social Life Survey of people between 18 and 59 years age, found that 15% men and 32% women lacked sexual interest for several months within the last year. SAD on the other hand is not that common. Both these disorders are found more commonly in women, with greater discrepancy being seen for SAD.

### Etiopathogenesis

It can be a functional issue, may be due to sexual identity reasons or stagnation in sexual growth. From a psychodynamic perspective, sexual dysfunction is caused by unresolved unconscious conflicts of early development. Diabetes and associated obesity, hypogonadism, obstructive sleep apnea, coronary artery disease, heart failure, renal failure, stroke and chronic infections can play a role. Many psychiatric medications can give rise to decreased sexual desire including antidepressants (selective serotonin reuptake inhibitors, norepinephrine serotonin reuptake inhibitors, tricyclic antidepressants, monoamine oxidase inhibitors) and antipsychotics.

## Diagnosis

There is difficulty in diagnosis and treatment of desire disorders because of confounding factors like comorbidities and combined subtype sexual disorders due to medical and substance-induced contributors. When assessing libido, many studies use the sexual desire (SD) domain of the International Index of Erectile Function (IIEF), i.e. IIEF-SD, which asks men about two libido-related questions: "Over the past 4 weeks, how often have you felt sexual desire?" and "Over the past 4 weeks, how would you rate your level of sexual desire?" The IIEF-SD questions can be used to diagnose mild, mild-to-moderate, moderate and severe dysfunction.[3] The Sexual Arousal, Interest and Drive (SAID) scale is another well-validated tool with patient reported outcomes, which measures and scores 5 items including sexual thought, arousal, interest and drive.[5] Serum testosterone should also be measured when evaluating these individuals as low testosterone affects desire. Normal physiological testosterone concentration ranges from 3 to 12 ng/mL. The apparent critical level for sexual function in males is 3 ng/mL.

## Nonpharmacological Treatment

Several nonpharmacological, psychological approaches have been used for the management of disorders of sexual desire/arousal

- *Psychotherapy:* This approach focuses on bringing awareness to unresolved conflicts and how they impact an individual's life. Even if there is an improvement, the sexual dysfunction often becomes persistent and autonomous, calling for implementation of additional techniques
- *Dual sex therapy by Masters and Johnson:* In this therapy, the couple along with one male and one female therapist (gay and lesbian couples may opt for same-sex therapists) meet together. And various steps of sexual act are enacted under the supervision of therapist
- *Cognitive behavioral therapy:* It is efficacious in the treatment of comorbid anxiety, depression, and other psychiatric disorders. Finally, analytically oriented sex therapy combines sex therapy with psychodynamic and psychoanalytic therapy and has shown good results.

## Pharmacological Treatment

Androgen supplementation in the form of intramuscular injections is a well-validated treatment for men with documented hypogonadism. Androgens are also available in many forms, including oral, sublingual, cream and dermal patch. It improves sexual desire in men with hypogonadism, but its role in men with normal hypothalamic-pituitary-gonadal (HPG) axis function is questionable.[5]

## Erectile Dysfunction

Erectile dysfunction is one of the most important, most researched and well-documented sexual dysfunctions in men with diabetes. ED is defined as a persistent inability to attain or maintain penile erection for sexual intercourse to be successful.[4]

### Epidemiology

According to the International Consultation Committee for Sexual Medicine on Definitions/Epidemiology/Risk Factors for Sexual Dysfunction, the prevalence of ED was 1–10% among men <40 years age, 2–9% in men aged 40–49 years; while the prevalence in men between 60 and 69 years and >70 years was 20–40% and 50–100%, respectively.[6] As per the Massachusetts Male Aging Study, men with diabetes showed a 3-fold increased probability of ED and 2-fold increase in age-adjusted risk of ED.[7] Men with diabetes tend to develop ED a decade earlier, which is more severe and is less responsive to oral medications with resultant decreased quality of life.[4] The worldwide prevalence of ED is estimated to rise to 322 million cases by 2025.[8] As per various longitudinal and cross-sectional studies, there is a strong association between cardiovascular (CV) risk factors and ED including diabetes, hypertension, dyslipidemia, smoking, sedentary lifestyle, metabolic syndrome, autonomic neuropathy, depression, poor health state and lower urinary tract symptoms.[2] Additionally, the presence of ED is associated with a significantly increased risk of CVD like stroke, coronary heart disease (CHD), and all-cause mortality.

### Etiopathogenesis

There is a multifactorial pathophysiology of ED in diabetes, consisting of hormonal, vascular and neurologic insults. Diabetic neuropathy may disrupt autonomic and somatic nerve functions essential for erection. There may be impairment of sensory impulses from penis to reflexogenic erectile center with reduced parasympathetic activity necessary for relaxation of corpus cavernosum smooth muscles.[2] Endothelial dysfunction in diabetes results in decreased bioavailability of nitric oxide (NO). Endothelial dysfunction can be due to accumulation of advanced glycation end products; impaired endothelial and neuronal NO synthesis, expression and activity; and increased levels of oxygen-free radicals that reduce the bioavailability of NO. It results in an imbalance between vasorelaxant and vasoconstrictive tone, ultimately favoring vasoconstriction. In overweight and obese men with diabetes, visceral adiposity-induced insulin resistance leads to a proinflammatory state resulting in decreased availability and activity of NO.

An increased risk of hypogonadism in diabetes with associated low serum testosterone levels further aggravates the problem.[9] Low testosterone reduces sexual desire and can lead to ED. The mechanisms of hypogonadism in diabetes include insulin resistance-mediated low levels of sex hormone-binding globulin (SHBG); increased aromatase activity in visceral adipose tissue with enhanced conversion of testosterone to estradiol; leptin resistance-mediated decreased secretion of luteinizing hormone (LH) and testosterone; increased inflammation with resultant suppression of gonadotropin-releasing hormone (GnRH) and LH; and the presence of antipituitary antibodies in men with diabetes.[2]

Presence of microvascular and macrovascular complications and endothelial dysfunction in diabetic men increases the risk of ED. Macrovascular disease manifests in the form of atherosclerotic damage in blood vessels reducing the penile blood flow. Concomitant intake of some medications including antihypertensive drugs (β-blockers, thiazides and spironolactone), antidepressants, and certain fibrates also have a deleterious effect on erectile function.[2] A moderate consumption of alcohol (≤7 alcoholic drinks per week and not more than 5% of the total daily caloric intake) may exert a protective effect on ED.[2]

## Diagnosis

Erectile dysfunction is diagnosed by questionnaires like International Index of Erectile Function-5 (IIEF-ED-5); a sum score ≤21 is indicative of the presence of ED.[1] The other assessments include questions regarding the patient's ability to penetrate (Sexual Encounter Profile 2 or SEP2) and have successful intercourse (SEP3), and a global assessment question (GAQ).

A complete workup requires evaluation of morning serum total testosterone (8-10 AM); SHBG and albumin levels to assess free and bioavailable testosterone; pituitary hormones (LH, follicle-stimulating hormone or FSH and prolactin).[10] Symptoms of hypogonadism may manifest at total testosterone levels less than 320 ng/dL and free testosterone levels <64 pg/mL.[10] One low value of total testosterone should be reconfirmed by repeat testing. Only the group of patients with low testosterone and symptoms pertinent to hypogonadism (weight gain, anxiety, fatigability, decreased libido, ED, depressed mood, decreased energy and decreased bone mineral density) with no apparent existence of other causes should be candidates for treatment.[5]

## Lifestyle Modification

Lifestyle changes including reduced caloric intake, a Mediterranean-style diet, and an increased physical activity lead to improvement of erectile function in the general male population. Healthy diet and physical exercise-mediated weight loss lead to amelioration of endothelial dysfunction, insulin-resistance, and the resultant inflammatory state due to diabetes and metabolic diseases.[1]

## Pharmacological Treatment

Pharmacological management consists of optimal metabolic control and medications targeting ED directly.
- *Glycemic control*: Optimal glycemic control improves erectile function. The Epidemiology of Diabetes Intervention and Complication (EDIC) Study demonstrated that with intensive therapy, there was a significant reduction in ED among men with diabetes for ≥10 years and microvascular complications, compared to those with a shorter duration of diabetes (1-5 years) and without complications.[11] However, the results have been conflicting in men with T2DM with regard to the impact of risk reduction interventions on ED
- *Phosphodiesterase type 5 (PDE5) inhibitors*: These are mainstay of treatment of ED. Worldwide sildenafil, vardenafil and tadalafil are commercially available; while udenafil and mirodenafil are used only in Korea. They act through the

nitric oxide/cyclic guanosine monophosphate (NO/cGMP) pathway. Sexual stimulation provokes the release of NO from cavernous nerves and endothelial cells. NO activates guanylate cyclase, which transforms guanosine triphosphate (GTP) to cGMP and triggers decreased intracellular calcium with subsequent relaxation of actin/myosin cross bridges and penile smooth muscle relaxation. Penile PDE5 mediates the conversion and deactivation of cGMP to Guanosine 5'-monophosphate.[12] PDE5 inhibitors block the inactivation of cGMP, leading to continuously elevated cGMP levels with resultant persistent smooth muscle relaxation. These drugs vary with respect to their time to onset and duration of action, but they show the same efficacy and safety profile in individuals with diabetes. Overall, men with diabetes have a somewhat poorer response to PDE5 inhibitors than men with ED of other etiologies. This is because of neuropathy and endothelial disease in diabetes that blunt the release of both neuronal and endothelial NO synthase.[12]

A randomized, placebo controlled trial, involving 268 men with diabetes and ED, demonstrated a dose-dependent improvement in erection in 56% of patients taking sildenafil compared with 10% of those in the placebo group.[13] In two different placebo-controlled multicenter studies, vardenafil 10 and 20 mg resulted in improvement in erection in 57% and 72% men, respectively compared to 13% men with placebo; and tadalafil 10 and 20 mg was associated with improved erections in and 56% and 64% of men, respectively in comparison with improvements in 25% among those in the control arms.[9,10]

Coronary heart disease is not an absolute contraindication for PDE5 inhibitors. But in patients with poorly controlled hypertension, unstable and severe angina pectoris, recent myocardial infarction, concomitant use of nitrates or nitrate donors and certain arrhythmias, particular caution has to be paid. Individuals with diabetes and underlying CVD should undergo detailed CV examination before initiating PDE5 inhibitor therapy[12]

- *Direct administration of vasodilators to the erectile tissue of the penis:* Commonly used agents include papaverine, phentolamine and prostaglandin E-1 (PGE1). Combinations of these agents are often used to reduce the adverse effects of each specific agent. Only PGE1 is approved by US-Food and Drug Administration (FDA). In a study of 300 men with intracavernosal PGE1 injection therapy in diabetics, 79% required ≤30 µg/dose and 72% remained satisfied with the initial dose during the 6 months follow-up period. The side effects included penile pain, penile nodule and priapism. A smaller study with 10 years follow-up demonstrated that men with diabetes tended to shift toward stronger agents (combination of alprostadil with papaverine and/or phentolamine), with decreased frequency of use. Men with type 1 diabetes mellitus (T1DM) stabilized their doses within 5 years and those with T2DM stabilized within 9–10 years[14]
- *Intraurethral administration of prostaglandin*: Medicated Urethral Suppository for Erections (MUSE®), a urethral prostaglandin suppository, is approved by US-FDA. Their side effects include urethral burning, pain and irritation of the sexual partner's mucous membranes[14]
- *Vacuum erection devices*: These may be useful in patients for whom injection or intraurethral therapy does not work. Possible local side effects include petechiae, a

feeling of having a cold penis, suboptimal erectile rigidity, and abnormal sensation of ejaculation[14]

- *Penile prosthetics*: These are the best alternative, when there is lack of efficacy or dissatisfaction with other modalities. Most contemporary prostheses are either hollow silicone cylinders that are inflated with saline via pump action or semirigid rods.[14] Prostheses have the highest satisfaction rates amongst all the modalities for treatment of ED with 95% satisfaction. The risk of prosthesis-related infections does not seem to be higher in men with diabetes. However, this is an irreversible surgery, where corporal tissue is permanently altered in a way that physiologic erections are no longer possible
- *Androgen replacement therapy*: Men with low levels of testosterone and symptoms of hypogonadism benefit from testosterone replacement therapy.[5] In addition to improvement of sexual dysfunction in men with hypogonadism, testosterone replacement is also associated with improved lean body mass and insulin sensitivity in men with diabetes and hypogonadism.[5] A variety of different testosterone formulations are available, including intramuscular injections, transdermal creams/gels, subcutaneous depots, and buccal tablets.

## Ejaculatory Dysfunction

Men with diabetes can also present with lack of ejaculation with sexual climax (anejaculation or retrograde ejaculation) and premature ejaculation. A coordination of three neurologic events gives rise to a successful antegrade ejaculation—seminal emission, bladder neck closure, and contraction of muscles of the pelvic floor (e.g. bulbocavernosus, ischiocavernosus, etc.).[15] In diabetic neuropathy, derangements of the nerves coordinating closure of the connection between the bladder and urethra may hamper normal ejaculation. Here the ejaculate is deposited in the innermost urethral portion of the urethra but there is no closure of connection between the bladder and urethra. Since the bladder neck is open, the ejaculate may revert backwards into the bladder during the muscle contractions that normally expel the semen from the penis. There may be total lack of seminal emission in most severe cases. This will have impact on fertility with other consequences and lack of full orgasmic enjoyment. Pharmacologic agents like anticholinergics, antihistamines and alpha-adrenergic agonists are used for treatment to close the bladder neck.[15] For fertility purpose, sperm may be retrieved from postejaculate urine and used for artificial insemination.

## FEMALE SEXUAL DYSFUNCTION

Diabetes has multifactorial detrimental effects on both psychological and physiological dimensions of female sexual function. Women may have hypoactive sexual desire, sexual pain disorder/dyspareunia, genital arousal or lubrication disorder, and orgasmic disorder.[16] As per newer and revised definitions by DSM-V, the sexual desire and arousal disorders have been grouped into the "female sexual interest/arousal disorder" category; whereas, vaginismus and dyspareunia have been combined into "genito-pelvic pain/penetration disorder" category.[17] Additionally, all of the sexual dysfunctions outlined in the DSM-V require minimum 6 months duration, and more precise severity criteria must be adhered to, in order to provide useful thresholds for making a diagnosis and for distinguishing transient sexual difficulties from more persistent sexual dysfunction.

## Epidemiology

Both T1DM and T2DM are associated with female sexual dysfunction (FSD). A recent meta-analysis of 26 trials consisting of 3,168 women with diabetes and 2,823 controls demonstrated that FSD is more frequent, and is associated with a lower Female Sexual Function Index (FSFI) score in women with diabetes than in controls.[18] In women with T1DM or T2DM, the odds ratio for risk of FSD was 2.27 [95% confidence interval (CI): 1.23–4.16] and 2.49 (95% CI: 1.55–3.99), respectively. Furthermore, when "any diabetes" (representing the two forms of diabetes together) is considered, the odds ratio for risk of FSD was 2.02 (CI: 1.49–2.72).

## Etiopathogenesis

The normal female sexual response needs the integrity of the sensory and autonomic nervous systems responding to erotic stimuli and the vasculature of external genitalia and vagina. The enhancement of genital blood flow and smooth muscle are dependent on the action of nonadrenergic/noncholinergic neurotransmitters, such as vasoactive intestinal polypeptide (VIP) and NO, as that in males. Diabetes may affect these integrated systems, leading to sexual dysfunction. The mechanisms described include hyperglycemia, infections, vascular and neurological damage, and hormonal disorders.[19]

Hyperglycemia reduces the hydration of the vaginal mucus membranes and increases the risk of genitourinary infections. The vascular and nerve dysfunction in diabetes may impair the sexual response by structural and functional changes in female genitalia such as impaired relaxation response of the vaginal tissue; reduced nerve-stimulated clitoral and vaginal blood flow; diffuse fibrosis of the clitoris and vaginal tissue; and reduction of the muscular layer and epithelial thickness in vagina.[19] Endothelial dysfunction and atherosclerotic damage may also be responsible for reducing clitoral engorgement and vaginal lubrication leading to decreased arousal and dyspareunia during sexual intercourse. Diabetic neuropathy may alter the normal transduction of sexual stimuli, thereby diminishing the triggered sexual response.[19]

Alterations in the levels of androgens, estrogens and SHBG can also contribute to FSD. Moreover, several associated endocrinopathies like thyroid disorders, polycystic ovary syndrome, and hypothalamic–pituitary dysfunction may further give rise to FSD.[1] Long-term complications of diabetes may also affect quality of life, health and relationship status, and a woman's self-image, generating a vicious cycle having detrimental effects on sexual performance and satisfaction.[16]

The common risk factors associated with FSD include aging, duration of diabetes, microvascular complications, obesity, hypertension, CVD, genitourinary disease, psychological disorders, depression, menopause, cancer, and other chronic diseases.[1] Limited social relations, cultural factors, employment status, financial difficulties, educational background, religious beliefs and lack of exercise represent the sociocultural risk factors of FSD.

## Treatment of Female Sexual Dysfunction

Therapeutic options for sexual dysfunction in women with diabetes include lifestyle changes, optimized diabetes management, psychotherapy, and selected medications when appropriate.

### Nonpharmacological Treatment

Individuals should adopt a healthy lifestyle with focus on adequate and balanced nutrition and increased physical activity. Psychological issues such as diabetes distress should be adequately addressed and depression, if present, should be clearly identified and managed. The Look AHEAD Sexual Dysfunction Ancillary study evaluated 229 sexually active women with T2DM and FSD. Intensive lifestyle intervention for 1 year was associated with significant improvement in the total FSFI scores across most of the FSFI domains. Additionally, they were more likely to experience a resolution in FSD, as compared with those in the control group (diabetes support and education group).[20] A multicenter randomized controlled trial of intensive lifestyle intervention in obese women with T2DM confirmed that women in the intervention group were more likely to: (1) remain sexually active at 1 year (83% vs. 64% for the intervention vs. control group, respectively); (2) improve specific domains of sexual function; and (3) obtain composite scores on the FSFI that were consistent with low risk for sexual dysfunction (28% of intervention patients vs. 11% of controls).[19] Further, optimized glycemic control reduces the risk of genitourinary infections and long-term micro- and macrovascular complications.

### Pharmacological Treatment

At present, transdermal or oral androgen replacement therapy is not approved by US-FDA for FSD; whereas for postmenopausal women, hormone replacement therapy is approved. PDE5 inhibitors acting via NO-mediated smooth muscle relaxation to increase vasodilatation might theoretically improve vaginal lubrication and vulvar engorgement. In a study of 28 women with T1DM, 100 mg sildenafil resulted in significant improvement in both subjective and objective parameters. Subjectively, arousal, orgasm and dyspareunia were improved in those taking sildenafil in comparison to baseline and compared to those taking placebo. Color Doppler ultrasonography revealed an increase in blood flow in clitoral arteries.[21] However, only few successes have been reported for the use of these agents, likely due to the inconsistencies observed between the physiological and psychological factors on sexual response or the low PDE5 levels noted in female reproductive system.

## CONCLUSION

Individuals with diabetes commonly have sexual dysfunction which can arise from a variety of neurological, vascular and hormonal derangements. The determinants of sexual dysfunction include glycemic control, age, duration of diabetes, psychological issues and CV risk factors, such as hypertension, dyslipidemia, overweight and obesity, metabolic syndrome, smoking and a sedentary lifestyle. Sexual problems related to diabetes also include reduced sexual desire, ED and ejaculatory dysfunction in men and a variety of sexual concerns in women. ED is seen in approximately 50% of men with T1DM or T2DM. ED/sexual dysfunction could also be the herald of vascular complications in diabetes. Significant ED is associated with diabetic retinopathy and increased CV morbidity. It would be wise on the part of diabetes care practitioners to screen for other complications, including retinopathy evaluation and CV assessment if ED is present. A detailed endocrine work-up including evaluation for hypogonadism and psychological assessment can help guide therapeutic choices.

Phosphodiesterase type 5 inhibitors are the first-choice agents in the management of ED although the failure rate is higher when compared to men who do not have diabetes. Second and third line options may be considered in case of PDE5 inhibitor failure. In addition to specific therapy aimed for various sexual concerns, management of underlying diabetes, and proper lifestyle modification would significantly improve sexual quality of life in people with diabetes.

## REFERENCES

1. Wild S, Roglic G, Green A, et al. Global prevalence of diabetes: Estimates for the year 2000 and projections for 2030. Diabetes Care. 2004;27:1047-53.
2. Maiorino MI, Bellastella G, Esposito K. Diabetes and sexual dysfunction: Current perspectives. Diabetes Metab Syndr Obes. 2014;7:95-105.
3. Montgomery KA. Sexual desire disorders. Psychiatry (Edgmont). 2008;5:50-5.
4. Kalra S, Balhara YS, Baruah M, et al. Consensus guidelines on male sexual dysfunction. J Med Nutr Nutraceut. 2013;2:5-18.
5. Rizk PJ, Kohn TP, Pastuszak AW, et al. Testosterone therapy improves erectile function and libido in hypogonadal men. Curr Opin Urol. 2017;27:511-5.
6. Lewis RW, Fugl-Meyer KS, Corona G, et al. Definitions/epidemiology/risk factors for sexual dysfunction. J Sex Med. 2010;7(4 Pt 2):1598-607.
7. Johannes CB, Araujo AB, Feldman HA, et al. Incidence of erectile dysfunction in men 40 to 69 years old: Longitudinal results from the Massachusetts male aging study. J Urol. 2000;163:460-3.
8. Ayta IA, McKinlay JB, Krane RJ. The likely worldwide increase in erectile dysfunction between 1995 and 2025 and some possible policy consequences. BJU Int. 1999;84(1):50-6.
9. Kapoor D, Clarke S, Channer KS, et al. Erectile dysfunction is associated with low bioactive testosterone levels and visceral adiposity in men with type 2 diabetes. Int J Androl. 2007;30(6):500-7.
10. Bhasin S, Cunningham GR, Hayes FJ, et al. Testosterone therapy in men with androgen deficiency syndromes: An Endocrine Society clinical practice guideline. J Clin Endocrinol Metab. 2010;95:2536-59.
11. Wessells H, Penson DF, Cleary P, et al. Effect of intensive glycemic therapy on erectile function in men with type 1 diabetes. J Urol. 2011;185(5):1828-34.
12. Gandhi J, Dagur G, Warren K, et al. The role of diabetes mellitus in sexual and reproductive health: An overview of pathogenesis, evaluation, and management. Curr Diabetes Rev. 2017;13(6):573-81.
13. Saenz de Tejada I, Goldstein I, Azadzoi K, et al. Impaired neurogenic and endothelium-mediated relaxation of penile smooth muscle from diabetic men with impotence. N Engl J Med. 1989;320(16):1025-30.
14. Nehra A, Jackson G, Miner M, et al. The Princeton III Consensus recommendations for the management of erectile dysfunction and cardiovascular disease. Mayo Clin Proc. 2012;87(8):766-78.
15. Clement P, Giuliano F. Physiology and pharmacology of ejaculation. Basic Clin Pharmacol Toxicol. 2016;119(suppl 3):18-25.

16. Sharma JB, Kalra B. Female sexual dysfunction: Assessment. Recent Adv Endocrinol. 2016;66:623-6.
17. American Psychiatric Association. Appendix. Highlights of changes from DSM-IV to DSM-5. In: Diagnostic and Statistical Manual of Mental Disorders, 5th edition. Arlington, VA: American Psychiatric Association; 2013.
18. Pontiroli AE, Cortelazzi D, Morabito A. Female sexual dysfunction and diabetes: A systematic review and meta-analysis. J Sex Med. 2013;10:1044-51.
19. Gupta L, Prakash S, Khandelwal D, et al. Diabetes and female sexual dysfunction. US Endocrinol. 2018;14: 35-8.
20. Wing RR, Bond DS, Gendrano IN, et al. Effect of intensive lifestyle intervention on sexual dysfunction in women with type 2 diabetes: Results from an ancillary Look AHEAD study. Diabetes Care. 2013;36:2937-44.
21. Caruso S, Rugolo S, Agnello C, et al. Sildenafil improves sexual functioning in premenopausal women with type 1 diabetes who are affected by sexual arousal disorder: A double-blind, crossover, placebo-controlled pilot study. Fertil Steril. 2006;85:1496-501.

# CHAPTER 22

# Reproductive Health in Diabetes

*Sambit Das, Sunil K Kota, Silver K Bahendeka*

## INTRODUCTION

Diabetes mellitus is a condition that affects almost all systems of the body. Hyperglycemia and the consequent metabolic derangements in both type 1 diabetes mellitus (T1DM) and type 2 diabetes mellitus (T2DM) affect the female and male reproductive systems alike. Other than male and female sexual dysfunction, diabetes can have a profound influence on hypothalamic-pituitary-gonadal (HPG) axis, ovarian function, semen quality and fertility. In this chapter, we discuss various aspects pertaining to reproductive health in men and women with diabetes, while sexual dysfunction is addressed in another chapter.

## REPRODUCTIVE HEALTH IN WOMEN WITH DIABETES

Diabetes can affect reproductive function throughout the lifespan of a woman, from menarche to menopause and also have an impact on the growing fetus during pregnancy.

### Reproductive Dysfunction in Women with Type 1 Diabetes Mellitus

#### Puberty and Menarche

Timing of menarche may be earlier or delayed in diabetes. Many studies have found that menarche was delayed in girls with T1DM, while others found no difference.[1] If the onset of diabetes is before puberty and there is uncontrolled hyperglycemia, menarche may be delayed as a result of hypogonadism and abnormal ovarian function.[2] Furthermore, significant weight loss and physiological stress before or at the onset of T1DM may contribute to a delay in menarche.[2] While delayed menarche may itself be a cause of concern for the child and parents, it is associated with poor accrual of bone mass and low bone mineral density.[3] Optimization of glycemic control along with adequate nutrition and physical activity is important for the maintenance of reproductive and bone health. Pubertal delay of 6 months to 1 year has been reported in 1980s and 1990s, but recent studies do not report similar trends, possibly due to intensive insulin regimens.[4]

Puberty is associated with significant insulin resistance and difficulty in maintaining glycemic control in girls, and this may in turn contribute to oligomenorrhea. Some fluctuations in glycemic control may occur during various phases of the menstrual cycle as well, with rising glucose levels noted during luteal phase.

## Menstrual Dysfunction

Menstrual dysfunction can manifest in up to 40% women with T1DM throughout the reproductive age group.[4] This may result from alterations at the hypothalamus, pituitary or ovaries due to hyperglycemia and/or insulin deficiency.

At one end of the spectrum, they may manifest a wide range of menstrual irregularities like amenorrhea, menorrhagia and oligomenorrhea, throughout their fertile years due to chronic abnormal metabolism associated with diabetes.[2]

Metabolic signals including leptin from adipose tissue, gastrointestinal tract and pancreas influence hypothalamic function and regulate energy balance as well as reproductive function. Persistent poor glycemic control, catabolic state and negative energy balance may lead to impaired activity of the gonadotropin-releasing hormone (GnRH) pulse generator by suppressing the expression of *KISS1*. This manifests as functional hypothalamic amenorrhea of varying severity that is likely to improve with optimization of glycemic control with insulin and maintenance of optimal energy balance.[4]

Alterations have been detected at the level of the ovaries as well including abnormal follicular growth, ovulation and oocyte maturation. With significant improvements in glycemic control over time, the prevalence of hypogonadotropic hypogonadism has declined. Insulin is also an important regulator of the HPG axis. Severe insulin deficiency has been associated with severe hypogonadism in animal models of T1DM, and this was partially ameliorated with insulin administration.[4]

## Polycystic Ovary Syndrome

Exogenous insulin therapy may be associated with supraphysiological systemic insulin concentrations, weight gain and insulin resistance.[5] In recent times, an increased incidence of polycystic ovary syndrome (PCOS) has been reported in women with T1DM.[4] PCOS phenotype may differ in women with T1DM, with milder hyperandrogenic features including hirsutism. Sex hormone binding globulin (SHBG) levels are preserved and free androgen levels are lower compared to PCOS without T1DM.

## Ovulation and Fertility

While ovulation rates have been reported to be comparable to controls, T1DM women have lower live birth rates.[4] This may result from several factors including lower rates of marriage, fewer attempted pregnancies, sexual dysfunction and long-term complications. In addition, menstrual irregularities are associated with increased cardiovascular (CV) risk and low bone mineral density and it is therefore, important to evaluate and address these issues. T1DM has also been associated with an earlier age of menopause in some but not all studies.

## Menopause

Women with T1DM can have early menopause partly because of premature ovarian failure and also because of the poor metabolic control. In a study by Dorman et al.,[6] women with T1DM were found to have a greater incidence of premature menopause.

## Premature Ovarian Insufficiency

Type 1 diabetes mellitus may be associated with autoimmune ovarian dysfunction and premature ovarian insufficiency. Premature ovarian insufficiency presents with the classic triad of amenorrhea, hypoestrogenism and elevated gonadotropins in women less than 40 years of age. T1DM and premature ovarian insufficiency may occur in polyglandular autoimmune syndromes 1 and 2. It is important to be aware of this association and there is a need for vigilance for other autoimmune, endocrine and nonendocrine disorders such as autoimmune thyroid dysfunction, adrenal insufficiency, pernicious anemia, vitiligo or connective tissue diseases.

# Reproductive Dysfunction in Women with Type 2 Diabetes Mellitus

## Puberty and Menarche

There are no published studies examining menarche in girls with T2DM. There is evidence to suggest that certain ethnic groups have greater insulin resistance and earlier menarche[7] but an association between lower age of menarche and T2DM is yet to be established. Earlier menarche could be a manifestation of hyperandrogenism and a forerunner of insulin resistance. It has also been associated with PCOS in adolescents and young adults.

## Polycystic Ovary Syndrome

Insulin resistance is one of the most important pathogenic mechanisms of both PCOS and T2DM. Hyperinsulinemia can directly stimulate ovarian androgen production and augments luteinizing hormone (LH)-stimulated and adrenocorticotropic hormone (ACTH)-mediated androgen production by increasing GnRH pulse amplitude and frequency leading to increased LH secretion and premature arrest of antral follicles.[8] In addition, the secretion of SHBG is inhibited, leading to increased bioavailable testosterone. Insulin resistance also is associated with increased insulin-like growth factor-1 (IGF-1) and decreased insulin-like growth factor binding protein-1 (IGFBP-1) secretion from the liver that further acts on the ovaries to increase androgen production. In turn, hyperandrogenism also contributes to insulin resistance and hyperandrogenic phenotypes of PCOS carry a greater metabolic and CV risk than nonhyperandrogenic phenotypes.

In this section, we briefly discuss management issues related to PCOS in women with diabetes. These aspects have been covered in detail in the Chapter "Glucocrinology of Female Reproductive System". Women with PCOS have a greater risk of glucose intolerance, overt diabetes and gestational diabetes. Therefore, periodic screening for dysglycemia is recommended. Pharmacological management of PCOS primarily includes oral contraceptives and antiandrogens that may have effects on glycemic control, blood pressure and lipids in women with diabetes, requiring close pharmacovigilance.

In addition, metformin is the first-choice drug in women with PCOS who manifest glucose intolerance or overt diabetes[9] as it reduces insulin resistance and may have modest benefits on hyperandrogenic features as well. Similarly, pioglitazone also has beneficial effects in PCOS and may be considered in women who do not tolerate metformin. However, the use of pioglitazone in women diabetes and PCOS is limited due to concerns of teratogenicity, fracture risk and weight gain.[10]

Glucagon-like peptide-1 (GLP-1) receptor agonists are associated with significant weight reduction and recent studies have explored their role in PCOS. A meta-analysis of seven short-term randomized controlled trials of GLP-1 receptor agonist liraglutide in women with PCOS demonstrated reduction in body mass index (BMI), waist circumference, Homeostatic Model Assessment of Insulin Resistance (HOMA-IR) and serum testosterone levels.[11] Sodium-glucose cotransporter-2 inhibitors may also have beneficial effects in PCOS and warrant further evaluation. However, while many antidiabetic agents may have beneficial effects on PCOS phenotype, adequate contraception is required in reproductive age group when using these drugs.

## Ovulation and Fertility

Diabetes per se is associated with menstrual irregularities and reduced fertility rates that can improve with optimized glycemic control. However, fecundability has been reported to be low in women with diabetes even when they do not have menstrual irregularities and the causes include ovulatory dysfunction, tubal and cervical factors.

Polycystic ovary syndrome is common in women with T2DM and is associated with chronic oligoanovulation. PCOS is a leading cause of female factor subfertility in infertility clinics. Obese T2DM women are three times more likely to experience infertility as a result of ovulation failure than women who have a normal BMI.[12] Diabetes may also coexist with thyroid dysfunction and both overt and subclinical hypothyroidism have been associated with reduced fertility.

## Menopause

Type 2 diabetes mellitus is the most common metabolic disease in the post-menopausal period.[13] Metabolic changes that occur with menopause may contribute to the development of diabetes, including increased visceral fat, reduced skeletal muscle mass, insulin resistance and reduced physical activity. In addition, the hypoestrogenic state is associated with dyslipidemia and endothelial dysfunction. All of these factors contribute to a significantly increased risk of cardiovascular disease in menopausal women.[14]

Perera et al.[14] found that use of low-dose hormone replacement therapy (HRT) in women with T2DM has no adverse effects on CV risk or metabolic control. In relation to timing of the menopause, overweight women with T2DM may undergo menopause later as it has been found that estrogen levels in these women reduce more slowly than in those who are underweight or of normal weight.[15]

## Contraception and Diabetes

Diabetes per se is not a contraindication for any type of hormonal contraceptive. However, associated factors such as the duration of disease, presence of micro- and macrovascular complications, severity of hypertension, prothrombotic risk, dyslipidemia and CV risk may influence the choice of hormonal contraceptives. In general, from a CV viewpoint, progestogen-only preparations are safer than estrogen-containing drugs.[16]

However, progestin-only pills are associated with irregular menstruation; so, if cyclicity is to be maintained, then low-dose estrogen-containing combined pills are preferred.[17] In a meta-analysis, there was no significant effect of low-dose combined oral contraceptives on glucose tolerance or lipid profile.[18]

The World Health Organization (WHO) recommended that the use of combined oral contraceptives be limited to nonsmoking, healthy women with diabetes who are 35 years or younger and who do not have hypertension, nephropathy and retinopathy.[19] Therefore, for younger women with diabetes, combined oral contraceptives may be the most appropriate form of contraception. The copper-containing intrauterine contraceptive devices are a useful choice in women with diabetes who have vascular disease, proliferative retinopathy and nephropathy.[19]

## Pregnancy and Diabetes

The prevalence of diabetes in pregnancy has been increasing due to several factors, including increasing maternal age at conception and rising prevalence of diabetes in younger women. The majority of cases of diabetes in pregnancy are gestational diabetes mellitus (GDM), with the remainder primarily pre-existing T1DM and T2DM.[20] The rise in GDM and T2DM is in parallel with obesity and insulin resistance. Hyperglycemia increases both maternal and fetal risk; therefore, close vigilance is required in women with diabetes in the preconception period, gestational period as well as postpartum period to optimize maternal-fetal outcomes.

### Preconception Period

Preconception counseling must be incorporated into routine diabetes care in all women, starting right from the onset of puberty. Family planning and contraception should be discussed. Preconception counseling should address the importance of good glycemic control of hemoglobin A1c (HbA1c) less than 6.5% for better fetal and maternal outcomes.[21] In addition, several medications for diabetes, hypertension and dyslipidemia may need discontinuation when a woman is planning pregnancy. In women with pre-existing T2DM, metformin can be continued while other antidiabetic medications should be replaced with insulin therapy. Similarly, angiotensin-converting enzyme (ACE) inhibitors, angiotensin receptor blockers, beta-blockers, thiazide diuretics and statins need to be discontinued before conception.

### Pregnancy

Diabetes is the most common medical problem to complicate pregnancy.[21] Pregnancy is associated with significant changes in glucose homeostasis, with increase in both insulin secretion and insulin resistance. These are discussed in the Chapter "Glucocrinology of Female Reproductive System". Uncontrolled hyperglycemia can lead to complications, including maternal, fetal and neonatal complications such as miscarriage, preterm delivery, maternal hypertension, operative birth, macrosomia, birth trauma and neonatal hypoglycemia.[22] Good glycemic control and frequent monitoring are the key to better maternal, fetal and neonatal outcomes. Though insulin is the gold standard for the management of hyperglycemia in pregnancy, glibenclamide[23] and metformin[24] can be used in certain circumstances with caution.

### Postpartum Care

In view of nutritional and immunological benefits of breastfeeding, all women including those with diabetes should be advised for exclusive breastfeeding. In addition, breastfeeding is associated with improvements in insulin sensitivity and leads to longer-term metabolic benefits to mother and the baby.[25] It has been shown that breastfeeding can prevent metabolic syndrome and future diabetes in the offspring. In women with pre-existing diabetes, glycemic control should be achieved with insulin during the period of breastfeeding.

## REPRODUCTIVE HEALTH IN MEN WITH DIABETES

Diabetes is commonly associated with male sexual dysfunction, and this has been discussed in the Chapter "Sexual Dysfunction in Diabetes". In addition, increased rates of hypogonadism have been reported in both T1DM and T2DM, and this has been attributed to functional hypogonadotropic hypogonadism. Diabetes may also affect spermatogenesis, sperm quality and fertility.

### Diabetes and the Hypothalamus-pituitary-testicular Axis

Men with diabetes can have functional hypogonadotropic hypogonadism.[26] Hyperglycemia and hyperinsulinemia may induce altered feedback at the level of the hypothalamus, leading to decreased secretion of LH and follicle-stimulating hormone (FSH). In addition, increased adiposity in diabetes may result in increased aromatase activity, with increased conversion of testosterone to estrogen and diminished testosterone levels. The increased estrogens, in turn, also exert a negative feedback effect on LH and FSH production, further suppressing the HPG axis.

Insulin activates protein kinase B (PKB), an important mediator of energy signaling in the brain.[27] In animal models, it has been seen that hyperinsulinemia increased GnRH pulsatility and stimulated LH secretion.[28] Therefore, both insulin resistance and insulin deficiency at the receptor level in men with diabetes may be contributory to lower GnRH pulse activity and the suppression of HPG axis. Insulin levels are also known to be correlated directly to circulating levels of leptin, an important molecule involved in maintaining energy homeostasis.

Furthermore, high circulating insulin levels inhibit SHBG synthesis in the liver. There is an inverse relationship between insulin levels and SHBG and, consequently, men with T2DM may have reduced SHBG levels. This is associated with reduced plasma levels of total testosterone and increased bioavailable estrogen.

There is ongoing debate about the role of testosterone replacement therapy in men with diabetes. While men with established persistent hypogonadism merit androgen replacement therapy, current evidence does not suggest that borderline low testosterone levels should be considered an indication for pharmacological management of hypogonadism. This has been discussed in the Chapter "Glucocrinology of Male Reproductive System".

## Puberty in Men with Diabetes

Various registries on T1DM have shown that the incidence of T1DM peaks at puberty. There is a bidirectional relationship between puberty and diabetes. On the one hand, metabolic decompensation in diabetes and functional HPG axis can lead to pubertal delay.[29]

On the other hand, diabetes control could be adversely affected by the physiological changes of puberty. Glycemic control deteriorates during puberty despite an increase in lean body mass. Development of insulin resistance has been attributed to the surge in growth hormone (GH) and sex steroids. A rise in insulin resistance increases insulin requirements in boys with T1DM during puberty and is often associated with wide fluctuations in glycemic control. It has been observed that an excessive GH secretion in T1DM during puberty has significant effects on ketogenesis. Adolescents with T1DM tend to develop metabolic decompensation very rapidly and may present with ketoacidosis. Behavioral changes during adolescence further contribute to poor glycemic control.[29]

## Diabetes and Spermatogenesis

Both T1DM and T2DM could have detrimental effects on male fertility, especially on sperm quality, such as sperm motility, sperm deoxyribonucleic acid (DNA) integrity, and ingredients of seminal plasma.

Diabetes has been associated with reduced spermatogenic cells, decreased seminiferous tubule diameter and greater seminiferous tubule atrophy. There is increased thickness of basal lamina in seminiferous tubules, accompanied by reduced sperm production and total size of seminiferous tubules.[30] Also, diabetes leads to reduction of Sertoli and germinal cells.

## Pathophysiological Mechanisms of Reduced Male Fertility

Maintenance of spermatogenesis in vivo and the fertility capacity of male sperm depend on glucose metabolism.[30] Sperm cells can effectively use several simple sugars such as glucose, fructose and mannose and generate adenosine triphosphate (ATP) from the catabolism of glucose to pyruvate and lactate by the glycolytic pathway enzymes. Sertoli cells produce lactate to maintain germ cell survival and this process has been shown to be predominantly under the control of the endocrine system, primarily sex steroids, FSH and insulin. An alteration in the ability of spermatozoa to utilize the substrates involved in ATP production would be expected to compromise sperm motility and subsequently fertility. Due to insulin resistance or insulin deficiency, men with diabetes have reduced cellular uptake of glucose mediated by glucose transporters. This supports an association of diabetes with disruptions in sperm metabolism and consequently subfertility or even infertility.

Reactive oxygen species (ROS) and free radicals can adversely affect the spermatogenesis. Hyperglycemia is associated with an increased production of free radicals in the mitochondria and may contribute to greater DNA damage. As ROS cause strand breaks in DNA and base modifications including the oxidation of guanine residues to 8-oxo-2'-deoxyguanosine (8-oxo-dG), 8-oxo-dG can serve as a sensitive biomarker of oxidative DNA damage.

Diabetes may also influence the epigenetic modification during spermatogenesis and this epigenetic dysregulation may be inherited through the male germline. Such epigenetic changes can be passed onto more than one generation, and it has been suggested that this may be associated with an increased risk of diabetes in the offspring.[30]

Optimization of glycemic control and metabolic health is, therefore, important to preserve reproductive function and fertility in men with diabetes. However, these issues are often overlooked in routine diabetes care. There is a pressing need for reproductive vigilance in the diabetes clinic.

## CONCLUSION

Reproductive health is an important concern in patients with diabetes, both men and women. The altered glucose metabolism, reduced insulin secretion and/or sensitivity, changes in body composition and leptin, SHBG levels and the reactive oxygen radicals can affect the HPG axis at any level. This is associated with significant concerns related to reproductive health including a higher incidence of functional hypogonadism, PCOS, sexual dysfunction and subfertility in women. The association of diabetes and reproductive dysfunction also creates unique management challenges. Optimized glycemic and metabolic control is important in improving outcomes in women with diabetes. Oral contraceptives need to be used with caution in women with diabetes due to the possibility of adverse metabolic effects. Many drugs used in diabetes management may need to be discontinued before pregnancy and during lactation.

In addition, men with diabetes may have functional hypogonadism, sexual and erectile dysfunction and reduced spermatogenesis or reduced sperm quality. While clearly established hypogonadism should be treated with androgen replacement therapy, optimization of glycemic control is important to improve reproductive health in men.

## REFERENCES

1. Strotmeyer ES, Steenkiste AR, Foley TP, et al. Menstrual cycle differences between women with type 1 diabetes and women without diabetes. Diabetes Care. 2003;26(4):1016-21.
2. Gaete X, Vivanco M, Eyzaguirre FC, et al. Menstrual cycle irregularities and their relationship with HbA1c and insulin dose in adolescents with type 1 diabetes mellitus. Fertil Steril. 2010;94(5):1822-6.
3. Schweiger BM, Snell-Bergeon JK, Roman R, et al. Menarche delay and menstrual irregularities persist in adolescents with type 1 diabetes. Reprod Biol Endocrinol. 2011;9:61.
4. Codner E, Merino PM, Tena-Sempere M. Female reproduction and type 1 diabetes: from mechanisms to clinical findings. Hum Reprod Update. 2012;18(5):568-85.

5. Codner E, Cassorla F. Puberty and ovarian function in girls with type 1 diabetes mellitus. Horm Res. 2009;71(1):12-21.
6. Dorman JS, Steenkiste AR, Foley TP, et al. Menopause in type 1 diabetic women: is it premature? Diabetes. 2001;50(8):1857-62.
7. Prentice P, Raine J. Menarche: onset and management in London schools. Arch Dis Child. 2011;96(1): 111-2.
8. Azziz R, Carmina E, Chen Z, et al. Polycystic ovary syndrome. Nat Rev Dis Primers. 2016;2:16057.
9. Naderpoor N, Shorakae S, de Courten B, et al. Metformin and lifestyle modification in polycystic ovary syndrome: systematic review and meta-analysis. Hum Reprod Update. 2015;21(5):560-74.
10. Valsamakis G, Lois K, Kumar S, et al. Metabolic and other effects of pioglitazone as an add-on therapy to metformin in the treatment of polycystic ovary syndrome (PCOS). Hormones (Athens). 2013;12(3):363-78.
11. Lamos EM, Malek R, Davis SN. GLP-1 receptor agonists in the treatment of polycystic ovary syndrome. Expert Rev Clin Pharmacol. 2017;10(4):401-8.
12. He Y, Tian J, Oddy WH, et al. Association of childhood obesity with female infertility in adulthood: a 25-year follow-up study. Fertil Steril. 2018;110(4):596-604.e1.
13. Wedisinghe L, Perera M. Diabetes and the menopause. Maturitas. 2009;63(3):200-3.
14. Perera M, Petrie JR, Hillier C, et al. Hormone replacement therapy can augment vascular relaxation in post-menopausal women with type 2 diabetes. Hum Reprod. 2002;17(2):497-502.
15. Rachoń D, Teede H. Ovarian function and obesity—interrelationship, impact on women's reproductive lifespan and treatment options. Mol Cell Endocrinol. 2010;316(2):172-9.
16. Altshuler AL, Gaffield ME, Kiarie JN. The WHO's medical eligibility criteria for contraceptive use: 20 years of global guidance. Curr Opin Obstet Gynecol. 2015;27(6):451-9.
17. Kalra B, Kalra S. Contraception in women with diabetes. J Pak Med Assoc. 2017;67(3):482-3.
18. de Melo AS, Dos Reis RM, Ferriani RA, et al. Hormonal contraception in women with polycystic ovary syndrome: choices, challenges, and noncontraceptive benefits. Open Access J Contracept. 2017;8:13-23.
19. World Health Organization (WHO). (2015). Medical eligibility criteria for contraceptive use. [online] Available from https://apps.who.int/iris/bitstream/handle/10665/181468/9789241549158_eng.pdf;jsessionid=A426A768F99C0CB88283FDFC9293604C?sequence=1. [Last accessed from April, 2019].
20. Downs JS, Arslanian S, de Bruin WB, et al. Implications of type 2 diabetes on adolescent reproductive health risk: an expert model. Diabetes Educ. 2010;36(6):911-9.
21. Coulthard T, Hawthorne G. Type 2 diabetes in pregnancy: more to come? Pract Diabetes Int. 2008;25(9):359-61.
22. Holmes VA, Young IS, Patterson CC, et al. Optimal glycemic control, pre-eclampsia, and gestational hypertension in women with type 1 diabetes in the diabetes and pre-eclampsia intervention trial. Diabetes Care. 2011;34(8):1683-8.
23. Sénat MV, Affres H, Letourneau A, et al. Effect of Glyburide vs Subcutaneous Insulin on Perinatal Complications Among Women With Gestational Diabetes: A Randomized Clinical Trial. JAMA. 2018;319(17):1773-80.
24. Priya G, Kalra S. Metformin in the management of diabetes during pregnancy and lactation. Drugs Context. 2018;7:212523.
25. Pereira PF, Alfenas Rde C, Araújo RM. Does breastfeeding influence the risk of developing diabetes mellitus in children? A review of current evidence. J Pediatr (Rio J). 2014;90(1):7-15.
26. Grossmann M. Low testosterone in men with type 2 diabetes: significance and treatment. J Clin Endocrinol Metab. 2011;96(8):2341-53.
27. Boura-Halfon S, Zick Y. Phosphorylation of IRS proteins, insulin action, and insulin resistance. Am J Physiol Endocrinol Metab. 2009;296(4):E581-91.
28. Burcelin R, Thorens B, Glauser M, et al. Gonadotropin-releasing hormone secretion from hypothalamic neurons: stimulation by insulin and potentiation by leptin. Endocrinology. 2003; 144(10):4484-91.
29. Chowdhury S. Puberty and type 1 diabetes. Indian J Endocrinol Metab. 2015;19(Suppl 1):S51-4.
30. Rato L, Alves MG, Socorro S, et al. Metabolic modulation induced by oestradiol and DHT in immature rat Sertoli cells cultured in vitro. Biosci Rep. 2012;32(1):61-9.

# Index

Page numbers followed by '*f*' figure; '*fc*' flow chart; and '*t*' indicate table respectively.

## A

Abdominal fat mass 186
Ablation treatments 123
Acarbose 199
Acetyl coenzyme A 29
Acid-labile subunit 232
Acinar 80
Acquired hypogonadotropic hypogonadism 102
Acquired immunodeficiency syndrome 165
Acquired lipodystrophy 254
Acromegaly 6, 11, 15, 128, 167, 195, 196, 237
   and cardiovascular risk 240
   clinical features of 196
   diagnosis of 17
   effect of treatment of 17
   progresses 240
Activated protein kinase 29
Addison's disease 32, 154, 170
Adenosine monophosphate 29
Adenosine triphosphate 13, 43, 73, 81, 296
Adipocyte 99
   hypertrophy 253
   myocyte crosstalk 29
   population 248
   secrete several proinflammatory molecules 249
   turnover 253
   white and brown dofferemces 249*t*
Adipokines 29, 261
   and enzymes 249
   levels 258
   physiological functions 250*t*
Adiponectin 111, 249, 250, 261
Adipose-derived stem cells 262
Adipose tissue 3, 54, 28, 108, 218, 248, 253, 291
   biopsy 259
   capacity, impaired 255
   circadian rhythm 251
   cytokines 112
   deposits and their physiological function 248
   distribution 254
   dysfunction 247, 251
      in diabetes 262*t*
   energy homeostat 250
   extracellular matrix expansion 255
   handling of acute nutrient flux 255
   health in diabetes 247, 248, 251
      assessment of 256
   clinical markers of 258
   effect of antidiabetic agents on 260
   radiological assessment of 258
   structural and functional changes of 253
   therapeutic strategies targeting 259
   inadequate vascularization of 255
   inflammation 255
   insulin resistance 252
   lipolysis 112
   pathogenesis of insulin resistance 252*fc*
   type 2 diabetes mellitus 252*fc*
Adrenal androgens 53, 56
Adrenal axis, abnormalities in 236
Adrenal cortical physiology in diabetes, changes in 65
Adrenal disorders in diabetes, vigilance for 76
Adrenal hyperplasia
   bilateral 64
   congenital 61, 65
   unilateral 64
Adrenal insufficiency 7, 63, 64, 130, 153, 158, 170, 176
   diagnosis of 236
   screening for 66
Adrenal medulla 76, 77
   constitutes 71
   glucose physiology in relation to 71
Adrenal tumor, surgical resection of 57
Adrenal-directed medical therapy 60
Adrenaline 73
Adrenergic
   receptors 72, 73
   symptoms 76
Adrenocorticotrophic hormone 14, 19, 53, 60, 68, 113, 178, 222, 228
Adrenovigilance in diabetes 65, 76
Advanced glycation end-products, formation of 266
Aging males' symptoms rating scale 104
Agouti-related peptide 12, 109
Alcohol 157
Aldactone, evaluation study 67
Aldosterone
   effects of 56
   primarily regulates 55
   producing adenomas 64
   producing adrenal lesion 243

Alkaline phosphatase 272
Alpha-glucosidase inhibitors 94
Alpha-interferon 194
Alpha-melanocyte-stimulating hormone 109
Alström syndrome 135, 136, 142, 143
Amblyopia 142
Amelioration of thyrotoxicosis 38
Amenorrhea 232, 291
American Association of Pediatrics 175
American Diabetes Association 184, 188
Amino acidemia 176
Amino acids 200
Amiodarone 239
Amiodarone-induced thyrotoxicosis 240
Amlexanox 263
Amylase 80, 83
Anabolic
    androgens 166
    hormone 81
Anakinra 261
Androgen
    deficiency 99
        in aging males 104
    deprivation therapy 99
        for prostate cancer 101
    excess in females 111$f$
    on female metabolism, effects of 110
    receptor 111
    replacement therapy 285
        compliance of 101
Androstenedione 56
Angiosarcoma 15
Angiotensin II receptor blockers 167
Angiotensin receptor blockers 210, 237, 239, 294
Angiotensin-converting enzyme inhibitors 210, 237, 239, 294
Angular cheilitis 202
Antepartum pituitary necrosis 239
Anthropometric measures 256
Antidiabetic medications, effect on 50$t$
Antihypertensive agents 166
Anti-inflammatory agents 42
Antiosteoporosis drugs 169
    on glycemic control 275
Antithyroid drugs 8, 37, 162, 169
Antithyroid peroxidase 31
Aortic root abnormalities 142
Apoptosis 253
Arcuate nucleus 12, 109
Artifactual hypoglycemia 149
Asian Indian phenotype 254
    characteristics of 254
Atherogenic dyslipidemia 278
Atherosclerosis 251
Auditory system 142
Autoimmune hemolytic anemia 143
Autoimmune hypoglycemia 152
Autoimmune polyglandular syndrome 135, 136, 141, 144$f$, 143, 144
Autoimmune thyroid disease 27, 34
Autonomic nervous system 71
Autonomic neuropathy culminates 93
Autophagy 256
    and metabolism 256
    deficient mice adipocytes 256
    science of 256
Axonal sensory neuropathy 142

## B

Bardet–Biedl syndrome 7, 15, 135, 136, 142, 143
Bariatric surgery 8, 260, 261
Basal bolus insulin therapy 63
Bathmotropic 72
Beckwith–Wiedemann syndrome 176
Beige adipocytes 249
Beta-adrenergic agonists 165
Beta-blockers 169, 194, 239, 294
Beta-cell
    adenosine triphosphate 180
    apoptosis 164
    cell insufficiency, stage of 86
Bicuspid aortic valve 142
Bile salt-dependent lipase 93
Biliopancreatic diversion 261
Bioimpedance absorptiometry 258
Birth asphyxia 177
Birth weight, very-low 179
Bisphosphonates 162, 169
Blood glucose
    concentration 82$f$
    self-monitoring of 63, 164
Blood pressure 258
    raised 124
    regulation 53
Blood-brain barrier 22
Blood-to-brain transport 208
Body composition 270
Body fat distribution, regulation of 110
Body mass index 62, 75, 169, 220, 247, 293
Body weight 257
Bone
    disease 45
        high-turnover 235
        low-turnover 236
    formation 274
    health
        antidiabetes medications, effect of 271, 272$t$
        effect of vitamin D 271
        in diabetes 265
        in type 1 diabetes mellitus 266
            factors leading to impaired 266
        in type 2 diabetes mellitus 267, 270
            factors leading to impaired 268
        interpretation 269
    metabolism parameters 51
    mineral density 8, 48, 221, 232, 265, 272, 274
        in type 2 diabetes mellitus 267

# Index

mineral health 51
mineral homeostasis 235
mineral metabolism 4, 41
morphogenetic protein-7 3, 44, 265
quality in type 2 diabetes mellitus 268
resorption, markers of 274
specific factors 274
turnover markers 48
Brain regions, diversity of 13
Brain-derived neurotrophic factor 15
Brainstem structures 13
Breast cancers 221
Bromocriptine 8, 9, 18, 60, 167, 225
Bromocriptine quick release 21
Bronchial carcinoids 199
Brown adipose tissue 12, 27, 28, 263
Brushfield iris spots 142

## C

Cabergoline 60, 162, 168
Calcium 42
Calcium and phosphate 265
Calcium-channel blockers 167
Canagliflozin 224
Capillary density 240
Carbimazole 37, 155, 162
Carboxyl ester lipase 136
Carboxylase 29
Cardiac rhythm abnormalities 241
Cardiomyocyte hypertrophy 240
Cardiomyopathy 241
Cardiovascular disease 3, 123, 188, 227, 239, 251, 272
    endovigilance in 238
    increased risk of 118
    treatment of 239t
    underlying 278
Cardiovascular events 67
Cardiovascular function 72
Cardiovascular risk for primary hyperaldosteronism 242
Cardiovascular system 142
Carnitine deficiency 176
Carotid intima-media thickness 241
Carpal tunnel syndrome 196
Catabolic phase 112
Catalytic conversion of glycogen 4
Catecholamine 71, 73, 76, 165, 200
    deficiency 155
    derivatives 262
    excess 155
    increase heart rate 72
    induced cardiomyopathy 241
    levels 175
    pharmacological use of 76
    producing tumors 241
    regulate glucose 72
    secreting tumors 74

Celiac disease 143
Cell, types of islets 80
Central glucose sensing, molecular mechanisms of 12
Central nervous system 11, 58, 68, 142, 148, 261
Ceramides 252
Cerebellar ataxia 142
Cerebral aneurysm 15
Cesarean section for fetal distress 177
Cholesteatoma 15
Chordoma 15
Chorea 142
Chronotropic 72
Circulating glucose 83
Cleft
    lip 177
    palate 177
Coarse facies 196
Cocaine-amphetamine regulated transcript 15
Cognitive behavioral therapy 281
Combined oral contraceptives 165
Complex syndrome 5
Conduction defects 142
Consortium for study of chronic pancreatitis 94
Continuous glucose monitoring 218
Continuous subcutaneous insulin infusion 218
Contraception and diabetes 294
Cori disease 157
Coronary artery disease 239
Corticotropin-releasing hormone 21, 68, 236
Cortisol 83
    deficiency 154
Counter-regulatory hormone deficiency 153
Cranial nerve palsy 196
Cranial radiotherapy 15
Craniopharyngioma 15
Cushing's disease 11, 19, 166, 197, 198
    clinical presentation 19
    diagnosis of diabetes in 19
    effect of treatment of 20
    management of diabetes in 21, 199
Cushing's syndrome 3, 6, 8, 54, 56, 129, 132, 167, 168, 194, 197-199, 211, 237, 240
    and cardiovascular risk 241
    clinical features of 198
    clinical phenotype of diabetes in 57
    glucovigilance in 59
    management of hyperglycemia in 61
    pathophysiology of secondary diabetes in 57
    screening for 66
    subclinical 57
Cycle adenosine monophosphate 5, 43, 54, 72, 284
Cyproterone acetate 116
Cystic fibrosis 85, 194
    related pancreatitis 87
Cytokine signaling, suppressor of 232
Cytotoxic T-lymphocyte-associated protein 4 144

## D

Daily living, activities of 188
Dead adipocytes promote insulin resistance 253
Debranching enzyme deficiency 157
Defective insulin
   action 139, 140
   secretion 137
Deficiency of phosphoenolpyruvate carboxykinase 157
Deficiency of pyruvate carboxylase 157
Dehydration, severe 187
Dehydroepiandrosterone 56, 166
   levels 66, 236
   secretion 186
   sulfate 69, 224
Denosumab 162, 169
Deoxyribonucleic acid 184
Diabetes 5
   and hyperthyroidism 37$t$
   and hypothalamus-pituitary-testicular axis 295
   and metabolic syndrome 104
      risk of 114
   and spermatogenesis 296
   clinical assessment of elderly 187
   epidemiology of secondary diabetes 193
   functional classification of elderly 188
   in acromegaly, management of 18
   in children and adolescents 181
   in postmenopausal women 117
   in Turner syndrome, screening for 116
   in women with PCOS 115
   in young, maturity onset 92
   incidence of 24
   management of fracture 49
Diabetes mellitus 41, 135, 144
   bone turnover markers in 49$t$
   classification of 194
   fibrocalculous pancreatic 182
      increased fracture risk in 267
   monogenic 182
   type 1 23, 27, 31, 32, 45, 48, 63, 64, 83, 135, 182, 193, 204, 205, 290
   type 2 14, 27, 32, 33, 46, 48, 85, 99, 100, 105, 135, 153, 165, 182, 193, 204, 205, 218, 253, 278, 290, 292, 293
   type 3c 87
   with unexplained hypoglycemia 66
Diabetes, pathogenesis of 193
Diabetes, specific factors 274
Diabetes, spectrum of 187
Diabetes, syndromes 7
Diabetes, treatment technologies 212
Diabetes, uncontrolled 65
Diabetes, underlying 201
Diabetic ketoacidosis 38, 224
Diabetic macrovascular disease 238
Diabetic vasculopathy 239
Diacylglycerol 252
Diastolic dysfunction 240, 253
Diazoxide 8, 170, 194
Digestive enzymes 80
Dilated cardiomyopathy 142, 241
Dipeptidyl peptidase-4 8, 9, 18, 50, 94, 164, 199, 222, 272
Disordered adipose tissue autophagy 256
Donohue syndrome 136, 139, 140
Dopamine 60, 200
   agonist 18, 20, 225
   receptors type 2 168
Dopaminergic tone 21
Dorsal motor nucleus 13
Double collecting system 143
Down's syndrome 7, 135, 136, 142, 194
DPP-4 inhibitors 50
Drospirenone 116
Dual energy X-ray absorptiometry 258, 274
Ductal adenocarcinoma 87
Dysglycemia 123
Dyslipidemia 6, 30, 196, 251
Dystonia 142

## E

Ectopic fat deposition 253, 256, 285
Empagliflozin 224
Endocardial cushion defects 142
Endocrine
   cells, clusters of 80
   component 80
   disease 6, 7
   disorder 4, 5, 161, 170
      underlying 194
   drugs 162
      beneficial effects on glucose metabolism 167
      detrimental impact on glycemic control 163
      on glucose homeostasis 162
   dysfunction, treatment of 170
   effects of drugs used for 239$t$
   factors in diabetes 6
   function 193
   gland 112
   health 123, 217
   metabolic milieu changes 174
   neoplasia: multiple, type 1 47
   pancreas activity 73
   perspectives 204
   Society Guidelines 104
   syndromes in diabetes 135, 136
   system 4, 41, 193
   therapy 8
      effects of 162
   vigilance in hypoglycemia 211
Endocrinology, canvas of 5
Endocrinopathy 194
   classification of 128
   with reversible hyperglycemia 202

# Index

Endogenous glucocorticoid excess 56, 167
Endogenous glucose production, source of 83
Endogenous hyperinsulinemia 7, 151
Endometrial 221
Endometrial cancer 118
Endoplasmic reticulum stress 252
Endoscopic retrograde cholangiopancreatography 89
Endothelial dysfunction 30, 123, 242, 251, 252, 283
Endothelioma 15
Endovigilance in
    chronic kidney disease 227
    diabetes therapy 217
    diabetic vasculopathy 227
Energy
    balance 109
    deficits 112
    expenditure, increased 29
    homeostasis, effects of estrogen on 109*fc*
Enhancer-binding protein alpha 248
Ependymoma 15
Epicanthal folds 142
Epidermoid 15
Epigenetic dysregulation 184, 297
Epigenetic programming 184
Epinephrine 8, 54, 72, 73, 76, 83, 200
Epithelial sodium channels 56
Eplerenone 67
Erectile dysfunction 282
    diagnosis 283
    epidemiology 282
    etiopathogenesis 282
    increased risk of 278
    lifestyle modification 283
    pharmacological treatment 283
Erythroblastosis fetalis 177
Estimated glomerular filtration rate 234
Estradiol 108
Estrogen 3, 231
    increase 109
    low doses of 183
    on metabolism, effects of 108
    receptor alpha 109
Ethanol 157
Euglycemia, maintaining 149
Euglycemic-hyperinsulinemic clamps 252
Exocrine antigens 93
Exocrine cells 80
Exocrine insufficiency 93
Exocrine pancreas, diabetes of 85
Exocrine pancreatic disorders 85
Exocrine pancreatic insufficiency 89, 93, 143
    in diabetes, risk of 92
    presence of 89
Exocrine pancreatic tissue 80
Exogenous glucocorticoid-induced diabetes 61
Exogenous insulin therapy 291
Extracellular
    collagen deposition 240
    fluid 55
    matrix 248
    regulated kinase 56

## F

Farnesoid X receptor agonists 262
Fast oscillations 81
Fasting blood glucose 168
Fasting plasma glucose 18, 44, 115, 124, 164, 185, 204, 258
Fatty acid 200
Fatty acid
    binding protein 248
    metabolism 176
    oxidation defect 7, 176
    trap 260
Fecal chymotrypsin 89
Fecal elastase-1 89
Female reproductive function 112
Female sexual dysfunction 285
    epidemiology 286
    etiopathogenesis 286
    treatment of 287
        nonpharmacological 287
        pharmacological 287
Fertilization 112
Fetal insulin secretion plays 174
Fibroblast growth factor-21 8, 228, 261, 262
Fibroblast growth factor-23 9, 41
Fibroblasts 248
Fibrocalculous pancreatic diabetes 90
Fibrocalculous pancreatopathy 85, 87, 194
Fibrosis and hypoxia 255
Follicle-stimulating hormone 104, 230, 231, 295
    evaluation of 104
Folliculogenesis 112
Food intake and energy balance 109
Forkhead box P3 144
Fracture risk
    assessment tool 273, 274
    in diabetes 48, 268*fc*, 273
        assessment of 273, 274*t*
    increased 48
Frank obesity 254
Free fatty acid 14, 16, 28, 55, 178, 195, 252
    induced insulin resistance 248
    trapping 248
Free thyroid hormone levels 220
Friedreich ataxia 7, 135, 136, 142
Frizzled-related protein-5 249
Fructose-1,6-bisphosphatase 54
Functional androgen deficiency 99

## G

Galactorrhea 196
Galactosemia 157, 176
Gallstone disease 251
Gamma knife radiotherapy 196

Ganglioneuroma 15
Gastric inhibitory polypeptide 3, 60, 166, 262, 272
   receptors 45
   secretion of 186
Gastrointestinal system 143
Gastrointestinal tract 291
Genetic
   defects of
      beta-cell function 194
      insulin action 194
      lipodystrophies 140
   syndromes 15, 194
      associated with diabetes 141
Genitourinary abnormalities 143
Geriatric diabetes 187
Germinoma 15
Gestational diabetes mellitus 46, 112, 184, 193
   diagnostic criteria 185t
   pregnancy planning and risk of 116
   risk of 183
   treatment targets 185t
Ghrelin 15, 111
Glucagon deficiency 155
Glucagon dysfunction 7
Glucagon facilitates 83
Glucagon levels 207
Glucagon secretion 55, 73
Glucagon-like peptide-1 58, 59, 60, 115, 157, 164, 186, 293
   receptor agonists 223
Glucagon-like polypeptide-1 3, 18, 199, 262, 272
   receptor agonists 36
Glucagonoma 6, 91, 194, 201
Glucagonoma syndrome 202
Glucagon-producing tumors 201
Glucocorticoid 8, 14, 53, 163, 170, 197
   deficiency states 176
   effects of 54t
      on glucose homeostasis 53
   excess 20
   exposure, long-term exogenous 64
   growth hormone 3
Glucocorticoid-induced
   diabetes, increased risk of 62
   hyperglycemia management of 62
   hyperglycemia minimizing 63
   hyperglycemia risk of 61
   protein kinase-1 56
Glucocorticoid-receptor antagonist 60
Glucocrinological
   considerations 34, 37t
   considerations hormone replacement therapy 118
   considerations treatment in Turner syndrome 116
Glucocrinology 3, 11
   adrenal cortex 53, 198
   adrenal medulla 71
   adrenals, new therapeutic avenues in 67
   bidirectional relationship 4
   concept of 161
   expanding frontiers 5
   female reproductive system 184, 292, 295
   framework 9
   historical perspectives 4
   neglected basics 5
   new beginning 10
   pancreas: historical perspectives 79
   reproductive system: female 108
   reproductive system: male 97
   scope of 6t, 9
   thyroid 27
Gluconeogenesis 83
Glucose and energy metabolism 28fc
Glucose brain of 76
Glucose counter-regulatory physiology 205
Glucose homeostasis 22, 43t, 54t, 56t, 67
   effect on 56, 162
   in children and adolescents 181
   in reproductive age 183
   role of insulin and glucagon in 81
Glucose lipid profile 294
Glucose metabolism 249
   regulation of 28
Glucose physiology 27
   during pregnancy 112
   in neonatal period 174
   in relation to
      adrenal cortex 53
      bone mineral metabolism 42
      female reproductive system 108
      hypothalamus and pituitary 11
      male reproductive system 98
      pancreas 80
Glucose, regulator of 123
Glucose sensing by pancreas 81
Glucose tolerance test 184, 294
Glucose transporter type 2 receptor mutations 157
Glucose transporter type-4 29, 43, 50, 54, 73, 98
Glucose-6-phosphatase deficiency 157, 176
Glucose-6-phosphate translocase deficiency 157
Glucose-6-phosphate transporter 54
Glucose-dependent insulinotropic peptide 255
Glucostatic theory 11
Glucovigilance in
   across stages of life 174
   childhood and adolescence 181
   disorders of
      adrenal cortex 56
      adrenal medulla 74
      female reproductive tract 113
   during pregnancy 184
   elderly 186
   endocrine therapy 161
   hypothalamic disorders 14
   male reproductive disorders 101, 102
   men with hyperprolactinemia 103
   menopause 117

# Index

neonates 174
pancreatic disorders 85
pituitary disorders 15
reproductive period 183
thyroid disorders 29
Turner syndrome 116
vitamin D deficiency 45
Glutamate dehydrogenase-1 176
Glutamic acid decarboxylase 144, 180
Glycated hemoglobin 188
Glycemic
  control 17, 167
    changes in 34
    effect of dopamine agonists on 21
    effects of therapeutic strategy on 59
    optimization of 297
    worsening of 37
  during menstrual cycle 112
  targets 212
Glyceraldehyde-3-phosphate dehydrogenase 266
Glycogen phosphorylase 157
Glycogen storage disease 7, 156-158, 177
Glycogen storage disorders 176
Glycogen synthase deficiency 157
Glycogenolysis 83, 175
Gonadal
  axis abnormalities in men 230
  hormones on metabolic health, effects of 127
  vigilance in diabetes mellitus 104, 118
Gonadotropin-releasing hormone 102, 113, 291
  amplitude of 230
Gonadotropins 101, 230
Graves' disease 30
Graves' ophthalmopathy 38
Graves' orbitopathy 38
Growth hormone 11, 102, 126, 164, 228, 232
  axis 23, 232
  deficiency 22, 164, 176
  on metabolic health, effect of 126
  releasing hormone 232
  replacement, effect of 22
  therapy 233
Guanosine triphosphate 284

## H

Hamartoma 15
Head trauma 15
Headache 196
Heart and estrogen 118
Hematological system 143
Hemochromatosis 85, 87
Hemodynamically stable 225
Hemoglobin A1C 44
  reduction in 105
Heparin 210
Hepatic gluconeogenesis, increase 54
Hepatic glucose
  output 73
  production 28, 73

Hepatic insulin resistance 30
Hepatic steatosis 143, 253
Hepatitis C virus 62
Hepatocyte nuclear factor 176
Hereditary fructose intolerance 7, 157, 158, 176
Hers disease 157
Hexokinase 176
Hirata disease 155, 169
Homeostatic model assessment of insulin resistance 293
Hormonal supplementation 123
Hormone
  binding inhibitor 33
  catabolism, abnormalities of 228
  deficiency 151, 176
  replacement therapy 117, 165
  secreting pituitary adenoma 25
Horseshoe kidney 143
Human immunodeficiency virus 165
Human leukocyte antigen 144
Human placental growth hormone 112
Huntington's chorea 7, 135, 136, 142
Hydrocortisone, formulations of 64
Hyperaldosteronism 240
  in T2DM 67
  primary 6, 64, 238
Hyperandrogenism 111, 112
Hypercalcemia 242
Hypercalciuria 269
Hypercortisolism
  on glucose homeostasis 60$t$
  on glycemic control 59
  resolution of 59
Hyperglucagonemia 93
Hyperglycemia 11, 33, 164
  and adverse pregnancy outcome 184
  endovigilance in refractory 193
  in neonates 178
    causes of 179$t$
  management of 75
  mechanisms of 20$f$, 54
  pathogenesis of 58$fc$
  prevalence of 89
  related to chronic growth hormone 16$f$
  screening for 59
  uncontrolled 195
Hyperglycemic emergencies 38
Hyperglycemic hyperosmolar state 187
Hyperinsulinemia 74, 269
Hypermetabolic state 38
Hyperparathyroidism 240
  primary 6, 238
  secondary and tertiary 235
Hyperplasia 253
Hyperprolactinemia 6, 11, 21
  chronic 21
Hypertelorism 142
Hypertension 123
Hyperthyroidism 3, 6, 30, 32, 38, 128, 194, 201, 240

and cardiovascular risk 242
and diabetes 37
and thyrotoxicosis 154
clinical presentation of 201
leads 30
Hypertrophic cardiomyopathy 142
Hypertrophic obstructive cardiomyopathy 241
Hypertrophy 253
Hypoactive sexual desire disorder 280
Hypoestrogenism 232
Hypoglycemia 38, 77, 169
　approach to 158
　associated autonomic failure 208, 209, 211
　causes 208
　classification of 214
　common causes of 151$t$
　consider risk factors for 211
　core element of 213
　development of 158, 208
　drugs useful in management of 170
　episode of 208, 212, 214
　evaluation of newborns for 177
　in diabetes 204, 205
　　elderly individuals 211
　　etiology of 209
　　impact of 208
　　improvement in insulin sensitivity 210
　　medical conditions 210
　　medications 209
　　pathophysiology of 206
　　treatment of 213
　in endocrinopathies 148
　incidence of 205
　increase risk of 63, 210, 234
　management of 177
　neurogenic manifestations of 207
　newborns at-risk for prolonged 177$t$
　pathological causes of 151
　prevention 204
　severe 207
　symptoms of 207
　unawareness 169
Hypogonadism 99, 130
　impact of symptoms questionnaire 104
　in males, treatment of 105
　screening for 104
　with diabetes, testing for 104
Hypogonadotropic 105
　hypogonadism: congenital 101
Hypoparathyroidism 47
Hypopituitarism 7, 11, 23, 25, 130, 153, 170
　part of 102
Hypothalamic
　arcuate nucleus 111
　control of pancreatic function 13
　dysfunction 15
　gonadotropin-releasing hormone 111
　nuclei
　　lateral 12
　　several 13

obesity 6, 15
　causes of 15
Hypothalamic-pituitary-adrenal axis 4, 24
Hypothalamic-pituitary-adrenal, increased
　activation of 65
Hypothalamic-pituitary-gonadal axis 4, 24, 97
Hypothalamic-pituitary-ovarian 108
Hypothalamic-pituitary-thyroid 4, 24, 33
Hypothalamic-pituitary vigilance in diabetes 23
Hypothalamus 30
　and pituitary 11, 229
　disorders of 11
　in glucose, role of 11
Hypotheses 92
Hypothyroidism 6, 7, 33, 125, 129, 170, 220, 229
　and diabetes 34
　　clinical presentation 35
　　effect on diabetic complications 35
　　levothyroxine treatment 35
　　prevalence of 34

# I

Iatrogenic hypoglycemia 206
Immune mediated diabetes syndrome 136
Immune system, cells of 45
Immunodysregulation 136
　polyendocrinopathy 143
Immunoglobulin E 144
Impaired glucose tolerance 30, 47, 195, 196
Inborn errors of metabolism 176
Incontinence, cerebellar ataxia 142
Incretin-based antidiabetic drugs 59, 199
Inflammation and hyperparathyroidism 232
Inflammation, chronic 123
Inflammatory bowel disease 143
Inflammatory cells 248
Infliximab 263
Inotropic 72
Insulin 8, 50, 166, 217, 272
　activates protein kinase B 295
　antagonistic effects in liver 28
　autoimmune hypoglycemia 169
　autoimmune syndrome 151, 152, 155, 169
Insulin gene 180
Insulin on bone, effects of 44
Insulin receptor gene mutation 176
Insulin receptoropathies 139
Insulin resistance 113$fc$, 183, 234, 253, 255, 256
　pathophysiological links with 113
Insulin resistance syndrome 139
Insulin resistance worsening 252
Insulin secretion 176
　and clearance 233
　biphasic 82$f$
　defect in 136
　mechanism of 82
Insulin sensitivity 168
　effects on 110
Insulin-induced hypoglycemia 24

# Index

Insulin-like growth factor-1  16, 48, 50, 60, 113, 221, 228, 232, 292
Insulin-like growth factor-binding protein  23, 232, 292
Insulinoma  91, 151
Insulin-regulated glucose transporter  98
Insulin-resistance syndrome  123
Intellectual disability  142
Interleukin-17  144
Interleukin-2 receptor alpha  144
Interleukin-6  228
International Association of Diabetes and Pregnancy Study group  184
International Diabetes Federation  124, 188, 257, 258
Interstitial fibrosis  240
Intestinal absorption  83
Intestinal lipase inhibitor  260
Intracellular accumulation  252
Intraurethral administration of prostaglandin  284
Intrauterine growth retardation  177
IPEX syndrome  143
Irregular pulsatile secretion  230
Irreversible myocardial damage  241
Islet antigen-2  144
Isoforms of estrogen receptors  109

## J

Jamaican vomiting sickness  157
Jaw malocclusion  196

## K

Ketoconazole  8, 60, 112, 200
Ketogenesis, effect on  296
Kexin type 9  167
Kidney disease, chronic  33, 220, 227, 230
    alterations in insulin/glucagon homeostasis  233
    clinical manifestations  233
    effect of  229$t$
    endocrine function in  228$t$
    gonadal axis abnormalities in women  231
    mechanism of  228$t$
    secondary diabetes due to endocrinopathies: effect on  237
    supplementation with ergocalciferol  235
Kinetics of insulin secretion  81
Klinefelter syndrome  7, 99, 135, 136, 142, 145, 194
    glucovigilance in men with  102

## L

Lactic acidosis, risk of  220
Langerhans  80
    islets of  83
Lanreotide  8, 60
Laparoscopic adjustable gastric banding  261
Laurence–Moon–Biedl syndrome  194
Leprechaunism  136, 139, 140

Leptin  15, 111, 249, 250, 261
Levofloxacin  162, 210
Levothyroxine  30
Lifestyle modification  259, 273
Ligand  72
Lipid
    abnormalities  168
    lowering drugs  167
    metabolism  123
    effect on  55
Lipocalin-2  3, 44
Lipodystrophic diabetes  136, 140, 142, 143
Lipodystrophy  7, 194, 254
Lipogenesis, promotion of  218
Lipolysis  175
Lipolytic enzyme  136
Lipoprotein lipase  248
    high-density  124, 258
    low-density  30, 125, 167
Lipotoxicity  251
Liraglutide  224, 260
Litchi-associated seasonal toxic encephalopathy  157
Liver
    and kidney diseases  155
    gluconeogenesis  112
    glucose output  3
    injury  253
    isoenzyme deficiency  157
Lorcaserin  8
Low libido  280
Luteinizing hormone  100, 113, 228, 231
    hypothalamic regulation of  111
    pulsatile release of  230

## M

Macroglossia  196
Macronodular adrenocortical hyperplasia  199
Macrovascular complications  89
Male fertility, pathophysiological mechanisms of  296
Male sperm, fertility capacity of  296
Malnutrition  236
Mammalian target of rapamycin  98
Massachusetts male aging study questionnaire  104
Maternal plasma glucose  174
Matrix metallopeptidase-13  266
Maturity-onset diabetes of young  136, 137, 143, 194
Mauriac syndrome  146
Meconium aspiration  177
Medicated urethral suppository for erections  284
Mediterranean-style diet  283
Medullary thyroid carcinoma, risk of  36
Megaloblastic anemia  143
Meglitinides  94
Melanin-concentrating hormone  12
Melanocortin 4 receptor  15, 29

**307**

Melanocyte-stimulating hormone 12
Membrane translocation of GLUT4 98
Meningioma 15
Menopausal hormonal therapy 118
Menopause 292, 293
Menorrhagia 291
Menstrual dysfunction 291
Menstruating women 183
Mesenchymal stem cells 248
Mesenchymal stem cells, apoptosis of 266
Metabolic acidosis 232, 236
Metabolic and storage diseases 156
Metabolic diseases, management of 247
Metabolic disorders 251
Metabolic economy 254
Metabolic health 217
　and higher cardiovascular 101
　on reproductive health, effects of 111
Metabolic regulation 3
Metabolic signals 291
Metabolic storage diseases 157
Metabolic syndrome 3, 44, 53, 67, 97, 99, 100, 104, 108, 118, 123, 183, 258
　and polycystic ovary syndrome: metabolic menace 131
　components of 126, 127
　criteria for 258
　diagnostic criteria for 124, 258
　in endocrinopathy 123, 127
　in endocrinopathy with hormone deficiencies 129
　in endocrinopathy with hormone excess 128
　PCOS overlap 131*f*
　prevalence of 117
Metaiodobenzylguanidine scan 76
Metformin 8, 50, 93, 199, 219, 220, 272
　activator of 5 220
Metformin
　associated lactic acidosis 219
　drug induced hyperprolactinemia 22
Methimazole 37, 155, 162
Methylene cyclopropyl glycine 157
Metreleptin 8, 169
Metyrapone 8, 60
Microarchitectural changes and bone strength 48
Micropenis 177
Mifepristone 8, 60, 162, 168, 200, 210
Mimic circadian rhythm 64
Mineral, crucial role in 265
Mineralocorticoid 53
　antagonists, effects of 67
　effects on glucose homeostasis 55
　receptor 56
Mitochondrial diabetes 7, 138, 139, 142, 143
Mitochondrial dysfunction 251
Mitogen-activated protein kinase 56
Mitotane 60
Mitral valves and myocardium 242
Monocyte chemoattractant protein-1 249

Monogenic diabetes 136, 139
　due to defective insulin secretion 136
　syndromes 135
Mood stabilizers 15
Motor neuropathy 142
Muscle weakness, progressive 142
Mutations 180
Mutations, single-gene 15
Myoblasts 248
Myocardial steatosis 253
Myocellular fat 253
Myoclonus and dementia 142
Myocytes 99
Myokines 29
Myopathy 196
Myotonia 142
Myotonic dystrophy 135, 136, 142

# N

Naltrexone-bupropion 8
Naltrexone-bupropion sustained-release 260
National Cholesterol Education Program Adult Treatment Panel III 257
National Health and Nutrition Examination survey 32
National Institutes of Health 114
Necrolytic migratory erythema 202
Neonatal
　diabetes 7, 136-138, 142, 178
　hyperglycemia in preterm and low birth weight infants 179
　hypoglycemia 175, 295
　　approach to 178*fc*
　　causes of 176
Nesidioblastosis 151
Net catabolic state 112
Neurodegeneration 142
Neuroendocrine tumor 201
Neurogenic symptoms 207
Neuroglucoprivation 76
Neuroglycopenia, onset of 206
Neuroglycopenic symptoms 206, 207
Neuroleptic malignant syndrome 225
Neuronal types 13
Neuropeptide Y 12
　expression of 109
　increased 29
Neutropenia 143
Niacin 167
Nicotinamide adenine dinucleotide 156
Nitric oxide 13
Nocturnal hypoglycemia 63
Nonalcoholic
　fatty liver disease 6, 251
　　beneficial effects in 221
　steatohepatitis 223
Nonhyperinsulinemic hypoglycemia 156
Noninsulin pancreatogenous hypoglycemia syndrome 152

# Index

Nonislet cell tumor hypoglycemia 153
Norepinephrine 8, 200

## O

Obesity 251
    and central obesity, diagnostic thresholds for 257t
    and diabetes 255
    drugs 260
Obstructive sleep apnea 196, 251
Octreotide 8, 60
    long-acting release 166
Oligoamenorrhoea 194, 291
Oocyte maturation 291
Optic atrophy 142
Oral contraceptive 183
Oral glucose tolerance test 17, 30, 88, 115, 168, 185, 195
Oral hypoglycemic agent 89, 158
Organic aciduria 157
Organic androgen deficiency 99
Organomegaly 196
Orlistat 8
Osilodrostat 60
Osmotic symptoms 37
Osteoblast-derived lipocalin-2 44
Osteocalcin 3, 9, 43, 44
    reduced secretion of 55
Osteokines in glucose homeostasis, role of 43
Osteoporosis 7, 48
    in diabetes, management of 274fc
    management of 273
    pharmacological management of 274
Osteoprotegerin 3, 43, 44, 49
Osteovigilance in diabetes 47
Ovarian steroidogenesis regulation of 111
Overnight dexamethasone suppression test 57
Overt diabetes 185
Ovulation 291
    and fertility 291, 293
Ovulatory dysfunction 112
Oxidation of guanine residues 297
Oxidative stress 252

## P

Palmitic acid-9-hydroxy stearic acid 262
Pancreas 54
    secretion from 73
Pancreatectomy 194
Pancreatic
    alpha-cells 28
    beta-cell function 28
        effects on 110
    cancer 85, 90, 194
        risk of 93
    cytokeratin 93
    defects in pathogenesis of
        type 1 diabetes mellitus 83
        type 2 diabetes mellitus 84
    diabetes 6
    disease 79, 194
    ducts 80
    enzyme replacement therapy 89
    fat 253
    hormones 80
    hypoplasia 179
    injury 85
    islets 28
    lipase 80
    vigilance in diabetes 91
Pancreatitis acute 85
Pancreatitis
    acute, risk of diabetes 92
    chronic 85, 87, 88
        risk of diabetes 92
    incidence of 222
    recurrent 85
    severe acute 87
    with antidiabetic drugs, risk of 93
Pancreatogenic
    causes of 87t
    diabetes management of 89
Paragangliomas 75
Parathyroid
    disorders 45
    hormone 3, 223
    system 41
Paraventricular nuclei 12, 109
Paroxysmal atrial fibrillation 240
Paroxysmal supraventricular tachycardia 240
Pasireotide 8, 18, 20, 60, 197
    worsens glycemic control 200
Peak bone mass 266
Pediatric endocrine society 175
Pegvisomant 8, 18
Penile prosthetics 285
Penis, erectile tissue of 284
Peptide hormones of brain 5
Periaqueductal gray 13
Perinatal stress 177
Peripheral arterial disease 37
Peripheral nervous system 142
Peritoneal dialysis 156
Permanent neonatal diabetes mellitus, cases of 180
Peroxisome proliferator-activated receptor
    delta 43
    gamma 50, 221, 222, 248, 262, 269
Persistent hyperinsulinemic hypoglycemia of infancy 158
Persistent hypoglycemia, management of 178
Phentermine-topiramate 8
    extended release 260
Phenylethanolamine N-methyltransferase 71
Pheochromocytoma 6, 74, 194, 200, 240
    and cardiovascular risk 241
    surgical treatment of 75
Phosphodiesterase type 5 inhibitors 283

Phosphoenolpyruvate carboxykinase 28, 54, 163
Phosphofructokinase 2/fructose
    bisphosphatase 2 54
Pinealoma 15
Pioglitazone 8, 37, 38, 199, 272, 293
    use of 63
Pituitary directed medical therapy 60
Pituitary disorders 14
Pituitary gonadotropin secretion 111
Pituitary in glucose regulation, role of 13
Pituitary macroadenoma 15
Pituitary tumors, treatment of 225
Plasma adrenocorticotropic hormone 236
Plasma c-peptide concentrations 158
Plasma glucose 175
    and free T4 30
    concentration in diabetes 206$t$, 207
    measurement of 180
    values 195
Plasma membrane 73
Plasminogen activator inhibitor-1 249
Pluripotent stem cells 99
Polycystic ovary syndrome 8, 98, 113, 114, 140, 143, 167, 183, 291-293
    effect of 115
    glucocrinological issues in management of 115
    pathogenesis of 113
    role of statins in 115
    use of antidiabetic medications 115
Polyendocrinopathy 136
Polyglandular autoimmune endocrinopathy 7
Porphyria 142
Positron emission tomography 152
Postpartum care 295
Postprandial blood glucose 168, 204
Postprandial reactive hypoglycemia 153
Potassium 55
Potassium channel 180
Prader-Willi syndrome 15, 136, 142
Preadipocytes 248
Preconception period 294
Pregnancy and diabetes 294
Premature ovarian insufficiency 292
    prevalence of 117
Primary hyperparathyroidism 47
Procollagen type 1 amino-terminal propeptide 49
Progesterone 3
Progestin
    on metabolism, effects of 110
    replacement study 118
Progestogen only contraceptives 116
Prognathism 196
Prohormone convertase-1 15
Proinflammatory
    adipocytokines 34
    cytokines 255
Prolactin 3, 14, 231
Prolactinoma 167
    treatment of 98
Pro-opiomelanocortin 12, 15, 29, 109, 111
Propranolol 169
Proprotein convertase subtilisin 167
Prostate cancer 99
Protein 123
    metabolism, effect on 55
    tyrosine phosphatase 144
Psychotropic drugs 15
Ptosis 142
Puberty and menarche 290, 292
Puberty in men with diabetes 296

## R

Rabson–Mendenhall syndrome 136, 139, 140, 142
Radioactive iodine uptake 219
Radioiodine ablation 8
Random plasma glucose 185
Reactive oxygen species 256, 297
Renal
    and genitourinary system 143
    cysts 143
    dysfunction 143
    dysfunction, progressive 143
    failure, end-stage 236
    impairment 234
Renin–angiotensin–aldosterone system 43, 55, 236
Renin–angiotensin system 66
Reproductive dysfunction 230, 231
    in women 290, 292
Reproductive health 297
    in diabetes 184, 290
    in men with diabetes 295
    in women with diabetes 290
Resistin 111, 249
Retinal dystrophy 142
Retinoic acid 20
Retinol-binding protein 4 249
Rogers syndrome 136, 138
Rostral ventromedial medulla 77
Roux-en-Y gastric bypass 261

## S

Salsalate 263
Sarcopenia 253
Sclerostin 44
Secrete pancreatic juices 80
Secretin-pancreozymin test 89
Selective estrogen receptor modulators 232
Sensorineural hearing loss 142
Serum thyroid-stimulating hormone 29
Serum trypsin measurement of 89
Sex
    hormone-binding globulin 111, 113, 220, 291
    levels 99
    steroids 186
    therapy, dual 281
Sexual
    arousal 104

aversion disorder 280
desire 280
   diagnosis 281
   epidemiology 280
   etiopathogenesis 280
   nonpharmacological treatment 281
   pharmacological treatment 281
dysfunction 7
   in diabetes 184, 278, 295
      major risk factors for 278
   in men with diabetes 280
   response cycle 279
      arousal/plateau 279
      desire/excitement 279
      orgasm 279
      resolution 280
Sheehan's syndrome 153
Sick sinus syndrome 241
Sildenafil 283
Sinus tachycardia 241
Sitagliptin 223
Skeletal muscle 3, 28, 29, 54
Skin and musculoskeletal system 143
Sleep disturbances 196
Small heterodimer partner 50
Sodium 55
Sodium-glucose cotransporter-1 inhibitors 30
Sodium-glucose cotransporter-2 inhibitors 48, 50, 94, 115, 188, 218, 224, 234, 260, 268, 272, 273, 274, 293
Somatostatin
   analogs 8, 18, 170, 197
   long-acting 166
   receptor ligands 166
Somatostatinoma 6, 194
Sperm motility 184
Spermatogenesis 184, 297
   impairment of 184
   maintenance of 296
Spironolactone 67
Statins 239
Steatohepatitis 143
Steatorrhoea 93
Steroidogenic factor-1 109
Sterol regulatory element-binding protein-1 248
Stiff-man syndrome 142
Strabismus 142
Stroke-like episodes 142
Sulfonylurea 8, 50, 94, 158, 179, 188, 218, 272
   receptor-1 176
Supraventricular tachycardia 241
Sympathetic nervous system 29, 68
Syndrome of inappropriate antidiuretic hormone 219
Syndromes associated with poor glycemic control 146
Syndromic diabetes
   classification of 142, 145
   diagnosing 145
Syndromic obesity 167

## T

Tactful glycemic control, principles of 212
Tadalafil 283
Teratoma 15
Testicular and erectile dysfunction 184
Testosterone 3, 98, 100, 101, 230
   enhances physical activity 99
   increases 99
   levels 99
   replacement 8
   therapy 105
   with glucose metabolism 98, 99*fc*
Thiamine-responsive megaloblastic anemia syndrome 136, 142, 143
Thiazides 194, 196, 294
Thiazolidinediones 50, 94, 188, 221, 260, 269, 272
   stimulate proliferator-activated receptor-gamma 38
Thrombocytopenia 143
Thyroglobulin 144
Thyroid
   and arterial hypertension 125
   and glucose intolerance 125
   and lipid metabolism 124
   and obesity 125
   disease 32
   disorders 27, 29
      associated with hypoglycemia 154
      prevalence of 32
      symptoms of 33
   dysfunction 4, 237, 239
      abnormalities 227
      effect of metformin on 36
      in patients 31, 32
   hormone 27, 154, 228
      analogs 262
      effect of 28
      excess 201
      on metabolic health, effect of 124
      receptors 27
      secretion of 240
   peroxidase 144
   stimulating hormone 8, 34, 144, 220, 229
Thyrotoxicosis 38, 167
Thyrotropin-releasing hormone 229
Thyrovigilance in diabetes 31
Thyroxine 229
Thyroxine-binding globulin 219
Tissue-specific effects on glycogen metabolism 55
Tissue transglutaminase 144
Toxic hypoglycemic encephalopathy 157
Toxic lipid metabolites 252
Trabecular bone score 275
Transient hyperglycemia 61
Transient hypoxia 175

Triglycerides, increased synthesis of 118
Triiodothyronine 34, 228, 229
Trimethoprim sulfamethoxazole 210
Trypsinogen 80
Tumor necrosis factor-alpha 34, 228, 249
Tumors 15
Turner's syndrome 7, 116, 135, 136, 142, 143, 145, 194

## U

Ultradian oscillations 81
United Kingdom Prospective Diabetes study 218
United States Food and Drug Administration 168
Upper airway obstruction 196
Upstream stimulatory factor-1 50
Uremic toxins 236
Urinary metanephrine levels 75

## V

Vacuum erection devices 284
Vardenafil 283
Vascular
    complications 266
    endothelial growth factor 266
    to extravascular space 228
Ventricular
    ectopic beats 240
    hypertrophy: left, echocardiographic criteria for 240
    tachycardia 240, 241
Ventromedial 109
Ventromedial nucleus 12

Visceral adipose tissue 248
Visceral adiposity index 258
Visfatin 249
Visual
    field defect 105, 196
    impairment 105
Vitamin D 3, 51, 265
    deficiency 6, 8, 42, 45, 271
    in glucose homeostasis, role of 42
    metabolism 235
Voltage-dependent calcium channels 82
Volumetric computed tomography 258
von Gierke disease 157

## W

Waist circumference 257, 293
Waist-to-hip ratio 257
Wasting syndrome 165
Weight loss 8, 202
Whipple's triad 148
White adipose tissue 27, 54
Wolcott–Rallison syndrome 143
Wolff–Chaikoff effect 229
Wolfram syndrome 7, 136, 138, 142
World Health Organization 294

## X

X-chromosome haploinsufficiency 116
Xp haplotype insufficiency 116

## Z

Zinc transporter 8 180